Evidence-biased Antidepressant Prescription

Michael P. Hengartner

Evidence-biased Antidepressant Prescription

Overmedicalisation, Flawed Research, and Conflicts of Interest

palgrave
macmillan

Michael P. Hengartner
School of Applied Psychology
Zurich University of Applied Sciences
Zurich, Switzerland

ISBN 978-3-030-82586-7 ISBN 978-3-030-82587-4 (eBook)
https://doi.org/10.1007/978-3-030-82587-4

Cover illustration: Clare Jackson / Alamy Stock Photo

This Palgrave Macmillan imprint is published by the registered company Springer Nature Switzerland AG.
The registered company address is: Gewerbestrasse 11, 6330 Cham, Switzerland

Contents

List of Tables

1

Introduction: How Did I Get Here?

Medicine is supposed to make progress, to go forward in scientific terms so that each successive generation knows more and does better than previous generations. This hasn't occurred by and large in psychiatry, at least not in the diagnosis and treatment of depression and anxiety, where knowledge has probably been subtracted rather than added. There is such a thing as real psychiatric illness, and effective treatments for it do exist. But today we're seeing medicines that don't work for ill-defined diagnoses of dubious validity. This has caused a crisis in psychiatry … In the rather ineffective drug treatments for depression known as the selective serotonin reuptake inhibitors (SSRIs)—the Prozac-style drugs—and in the triumph of such diagnoses as 'major depression' that exist more in the shadowland of artifact than in the world of Nature—academic psychiatry has a lot to answer for [1].

I believe that the enduring skepticism and distorted views about antidepressant drugs are due to the stigma of mental illness and prejudice toward the medical specialty responsible for its study and care. This historical stigma is perpetuated by lay and professional groups, who oppose the use and deny the efficacy of psychotropic medication for ideologic reasons or organizational biases. Psychiatry has the dubious distinction of being the only medical specialty with an anti-movement that is constantly challeng-

M. P. Hengartner, *Evidence-biased Antidepressant Prescription*,
https://doi.org/10.1007/978-3-030-82587-4_1

> ing and undermining the field. The other source of opposition comes from anti-scientific or anti-medical groups who draw the battle lines along whether medical or psychotherapeutic treatment modalities can or should be used … Doctors should not be fooled by the pharmacologic naysayers, and no patient with major depressive disorder should be denied the effective treatment that can be hugely beneficial for them [2].

The provocative critique by Dr Edward Shorter, a medical historian, and the typical defence of the drug-centred treatment approach in depression by Dr Jeffrey Lieberman, eminent professor of psychiatry and former president of the American Psychiatric Association (APA), illustrate nicely the controversial questions this book will address. Dr Shorter is by no means the only one who has questioned the validity (and utility) of our current definition of "major" depression, and the opposition to this ill-conceived diagnosis comes from psychiatrists, general practitioners (GPs), and psychologists alike [3–7]. How the concept of depression has changed over time and how this mental disorder—its putative aetiology (causation), phenomenology (experience), prevalence (frequency), course (trajectory), and disability burden (impairment)—is portrayed in contemporary scientific discourse and the media is the first main topic of this book.

Like Dr Shorter, many authors, again psychiatrists, GPs, and psychologists alike, consider the effectiveness of the SSRIs and other new-generation antidepressants poor and of doubtful clinical relevance in the average patient with depression [8–13]. My own analyses of clinical trials and my scrutiny of the scientific literature led me to similar conclusions [14–20]. Yet, I'm fully aware that the scientific evidence is ambiguous and that there is considerable variability in how the data can be interpreted. Like Dr Lieberman in his quote above, most psychiatrists, especially academic leaders in the field, resolutely dismiss negative conclusions regarding the effectiveness of antidepressants as ideologically biased anti-psychiatric propaganda devote of scrutiny and scientific justification and contend that these drugs are highly effective and safe in depression (see, for example [21–23]). These polarised and angry debates over the scientific evidence for (or against) antidepressants in depression are the second main topic of this book.

And then there is the pervasive influence of the pharmaceutical industry that has made billions of dollars in revenues with the marketing of both "major" depression as a brain disease and its putative cure, the new-generation antidepressants [9, 14, 24–26]. By necessity, every critical analysis of antidepressant prescribing for depression must thus address conflicts of interest and corporate bias in psychiatry and primary care medicine [9, 27–30]. This is the third main topic of this book.

The Inconvenient Truth about Scientific Research

Over my academic career, I went into different stages of belief and disbelief. I studied clinical psychology and psychopathology at the University of Zurich, Switzerland. Back in the early 2000s, we were taught about psychiatric diagnoses as if these were clear-cut natural disease entities. Our curriculum strictly followed the disorder categories outlined by the Diagnostic and Statistical Manual of Mental Disorders (DSM) of the APA. I can't remember that we ever had a critical discussion about the validity and utility of these diagnoses. The DSM was like a bible, an authoritative and definite resource that contains wisdom and ultimate knowledge. When a student asked something about a specific mental disorder, the professors typically answered that this is true or not *because* the DSM says so. The DSM was axiomatic, dogmatic, and conclusive. We also learned that antidepressants were safe and effective, and within my memory there never was mention of limitations or biases in the evidence base. The validity and reliability of most research findings was barely questioned. In general, we were taught about psychological experiments as if these provided definitive answers to fundamental questions of human being. Findings from seminal studies were often (not always) considered irrefutable truths about human behaviour, cognition, and emotion. I was taught that this is how humans think, behave, and feel because it has been confirmed in this or that study. I never considered that many, perhaps most of these studies, could be simply wrong.

I had my first doubts about the credibility (and quality) of research findings when I was conducting the statistical analyses for my master thesis. I had been working on a project about testosterone, sensation seeking, and fatherhood. I soon realised that data from such an observational study was prone to many biases and confounders. I also learned that removing one or two outliers, using different operationalisations of the same construct, and adding certain control variables to a statistical model could produce completely divergent results. I started to wonder if the authors of the seminal psychological studies we were taught in class also had come up with completely divergent results had they not deliberately chosen to analyse their data in a specific way. Could it be that they also ran multiple statistical models and then selectively reported the results that provided the neatest and most persuasive answer, that is, the results that confirmed their preconceived beliefs?

In Spring 2009, soon after I had obtained my Master of Science in clinical psychology and psychopathology, I started to work as a research associate at the Department of General and Social Psychiatry of the Psychiatric University Hospital of Zurich. I started my PhD project on the epidemiology of personality disorders under the supervision of professor of psychiatry Dr. Wulf Rössler, the then-director of the clinic, and Dr. Vladeta Ajdacic-Gross, a senior researcher at the department. My supervisors quickly noted that I was a talented researcher, and in late Summer 2010, in addition to my appointment as a PhD student, I was employed as a research associate for Dr. Rössler. We were mostly working on the data of the prospective Zurich Cohort Study, a community cohort study of young adults from the canton of Zurich followed over 30 years [31, 32]. The same year I also became a research associate for professor Dr. Jules Angst, former research director of the Psychiatric University Hospital of Zurich and lead investigator of the Zurich Cohort Study. One main research interest of Dr. Rössler were sub-clinical psychotic symptoms in the general population [33], so together with Dr. Ajdacic-Gross, I was examining if we could replicate the association between cannabis use and the occurrence of psychotic symptoms reported in the literature [34].

Again, I soon realised that different statistical approaches yielded conflicting results. The association between cannabis use and psychotic symptoms was not evidently clear from the outset, but I was told that I must search the data to find the "truth". Searching the data means to run various statistical models with changing definitions of predictor and outcome variables, checking the impact of different control variables on the results and thus deriving the "best" model. According to this exploratory approach, the "best" model is the statistical analysis that confirms your hypothesis. Thus, eventually we were able to demonstrate a prospective association between cannabis use and the occurrence of psychotic symptoms, and we published the results in a leading medical journal [35]. But was the "best" model necessarily the most accurate model? Did we really detect a true association, or did we rather adjust our statistical analysis until it confirmed our hypothesis (also referred to as data dredging or p-hacking)? As the saying goes, "if you torture the data long enough, it will confess to anything". It is now widely accepted that this is poor scientific practice that substantially increases the risk of false positive results, that is, statistical artifacts or chance findings [36–40]. But back in late 2010, as a PhD student, I simply did what I was told by my supervisors (and taught in university), even though it didn't feel right. I was not aware yet of the compelling scientific literature that strongly advised against such questionable research practices.

The publication of our cannabis-psychosis paper coincided with the proclamation of the replication crisis in psychology [41–44]. My intuition that psychological and psychiatric research, and by extension research in general, was often unreliable, irreproducible, and systematically biased towards spectacular but most likely false positive findings, became a prominently discussed hot topic. I was immediately intrigued by this flood of new research that exposed so many pernicious problems in contemporary psychological research. In my new position as research associate for Drs Rössler and Angst I prepared various research papers. I quickly gained experience in data analysis and I also acquired profound knowledge in statistics and research methodology. I dug deeper into the metascience literature and found deeply concerning evidence for what I have expected for so long, but never was told as a student and junior researcher. A large portion, presumably a majority, of research findings in psychology, psychiatry, and biomedicine, is most likely false or massively exaggerated [45–50]. I learned about p-hacking, the fabrication of statistically significant results [39], about the flaws and limitations of statistical significance testing [51], and about publication bias, the selective reporting of favourable (i.e. hypothesis-confirming) research findings [52].

In 2014, about a year after I had completed my PhD, I left the Psychiatric University Hospital of Zurich to assume a tenured position at the Zurich University of Applied Sciences. Metascience, research methodology, statistics, and the philosophy of science became my primary research interests. I started to write papers about methodological flaws and research biases and how these can easily produce false-positive results in biomedical and psychological research [53, 54]. I also wrote about the systematic biases in psychotherapy research [55]. But my biggest interest was in antidepressants for depression, and this preference changed my career fundamentally.

The Issue with Antidepressant Research

In my first year at the Zurich University of Applied Sciences I had been searching the scientific literature about publication bias in psychiatric research. This is when I opened Pandora's box, for when you search the literature on publication bias in psychiatry, among the first research papers you'll find are the seminal studies from the 2000s that demonstrated how selectively the results of antidepressant trials were published [56–58]. Next you'll discover how pervasively the pharmaceutical industry has corrupted academic medicine and that drug manufacturers systematically bias the scientific evidence so that their products appear more effective and safer than they really are [28, 59–62]. You will probably also learn about the various flaws in the contemporary definition of depression and other mental disorders [7, 63–65] and how mental disorders were misleadingly marketed by the pharmaceutical industry to increase the sales of psychiatric drugs [26, 27, 66, 67].

I have always been interested in the research of depression and have co-authored various papers on mood disorders and negative affectivity (see, for example [68–76]). I also have lived experience of depression as a young adult, when I was doing my military service. I didn't seek treatment back then and fortunately, my profound sadness, lack of interest and pleasure, and feelings of hopelessness that persisted for several weeks lifted soon after I was discharged from the army. After my recovery I flourished and, curiously, even felt emotionally stronger than before my depression episode. I gained a self-esteem and confidence I didn't have before. Later I learned that this phenomenon, that is, high functioning after full recovery from a depression episode, is a widely neglected topic, but it is presumably not that rare as most psychiatrists and clinical psychologists would think [77]. Thus, the concept and outcome of depression were interesting to me not only from a scientific perspective, but also from my personal life story. In 2017, finally, I published my first research paper on antidepressants for depression, a critical review of methodological limitations in clinical trials, selective reporting of research findings, and corporate bias in the evidence base [14].

This publication, and the many others that would follow, to my surprise (or naivety) also completely changed my research career and position within the scientific community. There were already several papers on these issues in the scientific literature, of which most were published in leading general medical and psychiatric journals (see, for example, [57, 78, 79]), and various books had been written about it (see, for example [9, 11, 80]). So I didn't think that my paper was really big news or that it would cause a stir. But I was proved wrong and in hindsight I also realise how naïve I was. Before long, other researchers contacted me and congratulated me on my first antidepressant paper. This is how I met Dr. Martin Plöderl, psychotherapist and senior researcher at the Christian Doppler Clinic, Paracelsus Medical University in Salzburg, Austria, who over time became a friend and close collaborator. Blog authors and journalists wrote and asked for interviews. With each additional paper on antidepressants I published there were more interview requests and invitations for talks at scientific meetings. Service users also wrote to me, mostly people harmed by antidepressants, who thanked me for my educational work on the risks of antidepressants and conflicts of interest in psychiatry. Soon I also communicated with influential researchers in this field, including, among others, Drs David Healy, Peter Gotzsche, Irving Kirsch, Joanna Moncrieff, Mark Horowitz, Janus Jakobsen, Tom Bschor, John Read, James Davies, and Giovanni Fava.

But there was not only delight and appreciation for my critical research on the benefit–harm ratio of antidepressants. Some people, especially psychiatrists, attacked me fiercely on social media, but also in their reviewer comments on articles I submitted for publication. Some accused me of spreading conspiracy theories and misinformation. Akin to Dr Lieberman in his blanket condemnation of researchers who question the clinical significance of antidepressants quoted at the beginning of this book [2], they alleged I was running an anti-scientific, ideologically biased crusade against psychiatry. My former PhD supervisor, Dr. Wulf Rössler, who also supported me as co-author on two controversial papers, once warned me that some leaders in the field would push back hard. He cautioned that by pursuing this kind of research I would soon make powerful enemies. He was right. There were times I felt exhausted and crestfallen, demoralised by insults on social media and irritating ad hominem attacks by anonymous reviewers.

I soon realised that the debate was highly polarised and hateful. Even scientific arguments could quickly turn into scathing and discrediting accusations. But there was also interest in my arguments and honest willingness to discuss the scientific evidence. A few debates were indeed constructive, especially when opponents were willing to discuss my scientific arguments instead of simply attacking me as a person for the kind of research I do. I also learned that many practicing psychiatrists and GPs were simply not aware of these pervasive issues that, to me, seemed so evident after my scrutiny of the literature. Some also admitted honestly to me, in confidence, that they were not allowed to raise these issues in the clinic, fearing disapproval and rejection from their colleagues and supervisors.

After I completed my habilitation (qualification for professorship and highest academic degree in Switzerland and various other countries) at the medical faculty of the University of Zurich, I gave my inaugural speech at the university in February 2019. I lectured about threats to evidence-based antidepressant prescribing. I detailed the selective reporting of efficacy and safety outcomes in antidepressant trials, which lead to a systematic overestimation of benefits and underestimation of harms. This is not just a provocative, misinformed opinion (as some psychiatrists had suggested), it is a well-established scientific fact consistently replicated over many years in antidepressant research [56–58, 81–83] and across various other therapeutic domains in general medical research [84–90]. The speech was attended by various colleagues from the Psychiatric University Hospital of Zurich, of which most were psychiatrists. After the talk, several came to me and confessed how concerned they were about these revelations. Never had they thought that the scientific literature was that biased and unreliable. Never during their training and continuing medical education had they heard about these seminal studies. I realised back then that this needs to change.

Since the publication of my first paper on antidepressants in 2017, I have given several talks at general hospitals, psychiatric clinics, and scientific conferences about the corruption of evidence-based medicine and systematically biased benefit–harm evaluations of antidepressants and other drugs. The reactions were always the same. The audiences, mostly physicians from various specialties and other healthcare providers (e.g. psychologists and social workers), were shocked about these findings. Quite often they were also embarrassed that they had been so ignorant about these pervasive issues. Several people asked me why I didn't write a book about it. I have long hesitated, as there are already several books and many research papers about the medical construct of depression, corporate bias, and antidepressant over-prescribing. However, obviously most practitioners, but also researchers, service users, advocacy groups and policymakers, are not aware of the multiple flaws in the way we define, diagnose, and treat depression. That's why I wrote this book on antidepressant prescribing in depression.

2

Antidepressants in Clinical Practice

All antidepressants available on the market increase the concentration of certain neurotransmitters (chemical messengers) in the brain, but how they exactly work in depression is poorly understood [91-93]. Based on their primary mechanism of action, antidepressant drugs can be broadly divided into five major classes. The monoamine oxidase inhibitors (MAOIs) prevent the breakdown of monoamines, predominantly serotonin, norepinephrine (noradrenaline) and dopamine, and thereby increase their availability in the synapse. The tricyclics increase the concentration of serotonin and norepinephrine by blocking their reuptake but also have potent antihistaminic and anticholinergic effects. The selective serotonin reuptake inhibitors (SSRIs) more selectively prevent the reuptake of serotonin, thus mostly increasing the availability of serotonin. The serotonin norepinephrine reuptake inhibitors (SNRIs) inhibit the reuptake of both serotonin and norepinephrine, thus primarily increasing the concentration of these two neurotransmitters. Finally, the atypical antidepressants are a heterogeneous class with different mechanisms of action, but to some degree all increase the concentration of serotonin, norepinephrine and/or dopamine (except the latest drug esketamine, approved in 2019, a chemical derivate of the anaesthetic and

M. P. Hengartner, *Evidence-biased Antidepressant Prescription*,
https://doi.org/10.1007/978-3-030-82587-4_2

popular street drug ketamine, which primarily acts on NMDA receptors [94]). The first-generation antidepressant drugs, the MAOIs and the tricyclics, were discovered in the late 1950s and introduced in clinical practice around 1960 [1, 95]. The SSRIs, SNRIs, and the atypicals form the broad class of new-generation antidepressants (sometimes SSRIs are also referred to as second-generation and SNRIs and atypicals as third-generation antidepressants). The SSRIs were introduced in the late 1980s and early 1990s and most SNRIs in the late 1990s and 2000s. The atypical antidepressants were introduced at various periods. Some entered the market in the 1980s and 1990s (for example bupropion and mirtazapine), and others only recently in the 2010s (for example vilazodone and vortioxetine). The generic and brand names of the most popular drugs from each class in the treatment of depression still on the market are shown in Table 2.1.

Most antidepressants were first approved for the treatment of depressive disorders and still are mostly prescribed for that condition [96-99]. Between the 1960s and 1980s, the MAOIs and tricyclics were predominantly prescribed by psychiatrists in psychiatric hospitals to patients with severe (melancholic) depression. With the advent of the SSRIs, which were safer in overdose and easy to use (achieving the optimal dose), antidepressants were increasingly prescribed in primary care by GPs for less severe forms of depression and for tension, stress symptoms, and anxiety [63, 93, 95]. Since the late 1990s, antidepressants also became popular treatments for anxiety disorders, sleep problems, and various non-psychiatric conditions, including pain disorders and menopause symptoms [96-100]. In the following I will explain in more detail how antidepressant prescribing for depression changed over time and then I will outline the issues of efficacy/effectiveness and the benefit–harm balance of antidepressants in depression.

Antidepressant Prescribing

The introduction of the SSRIs in the late 1980s led to a massive increase in antidepressant prescribing. In 1980, Americans filled about 30 million antidepressant prescriptions, in 2001 that number rose to a staggering

Table 2.1 Popular antidepressants for the treatment of depression still on the market

Class	Generic Name	Brand Name
MAOIs	Isocarboxazid	Marplan
	Phenelzine	Nardil
	Tranylcypromine	Parnate
Tricyclics	Amitriptyline	Elavil
	Clomipramine	Anafranil
	Doxepin	Sinequan
	Imipramine	Tofranil
	Nortriptyline	Aventyl
SSRIs	Citalopram	Celexa
	Escitalopram	Lexapro
	Fluoxetine	Prozac
	Paroxetine	Paxil, Seroxat
	Sertraline	Zoloft
SNRIs	Desvenlafaxine	Pristiq
	Duloxetine	Cymbalta
	Levomilnacipran	Fetzima
	Venlafaxine	Effexor
Atypicals	Agomelatine	Valdoxan
	Bupropion	Wellbutrin
	Esketamine	Spravato
	Mirtazapine	Remeron
	Trazodone	Trittico, Desyrel
	Vilazodone	Viibryd
	Vortioxetine	Trintellix

264 million prescriptions, making antidepressants the best-selling drug class of all [30]. At its peak in 1998, Eli Lilly's SSRI fluoxetine produced $2.8 billion in revenues [101]. In 1999, 3 of the top 10 best-selling pharmaceuticals in the US were SSRIs—fluoxetine, paroxetine, and sertraline—accounting for combined revenues of $6.7 billion [24]. Over time, newer antidepressants replaced them as market leaders. In 2006, the SNRI venlafaxine was the number 1 antidepressant and ranked 6th best-selling drug in the US with $2.3 billion in revenues and the SSRI escitalopram was number 10 with $2.1 billion in revenues (sertraline was number 15 with $1.8 billion in revenues) [102].

Due to their great popularity among both physicians and the public, antidepressants have largely replaced non-pharmacological interventions as first-line depression treatment. From 1987 to 1997, the proportion of

US outpatients with depression who were treated with antidepressants increased from 37% to 75%, while the proportion who received psychotherapy declined from 71% to 60% [103]. The proportion of outpatients receiving antidepressants remained constant at 75% from 1998 to 2007, but the proportion of outpatients receiving psychotherapy continued to decline and in 2007, a mere 43% of US outpatients with depression were treated with psychotherapy, often in combination with antidepressants [104]. Finally, in 2012/2013, a total 87% of US outpatients treated for depression were using antidepressants as compared to 23% receiving psychotherapy, of which the vast majority (79%) was additionally treated with antidepressants [105].

During the 1990s and 2000s, antidepressant prescription rates multiplied not only in the US [106, 107], but in all high-income countries, including European countries, New Zealand, and Australia [108-110]. For instance, in the UK adult population, antidepressant use increased from about 2–3% in the mid-1980s [111] to about 6% in 1995 and further to 13% in 2011 [112]. The most recent estimates from England indicate that in 2017/2018, in total 17% of the adult population used an antidepressant [113]. Most importantly, the majority of antidepressants are now prescribed for mild, minor and subthreshold depression [105, 114], which are the most prevalent forms of depression in the general population and in primary care [105, 115-117].

In most high-income countries, including the US, Australia, UK, Denmark, Sweden, and Germany, for about 15 years antidepressant use has also increased steadily in youth [118-121]. For instance, according to a population-based study from Sweden, 2.1% of female and 1.3% of male adolescents aged 12–17 years were on antidepressants in the year 2013, as compared to 1.1% and 0.6%, respectively, in 2006 [122]. In the UK, 3.2% of the youth population aged 15–19 was prescribed an antidepressant in 2012, as compared to 2.3% in 2006, whereas in the US the corresponding rates were 6.2% and 5.4%, respectively. Noteworthy is the marked discrepancy between countries: in Germany the rates were only 1.4% (2012) and 0.8% (2006), thus also increasing but many times lower than in the US [118].

In the last two decades, the rise in antidepressant prescribing was mostly due to increasing long-term use [112, 123-125]. In the US, from

2011 to 2014, 68% of antidepressant users aged 12 years and older had been taking the drugs for at least two 2 years, and about 25% had been taking the drugs for 10 years and more [107]. According to Mojtabai and Olfson [124], 7% of the US adult population had been on antidepressants for at least 2 years in the year 2009/2010, as compared to 3% in the year 1999/2000. In a large general practice study from the Netherlands, in the period 2005–2015, 44% of antidepressant users had been taking the drugs for 15 months and longer, as compared to 30% in the period 1995–2005 [126]. Finally, in England, as of 2018, altogether 52% of antidepressant users had been on the drugs continuously for more than 12 months [113], and according to a large general practice study in Scotland, 47% of adult antidepressant users were on the same drug for at least 2 years [127].

A third prescription trend that is worth mentioning is the growing rate of psychotropic polypharmacy. That is, antidepressants are increasingly prescribed in combination with other psychiatric drugs. In US psychiatric outpatient practice, from 1996 to 2006, 23% of adult antidepressant users were additionally prescribed sedative-hypnotic drugs (mostly benzodiazepines and Z-drugs), 13% were co-medicated with antipsychotics, and further 13% with a second antidepressant. The rate of polypharmacy had significantly increased from 1996 to 2006 [128]. Polypharmacy has also increased in youths. For example, in the Swedish population aged 12–17 years, polypharmacy in antidepressant users increased from 49% in 2006 to 70% in 2013. For the vast majority of youths using antidepressants, polypharmacy comprised co-medication with sedative-hypnotics and, considerably less so, with antipsychotics [122].

In sum, not only is an increasing proportion of the population prescribed antidepressants each year, people on antidepressants also use the drugs continuously for an ever-growing period and are increasingly co-medicated with other psychotropic drugs, especially sedative-hypnotics. Although antidepressants are increasingly prescribed for anxiety, insomnia, and non-psychiatric conditions (e.g. pain), another consistent finding is that, across countries and age groups, by far the most frequent treatment indication is still depression [96-99, 129-131].

Effectiveness of Antidepressants in Depression

Some readers may assume that the debate about the efficacy and safety of antidepressants is a recent phenomenon that started with the introduction and widespread prescription of the SSRIs. However, this is not true. Since they were first introduced in clinical practice around 1960, the benefit–harm ratio of antidepressants has been a controversial subject [93, 132]. In the mid-twentieth century the efficacy data of the first-generation drugs (i.e. MAOIs and tricyclics) was questioned just like the SSRIs and other new-generation antidepressants were (and still are) in the early twenty-first century (for recent critiques, see for example [18, 133-135]). For instance, in 1964, pioneering psychopharmacology researcher Dr Jonathan Cole reviewed the efficacy of the MAOIs and tricyclics, and overall, judged the scientific evidence far from being convincing:

> "The newer antidepressant drugs have now been used experimentally and clinically for approximately seven years. Their place in the physician's armamentarium is still far from clear, although many clinicians feel that the drugs are useful and effective. However, controlled clinical trials of these agents have not always led to unequivocally positive findings. Even when the findings have been favourable to the drugs under study, the differences between the efficacy of the drug and a placebo have not been as great as one might wish, or as one might have anticipated after reading published reports of uncontrolled trials" [136].

Up to this day, the main question for patients and prescribers still is: how effective are antidepressants for depression? Do most users really benefit? And how safe are the drugs? Although these questions seem straightforward and easy to answer, they're not. That's why after so many decades antidepressants have been on the market, there are still diverging opinions and fierce debates about their utility and whether benefits clearly outweigh harms [18, 133, 134, 137-140]. Take for instance the high-impact meta-analysis by Cipriani and colleagues published in 2018 in the leading medical journal *Lancet* [141], which, as of June 2021, has already been cited a stunning 1346 times according to Google Scholar.

For many psychiatrists, including Dr. Lieberman quoted at the beginning of this book, this study finally provided the ultimate answer that antidepressants are effective and safe [2]. Likewise, Dr. Carmine Pariante, spokesperson for the Royal College of Psychiatrists (RCP; the British psychiatric association), stated that this study "finally puts to bed the controversy on antidepressants, clearly showing that these drugs do work in lifting mood and helping most people with depression" [18]. Similar conclusions were drawn by many other vocal psychiatrists.

By contrast, some experts, including myself, drew much less optimistic conclusions from this meta-analysis, stressing that the data basically showed that antidepressants have at best very small and practically questionable therapeutic effects and that they benefit only a small minority of patients [18, 134, 140, 142]. According to Dr Nassir Ghaemi, professor of psychiatry at Tufts University School of Medicine, "This meta-analysis confirms the results of prior meta-analyses which found that antidepressants have small overall effects in 'MDD' [major depressive disorder] and do not provide major clinical benefit in general" [143]. And researchers from the Nordic Cochrane Centre, led by psychiatrist Dr Klaus Munkholm, wrote after their re-analysis of the data: "Taken together, the evidence does not support definitive conclusions regarding the efficacy of antidepressants for depression in adults, including whether they are more efficacious than placebo for depression" [13]. It's also important to differentiate between efficacy (treatment effects under controlled experimental conditions in preselected, narrowly defined trial participants) and effectiveness (treatment effects under "real-world" routine-care conditions in representative patient samples). That is, efficacy doesn't necessarily translate into effectiveness. What works in a tightly controlled experimental setting sometimes badly fails in messy real-world routine healthcare. But why do different experts arrive at such divergent, highly conflicting conclusions (i.e., antidepressants are clearly effective in most patients vs. antidepressants are minimally effective and benefit only a small minority of patients)? Antidepressants certainly have some treatment effects, but how meaningful are they? And how many patients truly benefit? In this chapter I will address these questions, though a definite answer is probably still not possible because the database consists almost exclusively of industry-sponsored, short-term efficacy trials with several methodological limitations [13, 54, 135, 144].

Drug Regulatory Assessments

Many psychiatrists argue that the therapeutic effects of antidepressant are clinically significant in depression, otherwise the drug regulators would not have approved them [145]. This is an appeal to authority, not a scientific argument. It also disregards how drug regulators like the US Food and Drug Administration (FDA) approve drugs and that different drug regulators may come to conflicting conclusions. For instance, before the FDA approved Eli Lilly's fluoxetine as an effective and safe antidepressant in late 1987, the German drug regulators had rejected Eli Lilly's new drug application for lack of efficacy and increased risk of suicidality in 1985 [146]. According to the assessment of the German drug regulators, fluoxetine was "totally unsuitable for the treatment of depression" [9]. Eli Lilly then obscured the increased risk of suicidality by re-coding suicidal events as "worsening depression" and "emotional lability", which is why later the FDA and also all other drug regulators, including the German agency, eventually approved fluoxetine [9, 147]. Reboxetine was approved by European drug regulators, suggesting its benefits outweigh harms, but the antidepressant was not approved in the US by the FDA, suggesting, conversely, that the drug is ineffective or harmful. Finally, nomifensine was approved as a safe and effective antidepressant by British drug regulators after a speedy review time of 10 months, but the FDA withheld its approval for several years as the data did not demonstrate efficacy. Eventually, after 72 months under review, the FDA also approved the drug despite questionable efficacy data, but within a year the drug was withdrawn from the market by the manufacturer for safety reasons [148, 149]. So, apparently, nomifensine had a very poor benefit–harm ratio, despite its rapid approval by the British drug regulators.

It is thus worthy of having a closer look at how the FDA and other drug regulators determine the efficacy of antidepressants. As summarised by Dr. Shorter, "Today, the FDA makes things easy. Rather than insisting that a new drug be superior to existing drugs, the agency permits the companies to test new products only against placebo. If you can beat sugar pills in your drug trial, you get your drug licensed" [1]. But it's even worse than that. Drug regulators don't even require that the new drug consistently beats placebo. In fact, the drug company can conduct as many trials as it wants and merely needs to demonstrate a positive result in two of them (sometimes in merely one trial). That is, a new drug may fail to be more effective than placebo in several adequately powered and well-controlled trials, but if at least two were positive (or partially positive), the license will be granted. This rather peculiar approach to assessing efficacy is based on the premise that when a drug fails to beat placebo in a controlled trial, the FDA determines that the trial lacked "assay sensitivity", that is, it was a failed and uninformative trial [150]. As aptly stated by Shorter referring to the controversial approval of sertraline, "This really involved almost bending over backward in order to avoid saying anything negative about sertraline [and other new-generation antidepressants]. This was the new FDA: When drugs fail, it is the trial not the drug that is at fault" [1].

This is intuitively problematic. Imagine that a new antidepressant failed to be superior to placebo in, say, four trials, but successful in two, this would mean that the trial success rate is only 33% (2 out of 6 trials). Would you deem a drug effective when it beats placebo in merely every third well-controlled and adequately powered clinical trial? Probably you will insist that this example is purely hypothetical and does not reflect the true regulatory situation. Unfortunately, it's not hypothetical. For instance, Pfizer submitted five placebo-controlled efficacy trials of its SSRI sertraline to the FDA for marketing approval. Sertraline was statistically definitely superior to placebo in one trial, a second trial was questionably positive (i.e. inconclusive statistical evidence), and three trials were definitely negative (i.e. sertraline did not beat placebo). So, success rate was 20% if you don't count the questionable trial as positive and 40% if you consider that questionable trial as positive. Indeed not really a favourable overall assessment. Of note, sertraline, which is one of the most widely prescribed antidepressants, also failed to demonstrate efficacy in most independently sponsored, well-designed post-marketing trials (see, for example [151–153]).

Or take citalopram, another very popular SSRI. Of five placebo-controlled efficacy trials submitted to the FDA for marketing approval, two were positive and three were negative, thus the trial success rate was only 40% [57]. Bupropion sustained-release, an atypical antidepressant, was approved even though the FDA reviewer considered all three placebo-controlled trials negative and the average treatment effect was only d=0.17, which is a marginally small treatment effect close to zero (d=0.0) [150]. But how is it that this drug was approved? Well, in that case the FDA decided that the immediate-release formulation had previously shown efficacy, thus a link could be made to the sustained-release formulation. At least the sponsor was not allowed to make efficacy claims for the sustained-release formulation, which is why the prescribing information stated "there are not as yet independent trials demonstrating the antidepressant effectiveness of the sustained-release formulation of bupropion" [150]. In other words, bupropion sustained-release was approved as safe and effective even though it failed to demonstrate efficacy. It only was granted a license because its sister drug, bupropion immediate-release, had demonstrated efficacy. There are various other antidepressants that were approved despite questionable efficacy data and unclear benefit–harm ratio, including reboxetine [82], vortioxetine [154] and, most recently, the controversial drug esketamine [155, 156].

Now, let's quickly discuss what the FDA considers a positive efficacy trial. "Positive" does not imply that a drug clearly works in the average patient or that its benefits are clinically (or practically) relevant. It merely means that the treatment effect was statistically significant in a controlled experimental setting in preselected (narrowly defined and thus unrepresentative) trial participants. People familiar with basic statistics will understand that this is not necessarily an indicator for robust, meaningful, and generalisable treatment effects. A statistically significant effect can be disappointingly small and fall short of clinical (or practical) relevance in the average patient [18, 150, 157]. Statisticians have repeatedly stressed that even the most trivial effects can reach statistical significance if sample size or measurement precision is high enough [158]. Neither does a statistically significant result imply that the treatment effect is necessarily true positive and replicable [51, 159, 160]. Are you confused now? It sounds rather technical and complicated, but it's in fact quite simple. Let me explain it briefly.

Imagine we want to test whether a new diet pill is effective. For it we carefully select a large sample of overweight people who are otherwise healthy and not using other medications. We also ensure that they have previously not shown a poor response to another diet pill. All participants are informed about the side effects of the new drug (e.g. tiredness, dizziness) and the exact study procedures. Those who consent to participate then enter the actual trial. Half of the sample is randomly assigned to the study drug and the other half to an inert placebo pill. The two pills look identical and both participants and the clinical investigators don't know who is taking the active drug and who is taking placebo, which is referred to as double-blind procedure. However, in reality, various participants will eventually correctly guess whether they take the active drug or placebo due to the presence or lack of side effects (referred to as unblinding). The participants are closely monitored and frequently tested for, say, 12 weeks. The primary outcome is the difference in body weight between treatment groups at 12 weeks and it is found that the diet pill has reduced weight by 200 grams relative to the placebo pill. This is the average treatment effect and a statistical test shows that it is statistically significant, meaning that the effect is unlikely due to mere chance (i.e. random variation) if, and only if, all assumptions of the statistical test are met. These assumptions are frequently violated though, thus in fact even a statistically significant effect could be due to chance [160]. So the average treatment effect of 200 grams is not even necessarily a true effect, despite a statistically significant result. And it could also be substantially overestimated due to methodological limitations, for example unblinding of trial participants. Assuming that people on placebo terminated the trial earlier because they correctly guessed that they received the inert placebo pill due to lack of side effects, it could well be that the tiny drug-placebo difference at study endpoint was a methodological artefact, that is, a false-positive effect due to inadequate handling of study dropouts and their missing data [161-163].

Nevertheless, according to the FDA and other agencies, the trial was positive, and the drug regulators would conclude that the investigational drug has demonstrated efficacy. If a second trial yields a similar result, and if there are no serious safety concerns, the FDA and other drug regulators will most likely approve the new drug. But would you consider such a drug truly effective? Would you risk various side effects for losing barely 200 grams weight? If you can't confidently answer these questions with "Yes", you understand that a statistically significant treatment effect does not imply clinical significance (or practical relevance), even when a second trial produced the same result. As demonstrated by van Ravenzwaaij and Ioannidis [164], the common regulatory approach to consider a drug effective based on two statistically significant trials provides rather poor evidential support, especially when the true treatment effect is weak, when sample size is modest, and when statistically significant results were obtained in a minority of trials (as is often the case in antidepressant trials). The authors thus state, "Medicines should only be endorsed if the evidence in favor of its efficacy is strong and consistent, but the reality provides a stark contrast to that ideal" [164].

The FDA made clear that it bases its decisions to approve a new psychiatric drug merely on whether a drug is statistically significantly better than placebo, and not on the magnitude of the treatment effect. That is, the FDA approves psychiatric drugs when they have any discernible effect at all relative to placebo, no matter how trivial that effect is, and even when a new drug is inferior to established antidepressants [1, 9, 150]. Dr. Leber, former director of the psychopharmacology division at the FDA once stated: "Now, again this brings up the old issue of size of treatment effect versus the existence of a treatment effect. And for purposes of approval we rely on the existence, the hypothesis testing whether or not it is there" [1]. Thus, any effect that is statistically discernible from zero, say 200 grams weight reduction as in the example above, qualifies as treatment efficacy. But the FDA and its advisory committee were of course aware that the average treatment effect of the new-generation antidepressants was quite disappointing. At various FDA advisory committee meetings it was acknowledged (and critically discussed) that the SSRIs were barely better than placebo and that they largely failed to demonstrate efficacy in psychiatric inpatients with severe (melancholic) depression, that is, those patients most in need of effective treatments [1, 9].

But despite underwhelming efficacy data, the SSRIs and other new-generation antidepressants were approved, for, according the FDA director Dr. Leber, "I think you have to understand that when we face an application, from a regulatory perspective, we are asked to face what the law requires us to do. We are obliged to approve an NDA [new drug application] unless our review finds that the drug is unsafe for use" [1]. This ultimately implies that the FDA approved the SSRIs and other new-generation antidepressants not because they were clearly effective in most patients, but because they were considered not harmful in most patients. But this doesn't necessarily prove that a drug is safe in use or that it conveys sustained benefits, for new psychiatric drugs are tested in small and selective samples over a very short period. In total, 43 new psychiatric drugs were approved by the FDA between 2005 and 2012. The median sample size in the pivotal efficacy trials was 432, of which a median of 231 received the investigational drug, and the median trial duration was a meagre 6 weeks (no trial lasted longer than 6 months) [165]. When the SSRIs and SNRIs were clinically tested in the 1980s and 1990s, the typical sample size in antidepressant trials was even smaller. In those years, the average number of patients per group was 84 for placebo and 85 for medication [166]. It is thus evidently impossible to detect rare but serious adverse drug reactions in such trials, especially harm resulting from long-term use. It is also impossible to determine whether the drug has any sustained benefits, that is, therapeutic effects lasting beyond the acute treatment period of 6–8 weeks.

The lenient criteria adopted by the FDA are of course not unique [167, 168]. Other drug regulators such as the European Medicines Agency (EMA) also have a permissive approval principle (i.e. statistically significant treatment effects against placebo in 1 or 2 small short-term trials or non-inferiority compared to approved drugs). Pignatti and colleagues [169] analysed 111 new drug applications submitted to the EMA and showed that 39% of drugs had marginal or no clinically relevant efficacy. However, marginal or no clinical efficacy did not influence whether an application was approved or not, indicating that a substantial portion of approved drugs were largely ineffective. Therefore, as recently concluded by Erhel and colleagues based on an analysis of EMA reviews of approved new psychiatric drug applications, "The evidence for psychiatric drug approved by the EMA was in general poor" [170]. Boesen and colleagues also criticised the designs for psychiatric drug trials recommended by both FDA and EMA. The authors concluded, "The EMA and FDA clinical research guidelines for psychiatric pivotal trials recommend designs that tend to have limited generalisability. Independent and non-conflicted stakeholders are underrepresented in the development phases and current guidelines emphasise trials with limited scope that may not offer much clinical value. EMA and FDA should reconsider their guideline development and find ways to promote greater involvement of the public and independent stakeholders" [167].

When the requirements for approval of new drugs are so low (or inadequate), it necessarily follows that a large portion of new therapeutic agents offer very little therapeutic benefit to the average patient treated in real-world healthcare settings [171, 172]. According to the German Institute for Quality and Efficiency in Health Care (IQWiG), 58% of all drugs approved in Germany between 2011 and 2017 had no added benefit (relative to established drugs on the market), and only 25% were judged to have considerable or major added benefit. The situation is even worse with respect to psychiatric drugs. Only 1 of 18 approved psychiatric drugs (6%) was shown to have a minor added benefit, all others had no added benefit [173].

Evaluation of Average Treatment Effects

The critical reader will thus certainly agree that a regulatory approval is insufficient to determine whether the treatment effects of antidepressants are clinically (or practically) relevant and whether benefits unequivocally outweigh harms in the average real-world patient, especially over the long-term. So how else can we evaluate the benefits of antidepressants? By looking exactly at those data that the drug regulators deem irrelevant, that is, how many antidepressant trials failed to demonstrate efficacy, and, most importantly, the size (or magnitude) of the treatment effect. And here is the pertinent scientific evidence.

The pooled data from placebo-controlled antidepressant trials with a typical duration of 6–8 weeks in adult patients with moderate to severe depression indicate that antidepressants are quite often not definitely better than placebo. Just about half of these efficacy trials found a statistically significant drug–placebo difference [57, 174], a finding confirmed by the FDA's own analysis [175]. That is, in every second clinical trial, the antidepressant drug failed to beat an inert placebo pill. This is worrisome and legitimately calls into question antidepressants' efficacy (and utility) in many patients prescribed these drugs. But then, why are so many patients treated with antidepressants getting better after a 6–8 week treatment trial? Many psychiatrists and GPs affirm that antidepressants are effective based on their clinical observation of improvements after treatment initiation, and this is also a common (although not evidence-based) reply to scientific debates about the questionable effectiveness of antidepressants (e.g. "in my clinical experience, antidepressants clearly work, I've witnessed it hundreds of times"). The answer is quite simple and straightforward: untreated depression symptoms often improve on their own after a few weeks, which is commonly referred to as spontaneous remission [176–180]. By consequence, even if a doctor would prescribe chocolate, dancing, or gardening, he/she would observe improvements in many patients [181, 182]. As detailed by Dr Hollon, "Depression is an inherently temporal phenomenon and most episodes will remit spontaneously even in the absence of treatment" [183]. Moreover, participants in an antidepressant trial receive a great deal of medical attention and psychosocial support, so frequent visits to physicians and a good therapeutic alliance, regardless of treatment provided, also have a considerable therapeutic effect [184-186].

But what about antidepressant trials in psychiatric inpatients with severe to very severe depression? It has been argued that people with severe (melancholic) depression improve less (or only slowly) without antidepressant treatment [187]; therefore, we would expect that the trial success rate is higher in this particular patient population. Unfortunately, the scientific literature provides no definite answer because patients with severe (melancholic) depression are rarely included in placebo-controlled trials. Most efficacy trials strictly exclude patients with acute suicidality [188], which is the strongest indicator of severe depression [189]. Most trials also exclude patients with comorbid disorders, both physical and mental conditions [188], even though comorbidity is another marker of severe depression [190]. Paradoxically (and, also concerningly), the efficacy of antidepressants in patients with severe to very severe depression thus remains largely unknown. Please bear this major limitation in mind when I guide you through the average efficacy estimates based on meta-analyses of clinical trials.

Pooled across trials, the response rate, defined as a symptom improvement of at least 50% from baseline, is about 50% for antidepressants [191] and 35–40% for placebo [192], thus producing a drug–placebo difference in response rates at the end of the acute treatment period of 10–15% and a rate ratio of about 1.2 to 1.4 [140, 193, 194]. This means that achieving a meaningful clinical improvement (i.e. response) is only 1.2 to 1.4 times more likely with antidepressants relative to inert placebo pills, which is a small clinical benefit (a rate ratio of 1 indicates no benefit). Likewise, based on these response rate differences, the number needed to treat is about 9, indicating that only 1 of 9 adults (11%) treated with an antidepressant achieve a good treatment outcome (i.e. response) that they would not have with a placebo pill. Conversely, this means that 8 of 9 adults (89%) treated with an antidepressant would have the same good outcome with a placebo pill but are unnecessarily exposed to the drug's side effects [18, 140]. Based on these established results for response rates it's evidently wrong to claim that antidepressants benefit most patients. In fact, the correct conclusion derived from these data is that they benefit only 1 in 9 patients, that is, 11% of all users. However, that's not a definite answer.

Response rates have serious limitations, since they are based on an arbitrary dichotomisation of continuous depression scores and capture only broadly defined improvements [13, 16, 195]. For instance, both patient A whose symptoms worsened by 20% (deterioration) and patient B whose symptoms improved by 49% (substantial improvement) are recorded as non-responders, although their treatment outcome is fundamentally different, whereas patient C whose symptoms improved by 50% (also a substantial improvement) is recorded as a responder, although his/her treatment outcome is almost identical to patient B (who is recorded as a non-responder). So, you see that classifying patients as responders and non-responders is a very imprecise and diffuse approach that largely misses the true individual treatment outcome. A much more accurate way to analyse antidepressant trials is therefore to examine the continuous depression scores at study endpoint, which denote exactly how well (or unwell) each patient was after acute treatment. Continuous depression scores also allow to determine to what extent a patient worsened or improved over the course of treatment. Continuous depression scores thus comprise much more information than response rates and also take into account that some patients' symptoms worsened (or remained unchanged) over the course of treatment.

According to the most widely applied depression outcome measure, the 17-item Hamilton Depression Rating Scale (HDRS-17; range 0 [no symptoms] to 52 points [most extreme symptoms]), the average symptom change on antidepressant from baseline to end of acute treatment is about 11 points, and the corresponding change on placebo is about 9 points, thus the drug–placebo difference at the end of the acute 6–8 week treatment period is only 2 points [13, 196]. On the Montgomery-Asberg Depression Rating Scale (MADRS; range 0 [no symptoms] to 60 points [most extreme symptoms]), another popular outcome measure, the average drug–placebo difference is 3 points [17]. The standardised effect size estimate derived from these drug–placebo differences is about d=0.3 for both scales [17, 57, 141]. There is little doubt that these are modest (or weak) effects, but how meaningful are they to patients? Are they trivial and not worth the side effects? Or else, are they small but important to patients, despite side effects? And, most importantly, does efficacy assessed in a controlled experimental setting translate into effectiveness in routine healthcare [20]?

Antidepressants have demonstrated modest efficacy in some clinical trials, but this does not necessarily imply that they are also effective in real-world clinical practice. Efficacy merely indicates that a treatment effect was statistically significant in a controlled experimental setting, no matter how practically relevant the effect size is. That is, a statistically significant effect is not necessarily meaningful. In fact, as detailed above, when sample size is sufficiently large and measurement precision adequate, even tiny effects that have no practical relevance whatsoever can reach statistical significance [15, 18, 158, 197]. Effectiveness, on the other hand, evaluates whether a drug can make a real difference in routine practice, where monitoring and clinical management are often poor. Therefore, to have a real impact in routine practice, an efficacy estimate established under optimal experimental conditions must reach a threshold that corresponds to a minimally important effect. So, what is this magical threshold where efficacy translates into effectiveness?

This question is again difficult to answer, for there is no agreed-upon threshold for a minimally important treatment effect. Nevertheless, according to the literature, it seems that treatment effects should be at least 3 points on both HDRS-17 and MADRS to be considered minimally important in real-world healthcare settings [20]. As detailed above, the average treatment effect according to meta-analyses of clinical trials is 2 points on the HDRS-17 and 3 points on the MADRS. Thus, in most users the effectiveness of antidepressants is presumably minimal (as assessed with MADRS) or doubtful (as assessed with HDRS-17).

Treatment effects are often transformed into standardised effect size estimates (commonly Cohen's d), but these estimates are also difficult to interpret. Per convention, effect sizes smaller than 0.5 are considered small and of doubtful clinical significance [143, 198]. Although this threshold is controversial [18], various studies indeed suggest that effect sizes smaller than 0.5 have very little or no practical relevance [199, 200]. In accordance, a recent Cochrane review on the efficacy of omega-3 fatty acids in depression found an effect size of 0.3 relative to placebo and concluded that "this effect is unlikely to be clinically meaningful" [201]. Note that, as detailed above, the average effect size of antidepressants in adult depression is also 0.3 [17, 57, 141, 198]. If researchers would apply the same assessment standard to antidepressants, then they would have to interpret the efficacy of antidepressants also as "unlikely to be clinically meaningful". Therefore, based on the clinical trial results, we cannot conclude with certainty that antidepressants have demonstrated clinically (or practically) relevant efficacy. In fact, it seems that the average treatment effect of antidepressants falls rather short of a minimally important effect. Please consider that due to a lack of consensus on a threshold for a minimally important effect, this is not a definite answer. So are there other ways to assess the effectiveness of antidepressants? Yes, there are, but they are also imperfect.

To evaluate the efficacy (or effectiveness) of antidepressants, we can also compare them to other depression treatments. In direct comparisons, antidepressants are equally effective as physical exercise and St. John's Wort (hypericum) [202, 203]. Many studies have further shown that antidepressants, both older and newer drugs, are equally effective as psychotherapy during the acute treatment phase [204–206], and this applies to both severe/melancholic depression and non-severe depression [205, 207, 208]. However, treatment discontinuation rates are significantly higher with antidepressants, suggesting that the benefit–harm ratio of pharmacotherapy is less favourable than that of psychotherapy, and in long-term studies, psychotherapy is consistently more effective than pharmacotherapy, indicating that psychotherapy has more sustained benefits than antidepressants [204–206, 209–212]. Finally, there is evidence that the combination of antidepressants and psychotherapy is more effective than psychotherapy alone during the acute treatment phase, but this is not consistently replicated when combination therapy is compared to psychotherapy plus pill placebo [204]. Moreover, long-term data (6 months and longer) indicate that combination therapy is not definitely superior to psychotherapy alone, suggesting that adding antidepressants to psychotherapy offers at best a marginally small long-term benefit over psychotherapy alone [204, 212, 213].

Long-term Outcomes

Given that most antidepressants are prescribed long-term (i.e. 6 months and longer), it would be extremely important to evaluate long-term benefits rather than merely 6–8 week acute phase results. In theory it's possible that antidepressants have substantial long-term benefits despite their modest (or poor) efficacy in the acute treatment phase. This is very unlikely though, given that, as detailed above, psychotherapy is superior to antidepressants in the long-term despite similar short-term treatment outcomes [214]. Nevertheless, let's briefly review long-term, placebo-controlled antidepressant trials. First thing to note is that, although there are hundreds of short-term antidepressant trials [141], there are almost no classic placebo-controlled long-term trials. A systematic review and meta-analysis of long-term SSRI trials found only 6 trials that lasted at least 6 months (specifically 6–8 months). While the effect on response rates was statistically significant and similar to that found in acute short-term trials, the authors failed to find a statistically significant effect on remission rates at 6–8 months [215]. Another systematic review compared acute treatment effects (at 8 weeks, based on 91 studies) to long-term treatment effects (at 20 and 24 weeks, based on 3 and 2 studies, respectively) and found that treatment efficacy was largely constant over time, but the long-term estimates were imprecise and could range from very small to moderate [216]. Thus, although there is clearly a lack of long-term efficacy studies, the literature does not indicate that long-term treatment effects are better than the small effects shown in short-term studies. Quite the contrary, according to various studies (both naturalistic and experimental), antidepressants' long-term effects are largely inexistent or even harmful [183, 217–221]. So let's look in more detail at sustained remission and let's address the question, whether antidepressants effectively prevent relapses in the long-term (also referred to as prophylactic effects).

According to two large real-world effectiveness trials that adopted an extensive medication algorithm, including switching and combination of drugs in case of non-response or partial response, less than 10% of adult patients with moderate to severe depression were in sustained remission after one year [219, 222]. Unfortunately, there was no placebo control group in these two trials, which is why we don't know if there was any benefit from the drugs' pharmacological action (improvements could also be due to spontaneous remission and/or psychosocial support). Nevertheless, the data indicate that less than 10% of patients who initiated antidepressant therapy did remit and remained well over a year. If these results are generalisable, they suggest that most patients with moderate to severe depression treated with antidepressants either do not remit despite extensive long-term pharmacotherapy (including medication switches and drug combinations) or eventually relapse after remission despite continued pharmacotherapy. In either case, this is undeniably a poor long-term outcome.

But it could be even worse. In fact, and as mentioned above, a growing body of evidence suggests that long-term antidepressant treatment may worsen depression, general mental health, and psychosocial functioning in some patients [183, 217, 220, 221, 223, 224]. It has been shown that repeated or prolonged antidepressant treatment may result in tolerance or loss of efficacy, which has also been referred to as tachyphylaxis

[223–226]. Patients who develop tolerance no longer have therapeutic benefits from antidepressant treatment (i.e. loss of efficacy), but often experience adverse drug effects and withdrawal symptoms that resemble mood disorder symptoms, including sleep disturbances, cognitive problems, hyperactivation, and affect dysregulation. As detailed by Dr. Vittengl, "antidepressant medications may recruit processes that oppose and eventually overwhelm short-term benefits resulting in loss of efficacy, resistance to retreatment, paradoxical effects, and withdrawal syndromes, perhaps via disruption of homeostatic control of monoamine neurotransmitters" [221]. Consequently, this condition is often labelled as treatment-resistant depression, which typically escalates in aggressive pharmacotherapy involving antipsychotics, lithium, and, more recently, esketamine [227].

Dr. Fava recently described the problems with long-term antidepressant treatment as follows: "if treatment is prolonged beyond 6 months, phenomena such as tolerance, episode acceleration, sensitization and paradoxical effects may ensue. The hidden costs of using the AD [antidepressant] may then outweigh their apparent gains, particularly when the likelihood of responsiveness is low" [218]. Such adverse effects of prolonged antidepressant treatment possibly also account for the fact that the combination of psychotherapy and antidepressants, despite being effective during acute treatment, provides no reliable long-term benefits over psychotherapy alone [183, 212, 213]. Therefore, to this day it's not clear whether long-term antidepressant treatment (also referred to as maintenance therapy) is, overall, an effective strategy to achieve sustained remission in depression [214, 228, 229]. As detailed by Dr Ghaemi, "[Antidepressants'] long-term prophylactic effectiveness in recurrent unipolar major depression remains uncertain" [230].

But wait, are there not dozens of relapse prevention trials, which, according to Nutt and colleagues, clearly demonstrate that "antidepressants have an impressive ability to prevent recurrence of depression … which makes them one of the most effective of all drugs" [22]? The readers familiar with the scientific literature might indeed wonder why I don't present the results of these relapse prevention trials, the main evidence putatively demonstrating long-term treatment benefits [231–233]. However, there is a simple and compelling reason not to consider the evidence of these studies. As detailed by many experts, including the authors of a recent Cochrane review and myself, relapse prevention trials are unreliable and systematically biased because they confound genuine depression relapse with withdrawal reactions [214, 215, 228, 234–239]. By consequence, these trials cannot inform about long-term treatment efficacy. I will thus discuss them in the chapter "Methodological biases".

Addressing Counterarguments

Of course, many psychiatrists (and likely also various GPs) will object to my evaluation of antidepressant efficacy and effectiveness. But in view of the compelling scientific evidence from the systematic reviews and meta-analyses detailed above, how do they defend the notion that antidepressants are clearly effective in some or even most users? So, let's consider their reasoning. A common counterargument is that some patients may derive substantial benefits from antidepressants while a larger portion has little or no benefit, which would invalidate evaluations based on average treatment effects [137–139]. While this is certainly a legitimate point, it's important to stress that if antidepressants are highly effective in a small subgroup of users, then, by necessity, they don't work in most users (otherwise the average treatment effect would not be so poor). Now you may object that if we prescribe antidepressants exclusively to this subgroup of patients, then they would work in most users. Unfortunately, it's not known whether antidepressants are more effective in some patient subgroups than others. Parallel-group clinical trials (here specifically a group of patients on antidepressant compared to a group of patients on placebo) can only estimate average treatment effects (i.e. the mean difference between antidepressant and placebo), since in such trials an individual participant receives either active drug or placebo, but never alternately both over repeated treatment periods [240]. For sure, changes in depression symptoms over the course of treatment differ between patients (some deteriorate, some have no meaningful change, some improve slightly, and others improve substantially), which is referred to as observed treatment outcome (or observed response). However, an observed treatment outcome is not exclusively due to the drug effect. In fact, more than 80% of the observed treatment outcome (i.e. symptom change over the course of treatment) are due to other factors than the drug's pharmacological effect [18, 140].

Based on a clinical trial it's thus impossible to determine whether inter-individual differences in symptom change among patients treated with an antidepressant were due to the drug's pharmacological effect (i.e. its biologically active ingredient), placebo effects, spontaneous remission, or other treatment effects, including the therapeutic relationship between physician and patient [184, 185] and comedication with sedative-hypnotic drugs, which are frequently prescribed in antidepressant trials [166, 241]. That is, not all people receiving a specific treatment improve equally. Someone's symptoms may decline rapidly, because the depression episode was improving anyway independent of treatment (i.e. spontaneous remission), while another person may even deteriorate because a stressful life event unrelated to treatment (e.g. separation from the partner or job loss) made the symptoms worse. Therefore, inter-individual differences in the observed treatment outcome don't imply that there is treatment effect heterogeneity, that is, inter-individual differences in drug effects [240, 242]. The only thing we can safely conclude from a parallel-group trial is that the average effect attributable to a drugs' pharmacological effect is the mean difference in outcome between the antidepressant and the placebo group. No more, and no less. So is there no way to determine whether antidepressants work better in some people than in others? There is.

If we can demonstrate that in a specific and clearly defined subgroup of patients (e.g. patients with severe anhedonia, specific personality traits or gen variants) larger drug–placebo differences are consistently shown across trials, then this would provide evidence for treatment effect heterogeneity. Such patient characteristics that reliably influence efficacy estimates are also referred to as treatment effect modifiers (or moderators). Alas, thus far no treatment effect modifiers have been found and there is no scientific evidence for treatment effect heterogeneity, suggesting that antidepressants' pharmacological effects on depression symptoms are largely similar across patients [243-246]. This sobering conclusion resonates with expert evaluations in general psychiatry and other medical specialties, which caution that personalised/precision medicine may fall short of expectations [247-251]. Therefore, unless proven otherwise, we must assume that antidepressants' treatment effects are largely similar across patients and that the average effect derived from meta-analyses is the best estimate for the benefits patients can expect from the drugs' pharmacological effect [244–246]. Does this conclusion also apply to melancholic depression?

Based on a few older studies, some researchers argued that antidepressants are more effective in patients with melancholic depression because these patients would improve poorly on placebo [187, 252, 253]. However, according to a recent meta-analysis, the melancholic depression subtype, relative to other subtypes, did not moderate the treatment outcome with antidepressants compared to placebo [207]. Another recent meta-analysis also failed to find higher efficacy estimates (i.e. drug-placebo differences) in patients with melancholic depression features compared to patients without such features [254]. Likewise, in a recent trial, both anhedonia and chronicity of depression (two features of melancholic depression [255]) did not predict treatment efficacy of sertraline against placebo [153]. It has also claimed that patients with severe/melancholic depression would benefit more from antidepressants than psychotherapy [187], but this assumption is not supported by meta-analyses of comparative clinical trials [207, 208]. According to the scientific literature, it's thus uncertain whether patients with melancholic depression benefit more from antidepressants than patients with non-melancholic depression.

Related to the point above, there is a widely accepted notion that antidepressants are more effective in severe depression than in non-severe depression (regardless of melancholic features), as for instance suggested by Kirsch et al. [198] and Fournier et al. [256]. However, these influential studies have subsequently been contradicted by many large individual-patient-data meta-analyses which found no association between efficacy and baseline depression severity [196, 257, 258]; for a review, see Plöderl and Hengartner [259]. A major shortcoming of these studies is that they quantify the severity of baseline depression according to scores on a depression rating scale. Such an approach to measure the severity of a depression episode may be inadequate or even misleading [260]. Moreover, as detailed above, I doubt that many patients with truly severe depression were included in antidepressant efficacy trials, given that acute suicidality, psychotic symptoms, and comorbid disorders are common exclusion criteria [188]. So, possibly, people with truly severe (serious) clinical depression could indeed benefit more from antidepressants than the average trial participant, but this hasn't been scientifically established yet. However, note that similar treatment effects in the moderate to severe range do not imply that antidepressants are equally effective at the lower end of the severity spectrum. But contrary to the upper end of the severity spectrum, the non-severe range is rather well researched. In patients with mild and minor depression, antidepressants consistently fail to beat placebo or watchful waiting [152, 261-264], which is why antidepressants are not indicated as first-line treatment in mild/minor depression [181, 232, 233].

Another popular argument is that, by switching antidepressants, better outcomes would be achieved than the small treatment effects demonstrated in efficacy trials [265]. This implies that in real-word routine practice, antidepressants would be far more effective than in clinical trials because doctors would switch the drug when patients initially don't respond. However, scientific evidence does not support this popular view. According to a comprehensive meta-analysis, switching to another antidepressant after initial non-response does not lead to a better treatment outcomes than continuing the same (ineffective) antidepressant [266]. That is, there is no convincing evidence from double-blind randomised controlled trials that switching to another antidepressant would yield better treatment outcomes.

Likewise, it has been suggested that the common clinical trial protocols with fixed dosing design (often including fixed low and medium doses) lead to an underestimation of antidepressants' true effectiveness [265]. As above, this argument implies that in real-word routine practice, by flexibly adjusting the dose (mostly dose increase after initial non-response), doctors would achieve better treatment outcomes than those observed in clinical trials. However, this assumption is scientifically completely unfounded. First of all, a meta-analysis by Papakostas and Fava showed that fixed versus flexible dosing did not influence clinical trial outcome [267]. Another meta-analysis found no dose–response relationship in SSRIs, indicating that efficacy (or inefficacy) of SSRIs is not a matter of fixed low, medium or high doses. However, high doses were associated with more side effects and therefore higher treatment discontinuation [268]. As confirmed by Furukawa and colleagues in another recent meta-analysis, flexible dosing (or titration) of SSRIs, venlafaxine or mirtazapine above the fixed minimum licensed dose does not increase efficacy [269]. In fact, as the authors conclude elsewhere, "For the most commonly used second-generation antidepressants, the lower range of the licensed dose achieves the optimal balance between efficacy, tolerability, and acceptability in the acute treatment of major depression" [270]. In accordance, two other recent meta-analyses demonstrate that dose increase (or escalation) as compared to unchanged dose after initial nonresponse does not improve treatment efficacy [271, 272]. Therefore, contrary to popular claims [265], there is absolutely no evidence from doubleblind randomised controlled trials that flexible dose increase (titration) would yield higher efficacy estimates than fixed low, medium or high doses. Increasing the dose does not add benefits, it merely produces more side effects [268, 270].

Finally, it could be argued that pooling all antidepressants together is inadequate since individual drugs differ in their pharmacological action and may thus produce distinct outcomes. It is certainly true that antidepressants differ in their psychotropic effects and side effect profile. For instance, most tricyclics, as well as trazodone and mirtazapine, have strong sedating effects, whereas the SSRIs and in particular the SNRIs have more activating effects [93, 273, 274]. However, SSRIs quite often also have sedating effects [274, 275], and all antidepressants—sedating and activating drugs—appear to cause emotional numbing (or blunting), that is, a reduction of both negative and positive emotions [276–279]. Bearing this in mind, let's examine whether there are meaningful differences in treatment efficacy between antidepressant drugs or classes. According to the scientific literature this doesn't seem to be the case, for comparative studies found only minor and unreliable differences in efficacy between drug classes and individual drugs [141, 280–282]. By contrast, various authors contend that the tricyclics are more effective than the new-generation antidepressants in patients with melancholic depression [1, 9, 253, 255, 283], but this view is controversial and not consistently supported by the scientific evidence [284–288]. Thus, it's still open to debate whether the tricyclics are more effective than the new-generation antidepressants, especially the SSRIs and SNRIs, in melancholic depression.

Efficacy in Minors, Old Adults, and Bipolar Depression

A particularly controversial issue is the effectiveness of antidepressants in children and adolescents [58, 289-291]. When pooled over all trials, including various unpublished studies, there is a questionable and at best marginally small benefit. According to a Cochrane review, the average treatment effect on the widely used Child Depression Rating Scale Revised (CDRS-R), which ranges from 17 to 113 points, was only 3.5 points. Remission rates increased from 38% to 45% for those treated with an antidepressant compared to placebo, with no differences between drug classes [292]. However, to this date not one paediatric antidepressant trial was positive on the prespecified primary efficacy outcome [293], and according to a seminal network meta-analysis by Cipriani and colleagues, only fluoxetine demonstrated efficacy across trials [294]. The most recent network meta-analysis by Hetrick and colleagues found moderate certainty evidence for the efficacy of fluoxetine, sertraline and escitalopram, and low certainty evidence for the efficacy of duloxetine. However, treatment effects were considered "small and unimportant", with drug–placebo differences of 2.6 to 3.5 points on the CDRS-R [295].

Given that the quality of evidence is mostly rated very poor [292, 294, 295], it's indeed questionable whether these minimal therapeutic effects are clinically meaningful and whether benefits outweigh harms in children and adolescents [58, 290, 291, 294]. Cipriani and colleagues thus concluded, "When considering the risk-benefit profile of antidepressants in the acute treatment of major depressive disorder, these drugs do not seem to offer a clear advantage for children and adolescents" [294]. Likewise, Hetrick and colleagues emphasised, "There remain important questions about the clinical effectiveness of these treatments and, even though they may reduce depression symptoms in comparison to placebo, the effects are small and unimportant … It is of concern that after 26 trials involving children and adolescents, we are still at a point where there are no trials that report convincing evidence of remission of a diagnosed major depressive disorder, or even of a substantial reduction in symptoms and that the quality of evidence remains low" [295].

The effectiveness of antidepressants is likewise uncertain in old adults with depression, for most drugs, especially the SSRIs, appear not definitely better than placebo [296, 297]. As detailed by Tham and colleagues, "on a group level, SSRIs might not be superior to a placebo in achieving remission and response during acute treatment of MDD [major depressive disorder] in this age group" [297]. Relatedly, antidepressants are often prescribed to treat depression in elderly patients with dementia, but they have little to no benefits in this population and can cause significant harms [298, 299]. For most old people with depression (with and without dementia), the benefit–harm ratio of antidepressants is thus likely unfavourable, especially in the long-term, given that the elderly are more susceptible to adverse drug effects due to frailty, comorbid disorders, and polypharmacy [300].

Finally, a last special case are antidepressants in bipolar depression, that is, manic-depressive disorder. This issue is also dealt with quickly. Although antidepressants are frequently prescribed in this condition [301], there is no conclusive scientific evidence that they are effective in bipolar depression [302-304]. In fact, the scientific evidence indicates that antidepressants are rather harmful in bipolar depression because not only do they fail to provide clear benefits, they can also worsen manic symptoms over the long-term [302, 305, 306]. Thus, according to Ghaemi and colleagues, "SSRIs like citalopram are not helpful to treat bipolar depression or to prevent it, and they may worsen manic symptoms if used long-term, especially in patients with a rapid-cycling course … Antidepressants should be avoided in bipolar depression" [305]. I will now turn to the issue of adverse treatment effects and a brief benefit–harm evaluation, focusing mainly on adult depression.

Adverse Effects and Benefit-harm Ratio of Antidepressants

As with any other medicine, antidepressants can have unintended adverse effects, typically referred to as side effects or adverse drug reactions, but a detailed account of safety and tolerability is beyond the scope of this chapter. Interested readers are referred to the literature [273, 275, 307]. In short, almost all antidepressants can and quite often do cause headaches and nausea early in the treatment course, but these side effects commonly disappear after a few weeks [273, 307, 308]. There are also various class-specific side effects. For instance, tricyclics cause marked anticholinergic side effects which are often persistent, including dry mouth, constipation, dizziness, confusion, sweating, and blurred vision. Activating drugs like SSRIs and SNRIs on the other hand more frequently cause an activation syndrome, which includes adverse reactions such as insomnia, nervousness, irritability, agitation, anxiety, and akathisia (extreme psychomotor restlessness) [273, 309, 310]. A rare but very serious side effect of the MAOIs is hypertensive crisis (a potentially life-threatening sudden increase in blood pressure following ingestion of certain foods or medications). Both MAOIs and tricyclics, but also various atypicals and SSRIs (especially paroxetine) rarely cause orthostatic hypotension (sudden drop in blood pressure upon standing), which can lead to falls and thus very serious injuries (including death), especially in elderly patients [307, 311, 312]. A rare but life-threatening side effect of the tricyclics as well as citalopram and escitalopram (two popular SSRIs) are cardiac arrhythmias which may lead to sudden cardiac death [313–315]. Various SSRIs and SNRIs can also cause abnormal bleeding, which, rarely, may result in brain haemorrhage (a type of stroke). They can also cause severe hyponatremia (extremely low sodium concentration in the blood causing confusion, seizures and coma), especially in elderly patients [275, 307, 316].

In addition, various antidepressant drugs rarely cause hepatoxicity (liver damage) [317] and there is mounting evidence that some antidepressants, especially SSRIs and SNRIs, may cause congenital malformations (birth defects) when women use them during early pregnancy [318–320]. A large body of evidence strongly indicates that activating antidepressants, relative to placebo, can cause suicidal ideation and behaviour in about 1–8% of adolescents and young adults with depression [292, 293, 321-324], which is possibly due to their propensity to induce agitation, aggression, disinhibition, and akathisia [9, 325, 326]. It is less clear whether antidepressants increase the risk of suicidal events in adult patients in general, as the evidence is inconsistent and may depend upon whether researchers focus broadly on suicidality (suicidal ideation and behaviour, including suicide attempts) or specifically on suicide attempts (both fatal and non-fatal). In any case, there is some evidence that antidepressants have no effect on suicidality or may even protect against suicidal ideation and behaviour in adult patients [323, 324, 327], but also evidence that they increase the risk of suicide attempts in this patient population [327–333].

A very frequent, but long under-recognised (and minimised) adverse effect of most antidepressants is sexual dysfunction [10, 334, 335]. When sexual dysfunction is systematically assessed in clinical trials, with some SSRIs and SNRIs, including the popular drugs fluoxetine, paroxetine, citalopram, sertraline, and venlafaxine, the rate of treatment-emergent sexual dysfunction is between 70 and 80%, as compared to only about 12% with placebo [336]. The rate ratio is thus roughly 6, meaning that patients on these specific drugs are about 6 times more likely to develop sexual dysfunction than patients on placebo (which reflects the rate attributable to the underlying depressive disorder). In addition, it's now officially acknowledged by drug regulators that, in some cases, antidepressant-induced sexual dysfunction can persist for indefinite time after treatment discontinuation [337, 338]. Another quite frequent adverse effect of many antidepressants [339], but especially with mirtazapine, paroxetine, and amitriptyline [340], is excessive weight gain following long-term use.

Finally, all antidepressants, to varying degree, cause neurophysiological adaptations after a few weeks of exposure (i.e., neurobiological changes due to the drugs' pharmacological action), especially receptor downregulation and desensitisation [223, 341–343]. These adaptations are best understood as a state of physical dependence (not to be confused with addiction [344]) and thus can cause withdrawal syndromes after treatment discontinuation or dose reduction in about 30–60% of users ranging from mild and short-lived to severe and long-lasting [345–349].

Common withdrawal symptoms include dizziness, vertigo, tremor, nausea, insomnia, fatigue, mood dysregulation, anxiety, panic, irritability, and agitation. Quite often, antidepressant withdrawal syndromes thus resemble a mixed anxiety-depressive disorder and are frequently misdiagnosed as relapse or a new emerging mental disorder when doctors are unfamiliar with physical dependence and withdrawal [350–352]. In some cases, antidepressant withdrawal can also trigger suicidal ideation and behaviour [353–356]. Even though severe and protracted antidepressant withdrawal has long been neglected and minimised [357, 358], it is now formally acknowledged by various medical organisations, including NICE [359] and RCP [360]. Nevertheless, research into protracted withdrawal is still very scarce and the syndrome and its treatment are poorly understood [354]. Although this listing of adverse effects is far from exhaustive, it illustrates nicely that antidepressants can cause various harms, including very serious and life-threatening adverse drug reactions.

Benefit–harm Balance

In sum, the efficacy of antidepressants is uncertain in children and adolescents and it appears that, if at all, only fluoxetine, sertraline, escitalopram, and duloxetine offer a minimal benefit [58, 292, 294, 295]. The efficacy of most antidepressants is also uncertain (and questionable) in older adult patients with depression [296, 297], including depression treatment in dementia [299]. Likewise, in adults with mild, minor, and subthreshold depression, the efficacy of antidepressants has not been established [261–263]. By contrast, antidepressants convey a small benefit over placebo with respect to improvement of depression symptoms in adults with moderate to severe depression [141], but the clinical significance (or practical relevance) of this effect is contested [10, 13, 17, 20]. On the other hand, all antidepressants can and do cause various harms. Some adverse effects are infrequent/rare but life-threatening (e.g. cardiac arrhythmias, liver damage) and others are frequent/common and persistent (e.g. sexual dysfunction, sleep problems) [273, 307, 339].

The proportion of adult patients who discontinue treatment due to lack of efficacy is higher with placebo, but discontinuation due to adverse events is higher with antidepressants [141, 193]. The difficult question now is, how do we balance therapeutic effects against adverse effects? Put differently, do benefits outweigh harms? As concerns both paediatric and geriatric depression as well as mild/minor depression in adults, the marginal and questionable benefits do not seem to outweigh harms. In these populations, I agree with Jureidini and McHenry who concluded, "We cannot be confident about which patients, if any, should receive antidepressants, but we can be confident that many people who are prescribed antidepressants should not be" [29]. In adults with moderate to severe depression, the overall assessment is more complicated and less clear. I don't support the view that antidepressants should not be used at all in these patients [133], but I agree with Dr. Fava, who stated "If we take into consideration the potential benefits, the likelihood of responsiveness, and the potential adverse events and vulnerabilities entailed by oppositional mechanisms, we would be inclined to target the application of AD [antidepressants] only to the most severe and persistent cases of depression for the shortest possible time" [218].

And here is how I evaluate the benefit–harm ratio. One approach to address this issue is to focus on treatment discontinuation due to any reason (all-cause discontinuation), which is assumed to balance benefit and harms and thus to provide a measure of overall treatment effectiveness. Although in antidepressant research this outcome is commonly interpreted as "treatment acceptability" [141, 361], in clinical research on antipsychotics for schizophrenia, for instance, all-cause discontinuation is an established measure of treatment effectiveness [362-364]. The logic behind this concept is quite simple and straightforward.

If an antidepressant drug is effective and has no or minimal side effects, a patient with depression will certainly not discontinue treatment because benefits (i.e. therapeutic effects such as improved mood and more energy) would clearly outweigh harms (i.e. adverse effects such as sleep problems and sexual dysfunction). A patient may also continue treatment despite a lack of clear benefits when the drug has no or minimal side effects, in the hope that the medication will eventually work. By contrast, if a drug is effective but has severe (intolerable) side effects, a patient may decide to discontinue treatment when the benefits do not outweigh the harms and a patient will certainly stop the medication if he/she experiences no benefits but considerable side effects. An inert placebo pill is pharmacologically inactive but has at least no side effects. People on placebo may still experience improvements in their condition though. This is not due to the action of the pill but the result of other factors (e.g. therapeutic relationship with the physician, spontaneous remission, effect of concomitant lifestyle changes, placebo effect). By consequence, when the drug is clearly effective and has minimal side effects, then the all-cause discontinuation rate will certainly be lower in people receiving the active drug than in people receiving the inert placebo pill. There would be no clear difference in all-cause treatment discontinuation between active drug and placebo when the drug has both minimal benefits and minimal side effects. No difference in all-cause treatment discontinuation is also expected to occur when a drug has substantial benefits but severe (intolerable) side effects. Finally, treatment discontinuation would likely be higher with the active drug compared to placebo if it has minimal or no benefits but severe (intolerable) side effects.

Now, let's have a look at all-cause treatment discontinuation in placebo-controlled antidepressant trials for both adult and paediatric depression. As you may have suspected, the all-cause treatment discontinuation rate does not differ between antidepressants and placebo [141, 193, 292, 294], suggesting that, on average, the small benefits do not clearly outweigh harms. This may sound controversial and perhaps you may find a good argument why this is not a fair assessment. However, please consider that all-cause treatment discontinuation is an established measure of treatment effectiveness in trials of antipsychotic drugs. Based on all-cause treatment discontinuation rates, leading schizophrenia researchers concluded that that the new-generation antipsychotic drugs (the so-called atypical antipsychotics) are, on balance, no more effective than the older (typical) antipsychotic drugs [364]. All-cause treatment discontinuation has also been applied to demonstrate that in the acute treatment phase, antipsychotics are more effective than placebo [362]. Thus, if we interpret the all-cause treatment discontinuation in antidepressant trials in the same way as it commonly is in antipsychotic trials, it follows that by balancing benefits and harms, antidepressants are no better than placebo. However, this is certainly not a definite answer, it's just one way to approach the difficult question whether the small treatment benefits of antidepressants outweigh their harms.

Alternatively, we can also ask antidepressant users how satisfied they are with their drugs. In a very large international survey, only 49% of patients with major depression receiving medication from a mental health specialist considered their treatment helpful, whereas in patients seeing a GP, 66% perceived their treatment helpful [365]. In an analysis of user ratings of duloxetine, escitalopram, vilazodone, and vortioxetine posted on three popular websites, 23% of users indicated they were very unsatisfied with the drugs, 11% somewhat unsatisfied, 16% were undecided, 21% somewhat satisfied, and 29% very satisfied [366]. Thus, corresponding with the results of the large international patient survey detailed above, just about half of users perceived their medication useful. According to an analysis of user ratings posted on www.askapatient.com, venlafaxine was rated positive by 49%, neutral by 19%, and negative by 31%, while fluoxetine was rated positive by 58%, neutral by 15%, and negative by 27% [276]. Finally, in another large international user survey, 61% felt that antidepressants improved their quality of life, 18% that their quality of life remained unchanged, and 21% that the medication worsened their quality of life [279].

These various studies consistently demonstrate that roughly 50–60% of all antidepressant users consider their medication helpful and perceive improved quality of life, whereas the rest of users (i.e. 40–50%) report a neutral or negative experience. Noteworthy, a significant minority of about 20% state being very dissatisfied with their antidepressants or that the medication harmed them. Put differently, these findings suggest that in 50–60% of antidepressant users the drugs' benefits seem to outweigh harms, in about 20–30% of users benefits and harms are balanced, while in 20% of users, harms outweigh benefits. But note that such subjective appraisals cannot accurately discriminate pharmacological effects from spontaneous mood improvement or worsening, placebo or nocebo effects, and other treatment effects (e.g. the patient–doctor relationship, comedication with sedative-hypnotic drugs). Nevertheless, two things are noteworthy. First, the proportion of users who state that they are satisfied with their antidepressants or who experience net benefits (50–60%) corresponds closely to the average rate of responders (at least 50% symptom improvement) for antidepressant groups in short-term clinical trials [191]. However, at least 80% of these responders get better for other reasons than the drugs' pharmacological effect [18, 140]. Second, the proportion of users who are very dissatisfied with their antidepressant or who perceive the drugs as harmful (20%) roughly matches the proportion of users who discontinue antidepressant treatment prematurely due to inefficacy or adverse effects (intolerability) in short-term clinical trials [367].

Finally, most physicians, including psychiatrists and GPs, are convinced that antidepressants are effective and safe [368–370]. Based on their clinical observations, to them "the effectiveness of antidepressants appears to be a no brainer" [371]. In accordance, a comprehensive study showed that 79% of psychiatrists recommend immediate treatment with an antidepressant to an outpatient with depression [372]. But would psychiatrists also take antidepressants if they personally had depression, that is, if they were the outpatient? No, surprisingly, most wouldn't, for according to the same study, only 39% of psychiatrists would immediately take an antidepressant if they personally had depression, while 61% would prefer watchful waiting [372]. Obviously, there is a striking discrepancy in what psychiatrists think is best for their patients and what they personally prefer if they were the patients. Perhaps then, the effectiveness of antidepressants isn't that clear to many psychiatrists after all. At least if they were personally affected by depression...

3

The Transformation of Depression

According to many authors, biomedical research and clinical practice are in crisis [29, 59, 171, 373–383]. Pressing problems include the commercialisation of the biomedical sciences, self-promotion and careerism at academic medical departments, systematic flaws in biomedical and clinical research, an abundance of industry-sponsored scientific studies mostly serving as marketing vehicles, the broadening of diagnostic boundaries, definition and branding of non-medical problems as new medical conditions, extensive screening in healthy low-risk populations, overtreatment and polypharmacy, managed care plans, and aggressive promotion of pharmaceutical drugs to both physicians and the public. Several of these now-all-too-common phenomena are subsumed under the concepts of "medicalisation" and "pharmaceuticalisation". Medicalisation refers to the process by which non-medical problems of human life, that is, social, behavioural, or bodily conditions, are defined in biomedical terms as illnesses and disorders, whereas pharmaceuticalisation defines the process by which these non-medical problems are treated or deemed to be in need of treatment with pharmaceutical drugs [375, 384]. Although distinctive, these two concepts overlap largely, and at the intersection they were merged into a new concept, termed disease mongering, which

M. P. Hengartner, *Evidence-biased Antidepressant Prescription*,
https://doi.org/10.1007/978-3-030-82587-4_3

Moynihan and colleagues define as "widening the boundaries of treatable illness in order to expand markets for those who sell and deliver treatments" [385].

Medicalisation and pharmaceuticalisation lead to overdiagnosis, which means "making people patients unnecessarily, by identifying problems that were never going to cause harm or by medicalising ordinary life experiences through expanded definitions of diseases" [386]. The main drivers of overdiagnosis thus are overdefinition and overdetection of disease. Overdiagnosis also includes the detection of abnormalities or bodily states not related to disease, that is, false-positive diagnoses [387]. Another consequence of medicalisation/pharmaceuticalisation is medical overuse, which is defined as "care in the absence of a clear medical basis for use or when the benefit of therapy does not outweigh risks" [387] or, simply put, "the provision of medical services for which the potential for harm exceeds the potential for benefit" [374]. Medicalisation and pharmaceuticalisation also affect the economy. While the major pharmaceutical companies represent the most profitable industry sector [388], healthcare systems are increasingly unsustainable and unaffordable [374, 389].

In psychiatry, both medicalisation and pharmaceuticalisation are closely related to a third process that started simultaneously and developed in tandem with the former: biological reductionism [390–394]. Biological reductionism in psychiatry describes the causal attribution of complex psychological problems, that is, problems in thinking, behaviour, motivation, and emotion, to unproven (and ill-defined) biological processes, mostly faulty brain functions [395, 396]. These three intertwined developments—medicalisation, pharmaceuticalisation, and biological reductionism—led to a fundamental transformation of the concept and treatment of depression. In the following chapter I will outline how medicalisation and pharmaceuticalisation led to a redefinition of depression and a shift in diagnosis and treatment. I will first describe the process of overdefinition and then I will turn to the process of overdetection but note beforehand that the two are related and often go hand in hand. I will then critically discuss whether we are facing a true depression epidemic that purportedly led to a serious public health crisis [397]. Biological reductionism is a byproduct of the biological revolution in psychiatry and the ensuing aggressive marketing of psychiatric drugs. In the domain of depression, a major driver of this development was the chemical imbalance (serotonin) theory. I will discuss these issues in the last section of the chapter and conclude with a brief synopsis.

Medicalisation and Pharmaceuticalisation

Overdefinition of Depression

In the post-World-War era and until the 1970s, depression was considered a severe but rare disorder mostly treated in psychiatric hospitals but rarely in primary care practices and psychiatric outpatient services [1, 63]. Many experts differentiated between endogenous/melancholic depression and reactive/neurotic depression, whereas others saw these different clinical presentations not as distinct types of depression but rather as different manifestations of severity, with melancholic depression denoting the most severe manifestation of depression [1, 398]. Endogenous/melancholic depression was characterised by the complete absence of mood reactivity, profound anhedonia (i.e. lack of interest and pleasure), psychomotor retardation, somatic symptoms (e.g. sleep problems and lack of appetite), suicidal thoughts, and psychotic symptoms (e.g. delusions and hallucinations). By contrast, reactive/neurotic depression was typically less severe and presented primarily with sadness, loss of interest, and feelings of guilt and worthlessness.

In any case, depression was considered predominantly self-limiting and to have a good prognosis. Most experts of the time affirmed that the great majority of depressed patients, that is, up to 80%, would recover after some time, even without treatment [63, 132, 399]. For instance, in 1961, Dr Leyburn wrote in the *Lancet* that "most depressed patients get better anyway and the patients who improve after one has prescribed tablets have done so *post hoc* but not necessarily *propter hoc*" [400]. Likewise, in 1964, Dr Kline wrote in *JAMA*, "In the treatment of depression one always has as an ally the fact that most depressions terminate in spontaneous remission. This means that in many cases regardless of what one does the patient eventually will begin to get better" [401]. And another eminent expert of that time, Dr Cole, also writing in *JAMA*, stated "depression is, on the whole, one of the psychiatric conditions with the best prognosis for eventual recovery with or without treatment. Most depressions are self-limited" [136]. As I will detail below, this widely accepted notion of depression changed dramatically between the 1970s and 1990s [1, 9, 63, 399]. But how did that happen? How did a rare disorder with mostly good prognosis (even when left untreated) suddenly became a global public health crisis [397]?

During the 1950s and 1960s the most prevalent mental health problems were stress, anxiety, tension, and insomnia, subsumed under the broad diagnostic category of neurotic disorders [63]. These problems were considered consequences of the strains of everyday life (i.e. problems of living) and they were often treated with tranquilizers by GPs. Antidepressants were mostly prescribed by psychiatrists and were reserved for the most seriously ill inpatients (i.e. hospitalised patients) with melancholic depression. Moreover, drugs were merely seen as aids and not as curative treatments. At that time psychiatry was largely dominated by psychoanalytic thinking, and the predominant opinion was that true recovery from serious mental illness was only possible with psychotherapy. But soon psychoanalysis came publicly under criticism for controversial concepts like the "schizophrenogenic mother", while psychiatric diagnoses based on psychoanalytic theory were found to be utterly unreliable and to have no scientific basis. Moreover, psychiatry was perceived by many stakeholders as oppressive and coercive. The profession was thus confronted with serious charges that threatened both its authority in the mental health field and its legitimacy as a scientific medical discipline [393]. In the words of Dr. Horwitz, "Psychiatry was under attack from many fronts, including the libertarian right, the Marxist left, and feminists, all of whom focused on its perceived suppression of individual freedom" [63]. There was also discontent within the profession. Many biologically oriented psychiatrists felt that psychoanalytic theory and the reigning psychosocial models were disadvantageous to psychiatry as a medical speciality and thus threatened the profession's authority and scientific credibility.

Starting in the 1970s and culminating in the 1980s, these factors, coupled with changes in health policy, set in motion a dramatic and fundamental transformation of the profession [63, 393, 394]. Psychoanalysis vanished, biology flourished, and psychosocial models were gradually replaced by biomedical models. The neurosciences and psychopharmacology became influential drivers of the biological revolution and depression was their main target, as anxiety and stress-related disorders were too closely connected to psychoanalytic theory and psychosocial models. The emerging new position in mainstream psychiatry was that depression was fundamentally a biomedical condition. It was further posited that depression was under-recognised and undertreated and that many anxiety and stress-related disorders were in fact depression episodes and thus should be treated with antidepressants [1, 9]. And so, by expanding into the diagnostic realm of the neurotic disorders, depression morphed from a rare but severe disorder to a relatively common but highly heterogeneous disorder of varying severity and diverse clinical presentation [4, 63]. Inherent in this transformation was also the growing medicalisation of social and interpersonal problems. Various psychosomatic symptoms that were previously seen as normal stress reactions to problems of living were now increasingly conceptualised as symptoms of biomedical conditions, especially brain disorders [63, 399].

The pharmaceutical industry was of course not inactive in this fundamental transformation [5, 93]. From the 1960s on, the pharmaceutical companies manufacturing antidepressants sought to educate GPs about the importance of unrecognised (masked) depression in primary care patients in order to increase the antidepressant market, which until then was largely restricted to inpatients treated in psychiatric hospitals. For instance, the huge success of amitriptyline during the 1960s and 1970s was in part the result of skilful marketing by its manufacturer Merck. Psychiatrist Dr. Frank Ayd had conducted one of the key clinical trials of amitriptyline for Merck and in 1960 had already published an article about amitriptyline for depression [402]. Merck then approached Ayd and suggested to him "that he write a book to help other clinicians, especially those in general practice, deal more effectively with patients suffering from depression" [393]. He agreed and in January 1961 he published his book *Recognizing the Depressed Patient: With Essentials of Management and Treatment*. The book quickly became a bestseller and sold 150,000 copies, of which 50,000 copies were purchased by Merck and distributed worldwide to GPs to promote the use of amitriptyline [393, 403]. So the increased prescribing of amitriptyline by GPs was largely due to skilful pharmaceutical marketing rather than increased treatment need.

Another example. In 1974, Ciba-Geigy (now Novartis), the manufacturer of imipramine and clomipramine, organised a scientific meeting at St Moritz, a noble ski resort in the Swiss mountains. This event—labelled "depression in general practice"—was attended by most European depression specialists of the time. Main topics of the meeting were to discuss the recognition and diagnosis of depression, the detection of masked depression, and the pharmaceutical treatment of depression in primary care. A main objective of Ciba-Geigy was to pave the way for its new tetracyclic antidepressant drug—maprotiline (Ludiomil)—to enter the huge market of primary care [404]. For it, Ciba-Geigy actively constructed and promoted "masked" depression as a new indication for antidepressants. As Gerber and Gaudilliere note, "Ciba-Geigy's marketing strategy gradually shifted from a focus on isolated products to the promotion of diagnostic categories and prescription practices. Accordingly, the new profiling of Ludiomil as an antidepressant with anxiolytic properties specially designed for the treatment of mild or masked depression in general practice started in 1973. This strategy was advanced through a second symposium in St. Moritz, the entire purpose of which was to discuss masked depression" [404]. With these meetings and other marketing actions, including educational brochures handed out to GPs, "Ciba-Geigy aimed to establish a unified depression as indication for general practice by combining a (relatively) specific set of targeted symptoms with a program of replacing tranquilizers with antidepressants, requiring the promotion of new diagnosis habits" [404]. This was also the time when the pharmaceutical industry began to collaborate closely with influential psychiatrists (mostly professors, chief physicians and medical directors) by paying them handsome sums as consultants and speakers, a group now routinely termed "key opinion leaders" [405, 406]. The fundamental role of key opinion leaders in the creation and expansion of antidepressant markets will be discussed in more detail below and in the chapter "Conflicts of Interest". For now, we note that the pharmaceutical industry has made great efforts to broaden the concept of clinical depression and to promote antidepressant prescribing in primary care.

Meanwhile, the World Health Organization (WHO) announced in 1974 that in various countries about 20% of the population has depression symptoms and worldwide about 3–4% of the population could have clinical depression [407], a prevalence rate that was at least 10 times higher than previously estimated [9, 30]. In accordance with the pharmaceutical industry, the WHO called for an unified classification of depression and a standardised symptom-based assessment. The same goal was also pursued by the APA, which wanted to shift the classification of mental disorders from a diagnostic system based on psychoanalytic theory to a purely descriptive classification system decoupled from aetiology [63, 393]. The idea was that categorising mental disorders based on symptoms and behavioural signs would improve diagnostic reliability and thus finally enable to find the biological causes of mental disorders.

As a result, in 1980 the APA published its fundamentally revised new diagnostic manual of mental disorders, the DSM-III [408]. Its symptom-based diagnosis of depression was so broad and overinclusive that already after two weeks of sadness and diminished interest/pleasure, along with common but unspecific stress-symptoms such as sleep problems, lack of appetite, fatigue, and decreased concentration, a person could be diagnosed with "major" depression. The typical features of severe (melancholic) depression, that is, lack of mood reactivity, marked anhedonia, psychomotor disturbances, suicidality, and psychotic symptoms were no longer deemed necessary to diagnose depression. The new diagnostic criteria of depression set forth by the DSM-III remained largely unchanged in its successor versions, the DSM-IV (1994) and DSM-5 (2013), and also lay the foundation for the diagnostic criteria established in the ensuing revision of the diagnostic manual of the WHO, the ICD-10 (1992). But the new definition of depression (and other diagnoses alike) was not based on empirical evidence, it was created by "voting and consensus" [409]. According to Ghaemi and colleagues, "MDD [major depressive disorder] was a political compromise in DSM-III, grafted onto science, as documented in a recent history based on the minutes of the DSM-III committees" [4].

A brief critique of the DSM-III and its revisions is therefore warranted at this place, for it was an important driver of antidepressant prescribing in the following decades, especially in primary care. Although the DSM-III replaced the unscientific psychoanalytic diagnostic concepts, the validity and utility of its descriptive symptom-based diagnoses, including "major" depression, has been criticised widely [7, 64, 399, 409–413]. According to Ghaemi and colleagues, "As a single unified construct, MDD [major depressive disorder] has less and less scientific validity, yet it persists largely unchanged through each successive revision of DSM" [4]. The main issue is that different DSM diagnoses fail to delineate natural disease entities with distinct aetiologies. It has also been stressed that various diagnoses, e.g. depression, social anxiety disorder, and generalised anxiety disorder, fail to differentiate truly dysfunctional/pathological mental states from normal human variation and adaptive responses to critical life events and more enduring problems of daily living. This, so many authors argue, resulted in the systematic overmedicalisation of ordinary distress, unhappiness, sadness, anxiousness, and shyness [3, 5, 410, 414–417].

Dr. Robert Spitzer, chair of the taskforce that created the DSM-III, later admitted that "we made estimates of the prevalence of medical disorders totally descriptively, without considering that many of these conditions might be normal reactions which are not really disorders, because we were not looking at the context in which those conditions developed" [418]. Even the US National Institute of Mental Health (NIMH) has criticised the DSM for its lack of validity and in April 2013, its then-director Dr. Thomas Insel announced that the NIMH is "re-orienting its research away from DSM categories", for "patients with mental disorders deserve better" [419]. It is also worthy of note that the main objective of DSM-III was to improve the reliability of diagnoses, that is, whether two independent clinicians would ascribe the same diagnosis to the same person. But was the new diagnostic manual and its successor versions successful in this regard? Mounting evidence indicates that it failed to achieve this goal, given that the test-retest interrater reliability, that is, the agreement between two clinicians that independently diagnose the same patient, appears to be modest, and with respect to some diagnoses, even utterly poor [420, 421]. Major depression also belongs to the latter group of diagnoses with very low reliability [422].

Finally, the transformation of depression and the expansion of the antidepressant market was facilitated by another important factor: the demise of the best-selling tranquilizers of the 1960s and 1970s, the benzodiazepines [9, 63, 399]. By the 1980s, these sedative and anxiolytic drugs were shown to be addictive and dependence-forming, limiting them to short-term use [423]. This brought the benzodiazepines in disrepute and made antidepressants a formidable treatment choice for the various problems of living that were previously seen as neurotic (stress) reactions but which, subsequently, with the introduction of the DSM-III largely fell under the new diagnosis of major depression [4, 63]. The takeover of the benzodiazepines by the antidepressants in the neurosis marketplace was further facilitated by the introduction of the SSRIs in the late 1980s, which were better tolerated and safer in overdose than the older antidepressants and, contrary to the benzodiazepines, touted as non-addictive and not dependence-forming [1, 9]. As summarised by Dr Shorter, "Major depression served the then-nascent field of biological psychiatry in the way that psychoneurosis had once served psychoanalysis. And drugs supposedly specific for depression focused the optic: If all you have are antidepressants (given that by the early 1970s the benzodiazepines had been declared terribly addictive), everything you see looks like depression. If all you have is a hammer, everything looks like a nail … Bottom line: Major depression doesn't exist in Nature. A political process in psychiatry created it" [1].

Overdetection of Depression

In the late 1980s and early 1990s, several large-scale depression awareness campaigns were conducted. Here I will briefly describe the two best known of them, the Depression Awareness Recognition and Treatment (D/ART) program in the US and the Defeat Depression campaign in the UK. D/ART was initiated by the NIMH in collaboration with the APA and the pharmaceutical industry [424]. According to the NIMH, depression was poorly recognised and undertreated. Its main objective, therefore, was to "alert health professionals and the general public to the fact that depressive disorders are common, serious, and treatable" [424].

The Defeat Depression campaign [425] was launched in the UK (1992–96) by the Royal College of Psychiatrists (RCP) together with the Royal College of General Practitioners (RCGP) and it was partly funded by the pharmaceutical industry [426]. The aim and result of the Defeat Depression campaign was summarised as follows by the lead authors [425]:

> "An informational media campaign directed toward the general public was successfully undertaken. Leaflets, books, and audiotapes were also prepared and distributed to the public. Multiprofessional conferences on specific aspects of depression were organized. An extensive program of general practice education included consensus conferences and statements, recognition and management guidelines, training videotapes, and other publications. Public attitudes were found to be relatively favorable, except attitudes toward antidepressants, which were viewed as addictive. A general consequence of the campaign was the development of much additional public material and professional education not directly originating from the campaign".

According to Medawar [132], "The Defeat Depression campaign focused in particular on what the organisers believed were widely-held misconceptions. One concerned the public's failure to recognise the value of drug treatment. Another was the general failure to recognise depression for the complex and hidden disease it may be". I will return to these campaigns later, but for the moment I want to focus a bit more on the influence the pharmaceutical industry exerted on the public perception and recognition of depression. The drug companies were more than eager to support these large depression awareness campaigns in the US and the UK and they also launched their own information campaigns about depression (and later also about anxiety disorder), for they had long recognised that to expand drug markets (i.e. to sell more drugs), they need to market the diseases for which they provide drugs [66, 427–429]. These marketing strategies have also been referred to as "disease mongering" and "condition branding" [430–432]. Indeed, the industry is willing to invest a lot of money in disease marketing. From 1997 through 2016, spending for direct-to-consumer awareness campaigns—unbranded advertising promoting a disease without mentioning the drug or indication—increased from $177 million to $430 million in the United States [433].

As detailed above using the example of masked depression in primary care, the pharmaceutical industry strongly supported the widening of the diagnostic boundary of depression as it proved to be an exceptional marketing opportunity to increase antidepressant sales [404]. But the most precious gift was probably the introduction of DSM-III in 1980, which defined depression so broadly and overinclusively that it was possible to impose a depression diagnosis on a large population of healthy people who were just acutely distressed or unhappy [3, 63, 434]. As detailed by Ghaemi and colleagues, "Some people, if not most, do not have diseases; they suffer from being human beings. Their suffering is the same as everyone else's: being unhappy because of the limits and traumas of life. This experience is the existential aspect of all human suffering, and specifically of depression" [4].

Unsurprisingly, the pharmaceutical industry did not care about the fuzzy boundary between normal negative emotions and disordered (dysfunctional) emotions. It swiftly seized the unique opportunity provided by the DSM-III to market depression as a common, chronic, and severe disorder that often remains undetected and untreated, in particular in primary care [9, 132, 399]. The introduction of the various SSRIs in the late 1980s and early 1990s (i.e. patented, costly new drugs competing for market share) gave the industry further impetus. As a result, depression, and later the anxiety disorders, became extremely lucrative brands that were aggressively promoted through awareness campaigns and related marketing strategies to sell antidepressants. Applbaum summarises this marketing plan as follows:

> "Combined marketing and R&D [research and development] divisions created and publicized research to demonstrate the efficacy of the drug; obtained academic 'key opinion leader' (KOL) endorsements for professional audiences (people whose careers and pocketbooks improved simultaneously); aired celebrity spokespeople and advertising to educate the lay public about the disease; lavishly funded antistigma campaigns; promoted among family doctors the use of abridged depression questionnaires and educated, and thus empowered, these doctors (and eventually their non-

> MD assistants) to look for telltale signs of depression and treat it; enrolled (in some cases, also bankrolled) the support of patient advocacy groups and solicited testimonials from among them; generated certified guidelines formulated and endorsed by psychiatrists in the employ of industry, to be adopted by hospital formularies and public insurance programs; took a lead role in determining the curriculum and scientific programs at continuing medical education programs and professional congresses; designed Web sites with diagnostic self-tests encouraging consumers along the path from self-diagnosis to the request for medication at the doctor's office—a request most often honored; dispatched the MR [marketing representative] brigades; and so on". [27]

Nowadays, the internet facilitates to directly reach large parts of the general population, and thus potential antidepressant users (i.e. consumers), in no time at almost no costs. One example among many is a digital pamphlet titled "Depression: A Global Crisis", published by the World Federation for Mental Health and sponsored by the pharmaceutical companies Lundbeck, Eli Lilly, and Otsuka. The document stresses the tremendous global burden of depression, advices the public how to recognise depression, and calls for comprehensive treatment, especially with antidepressants. Among others, the document asserts that "Depression and other common mental health problems that present in primary care, no matter how mild, contribute significantly to the burden of disability and lower the quality of life people enjoy. Common mental health problems have been associated with substantial impairment in health-related quality of life, even in those with sub-threshold illness. This suggests that primary care should address even the mildest forms of illness through improved access and early diagnosis" [397]. I will later detail whether these claims are scientifically accurate.

Promotion of depression self-diagnosis via brief symptom checklists and screening instruments play an integral part of industry-sponsored depression marketing campaigns. Depression screenings directly take advantage of the broad and overinclusive diagnostic criteria and further exploit the unspecificity of various "depression symptoms", for example, sleep problems, fatigue, difficulty concentrating, or lack of appetite, which overlap greatly with normal reactions to stressful life events such as having a newborn, going through a divorce, or experiencing a high workload. Screening instruments are designed to correctly detect as many people with depression as possible, meaning their sensitivity is high. This comes at the price of low specificity, meaning that they often classify healthy people as ill (also referred to as false-positive detection). Perhaps the most popular depression screener is the PHQ-9 [435], which was funded by Pfizer, manufacturer of sertraline and since the acquisition of Wyeth in 2009, also of venlafaxine and desvenlafaxine. The PHQ-9 is a freely available self-report instrument that measures the severity of all 9 symptoms of depression over the last 2 weeks based on DSM criteria, that is, (1) depressed mood, (2) loss of interest or pleasure, (3) sleep problems, (4) fatigue or lack of energy, (5) lack of appetite or overeating, (6) feelings of worthlessness or guilt, (7) concentration difficulties, (8) speaking slowly or being restless (psychomotor retardation or agitation), and (9) suicidal ideation or behaviour. Each symptom is rated on a 4-point scale ranging from 0 (not present at all) to 3 (present nearly every day). The total score can thus range from 0 to 27; scores of 1–4 are rated as minimal depression, 5–9 as mild depression, 10–14 as moderate depression, 15–19 as moderately severe depression, and 20–27 as severe depression [435].

The questionnaire weighs all symptoms equally and ignores context or circumstances. It follows that someone can attain rather high "depression" scores even without reporting low mood and loss of interest/pleasure (anhedonia), the core symptoms of depression. Further note that symptom severity is assessed via frequency or persistence of symptoms, and not via perceived burden or distress. High frequency or persistence of symptoms does not necessarily imply high severity. Having troubles falling asleep almost every day certainly has a different clinical importance than having suicidal thoughts almost every day, but the questionnaire treats them the same (both add 3 points to the total score). But the most serious flaw arguably is the neglect of context. Fatigue, sleep problems, lack of appetite, and difficulties concentrating that develop as part of life circumstances (e.g. having a newborn), a general medical condition (e.g. an endocrine disorder), or as consequence of a medical treatment (e.g. chemotherapy) have a completely different meaning than when they result from a deep-seated unhappiness with one's life. Only in the latter case they are likely to be symptoms of a depressive disorder.

Depression screening instruments are frequently used in epidemiological research as simple and cost-efficient alternatives to expensive and time-consuming diagnostic interviews. However, for the reasons detailed above, their application results in overdetection and misclassification [436]. A comprehensive meta-analysis has recently confirmed that the PHQ-9, the most popular depression screening instrument, overestimates the prevalence of depression by a factor of two. According to the PHQ-9 the prevalence rate of depression in primary care and community samples was 25%, whereas the more reliable semi-structured diagnostic interviews produced a prevalence rate of 12% [437]. It has also been shown that the PHQ-9 significantly overestimates the severity of depression, that is, the screening instrument "is overinclusive in classifying patients with severe depression, and correspondingly underinclusive in classifying patients with mild depression" [438]. Public mental health policy and treatment decisions should therefore not be based on the misleading results of screening instruments such as the PHQ-9, but unfortunately, their misapplication (and misinterpretation) is all too common.

For instance, in a recent German study of primary care patients, the researchers deduced depression diagnoses from the Depression Screening Questionnaire (an instrument similar to the PHQ-9) and then, unsurprisingly, found that many screen-positive cases were not diagnosed by their physician with a depressive disorder [439]. This naturally follows from the inadequate diagnostic validity of screening questionnaires and their poor positive predictive value, that is, the proportion of people with a positive test result who actually have the disorder [436, 437, 440]. Fortunately, a skilled GP will not diagnose major depression in all screen-positive cases and by consequence will not treat patients for a non-existent depressive disorder. Although the authors acknowledged in the study limitations section that a screening questionnaire "has limitations regarding the correct classification of patients with depression", they disregarded this major flaw when interpreting their findings, stating that primary care physicians often failed to correctly diagnose depression and that depression was thus undertreated [439]. Ignorant of the poor diagnostic validity of screening questionnaires, they even concluded that their study "indicates a need to improve general practitioners' ability to diagnose these conditions and determine the indication for treatment" [439]. This bold conclusion is unsubstantiated and misleading. It is also insulting to GPs to question their diagnostic proficiency and treatment decisions based on an inadequate screening questionnaire.

But are depression-screening instruments at least useful in clinical practice? Not really. According to the scientific literature, their application provides very limited benefits, if at all. Most importantly, in general medical practice, depression screening instruments have not been shown to improve the outcome of depression [441, 442], but may result in overdiagnosis and overtreatment [443]. As summarised by Thombs and Ziegelstein [444],

> "There are some conditions, like diabetes mellitus, that almost always require screening or other special laboratory testing to diagnose. Depression is not one of those conditions. Primary care providers are expected to have the necessary knowledge and expertise to diagnose and treat common health conditions like depression, and if they do not, they should obtain it. Indeed, a lack of knowledge is no excuse for using a screening tool with unacceptable test characteristics on all patients, and the best available evidence suggests that doing so would likely lead to more harm than good. Screening is not a substitute for good medical care".

But despite a clear lack of supporting evidence, depression-screening instruments are aggressively marketed by the pharmaceutical industry and strongly endorsed by various leaders in the field as economic case-finding tools [445, 446]. That the industry has strong vested interests in the routine application of depression screenings is understandable from a commercial point of view, given that screening instruments may propel overdiagnosis and overtreatment [443]. But why mental health professionals praise (and endorse) their use is less clear. Perhaps they are simply not aware of the limitations and negative consequences of routine depression screenings in primary care.

In his book *Bad pharma*, Dr Ben Goldacre describes how in 2010, Eli Lilly (manufacturer of the antidepressants fluoxetine and duloxetine) launched a new depression-screening test on the popular medical information website WebMD [428]. The test was introduced with the heading: "Rate your risk for depression: could you be depressed?" Similar to Pfizer's PHQ-9, the test consisted of ten questions that assessed the various depression symptoms (e.g. "I feel sad or down most of the time", "I feel tired almost every day", "I have trouble concentrating"). Now, even if you answered every single question with "No", the test yielded the response: "You may be at risk for major depression". It went on to explain a few things, including "You replied that you are feeling four or fewer of the common symptoms of depression. In general, people experiencing depression have five or more common symptoms of the condition. But every individual is unique. If you are concerned about depression, talk with your doctor". Well, of course many people will get concerned when a screening test placed on a respected medicine website tells them that they are at risk of major depression! What Eli Lilly basically says to the thousands of readers of WebMD is that even when they are absolutely not depressed, they may still have the condition and thus it would be better to visit a doctor (who, with good chance, will pre-emptively prescribe an antidepressant). At least the funding of the test was declared on the page, but you certainly grasp the absurdity and hazardousness of this utterly flawed "screening test" that is nothing more than a disease-mongering marketing tool for antidepressants [428]. We don't need to wonder why depression became an epidemic and why antidepressants are massively overprescribed in mild and subthreshold depression when such flawed screening instruments are widely in use.

Health organisation, academic psychiatrists, patient advocacy groups and the pharmaceutical industry, often in close collaboration, have launched programs and campaigns that have undeniably contributed to the overdefinition and overdetection of depression, resulting in overdiagnosis and unnecessary antidepressant use in many people with normal emotional reactions to loss, stressful life events, and common problems of everyday life [3, 5, 434, 447]. Depression awareness campaigns like the UK Defeat Depression campaign and other educational materials were specifically directed at GPs and the general public to increase the recognition and detection of depression. My impression, in accordance with various other authors [9, 132, 399, 448, 449], is that these programs overreached and thus had serious negative consequences. Many, perhaps most, people now diagnosed with depression in primary care don't even meet the liberal DSM-criteria for major depression [117]. This was confirmed by a comprehensive meta-analysis by Mitchell and colleagues published 2009 in the leading medical journal *Lancet* [450]. The results showed that for every 100 unselected primary care patients, there were more false positive depression diagnoses (n = 15) than either missed (n = 10) or correctly identified cases (n = 10). Thus, although GPs did not detect depression in some people (presumably milder, self-limiting episodes not in need of treatment [451]), a larger number of people were diagnosed with depression even though they didn't have clinical depression. This is presumably also due to legal reasons, because in many countries insurances only cover (or pay for) mental health services and sick leave when a respective psychiatric diagnosis has been issued.

As one GP gloomily put it in a large qualitative study, "people come along to see us with all sorts of problems that are not illnesses. People come in with unhappy relationships. They are unhappy at work. They have problems with their neighbours. They are generally dissatisfied with life and they expect the GPs to do something about this, which obviously we can't but we can label it as depression and medicate them. Whether that's actually doing anyone any good in the long run is arguable" [452]. And another GP stated "We've been hounded for so long that we were missing depression now we're, in a way, perhaps we're over diagnosing or perhaps we're treating more mild depression that in the past people would just have got on with. I mean, it then becomes quite subtle whether or not somebody's degree of unhappiness is tipping them into a mild depression or is it just life, and that's a bit of a fine line" [452]. Finally, Dr Derek Summerfield, a practicing psychiatrist and senior lecturer, summarised the "depression epidemic" and "mass prescribing" of antidepressants as follows:

> "My patients' presentations often bear out the reality that life in the UK is getting harder: the fortunes of the haves and have-nots are diverging, the fabric of the welfare state thins, employment entitlements grow precarious. The Archbishop of Canterbury calls our economic model 'broken'. Many people receiving a diagnosis of 'depression' might be more authentically seen as carrying generic social suffering. The doctor can do little about the

patient's social predicament, but feels she must do something and so prescribes an antidepressant by reflex. This 'epidemic' of depression lets the neoliberal political and economic order off the hook". [453]

In conclusion, depression, as currently defined, is often (not always) a normal emotional reaction to societal problems (e.g. job strain, financial hardship, inequality, unemployment, marital difficulties) rather than a genuine biomedical condition (i.e. bodily disorder or disease). In this respect, the mass prescribing of antidepressants is presumably best conceived as an inadequate (or desperate) medical solution to pervasive socio-economic problems [454]. Research findings, in line with the perception of many practitioners, further indicate that normal sadness and unhappiness are frequently misdiagnosed as clinical depression, thus many people (not all) are unnecessarily prescribed an antidepressant from which they most likely don't benefit [3, 5, 117, 414, 447, 453, 455]. As cogently summarised by Dr. Roger Mulder,

"Major depression is not a natural entity and does not identify a homogenous group of patients. The apparent increase in major depression results from: confusing those who are ill with those who share their symptoms; the surveying of symptoms out of context; the benefits that accrue from such a diagnosis to drug companies, researchers, and clinicians; and changing social constructions around sadness and distress. Standardized medical treatment of all these individuals is neither possible nor desirable". [410]

Digression: The Medicalisation of Shyness and Anxiousness

In parallel with the medicalisation of unhappiness and sadness [3, 5, 447], several authors also noted a medicalisation of shyness and anxiousness as reflected in the diagnostic labels of social anxiety disorder (social phobia) and generalised anxiety disorder [385, 415, 427, 429, 456]. Unlike depression, the increased awareness (and popularisation) of these two diagnoses during the 1990s was not born on the widespread professional perception that they were under-recognised and undertreated, but largely resulted from clever disease marketing by the pharmaceutical industry in order to broaden antidepressant markets. The industry-sponsored anxiety campaigns started shortly after the introduction of paroxetine (brand name: Paxil) in 1993. When this SSRI was first approved for major depression, its manufacturer SmithKline Beecham (now GlaxoSmithKline) was faced with a saturated depression market largely dominated by its competitor Eli Lilly (fluoxetine, launched 1988). Moreover, before GlaxoSmithKline introduced paroxetine, in 1992, its rival Pfizer had just launched its depression marketing campaign for sertraline. GlaxoSmithKline's marketing strategy was thus to position its antidepressant as an anti-anxiety drug and to enter the new market of the various anxiety disorder diagnoses [427]. The company thus requested the approval of paroxetine for social anxiety disorder (SAD; granted in 1999) and, a bit later, for generalised anxiety disorder (GAD; granted in 2001).

In the early 1990s, before paroxetine was marketed as an anti-anxiety drug, both SAD and GAD were considered extremely rare. They were little known in public, and infrequently diagnosed in clinical practice (remember that the anxiety conditions were largely redefined as depressive disorders during the 1970s [63]). This situation changed drastically in the late 1990s. "GlaxoSmithKline has spent millions of dollars to raise the public visibility of SAD and GAD, by sponsoring well-choreographed disease awareness campaigns. The pharmaceutical company's savvy approach to marketing SAD and GAD, which relied upon a mixture of 'expert' and patient voices, simultaneously gave the conditions diagnostic validity and created the perception that it could happen to anyone" [427]. By the early 1999, a particularly successful SAD media campaign widely publicised the catchy slogan "imagine being allergic to people". This disease awareness campaign was officially run by the Social Anxiety Disorder Coalition, a patient advocacy group created and marketed by GlaxoSmithKline [429]. In a press packet given to journalists, GlaxoSmithKline further claimed that SAD "affects up to 13.3% of the population", or 1 in 8 Americans, and that it is "the third most common psychiatric disorder in the United States, after depression and alcoholism", even though the DSM-IV gave much lower prevalence estimates [429].

In the GlaxoSmithKline "Business Plan Guide" from 1998 sent to its sales representatives, it was stated, "The launch of Social Anxiety Disorder is quickly approaching and preparations are underway … It is important that we prepare ourselves to take full advantage of the opportunity Social Anxiety Disorder provides to differentiate Paxil, grow our market share and achieve our super bonus goal of passing Zoloft and attaining $1.5 billion in sales. Let's get psyched!" [29]. The aggressive marketing of SAD was indeed extremely successful. "In the two years preceding Paxil's approval, fewer than 50 stories on social anxiety disorder had appeared in the popular press. In May 1999, the month when the FDA handed down its decision, hundreds of stories about the illness appeared in U.S. publications and television news programs, including the New York Times, Vogue, and Good Morning America" [429]. The same marketing strategy, referred to as disease branding (marketing a condition to sell drugs) was shortly after repeated for GAD and was equally successful. In the year 2000, GlaxoSmithKline invested in total US$92 million in direct-to-consumer advertising for paroxetine, which was the fourth highest amount spend for any prescription drug in that year [457]. The money was well invested, as it helped to make paroxetine the number 1 antidepressant on the market and number 6 of all drugs in terms of prescriptions by 2002 [427].

The marketing of "unrecognised" disorders (like masked and mild depression, social anxiety disorder, and generalised anxiety disorder) as a means to enhance prescription drug sales would not be possible without the help of prominent physicians acting as "product champions" or "key opinion leaders" for the pharmaceutical industry [29, 405, 406]. Among the experts paid by GlaxoSmithKline to enhance the awareness of SAD and GAD were prominent key opinion leaders such as professors Drs. Nemeroff, Gorman, Liebowitz, Ballenger, Davidson, Dunner, and Hirschfeld [30, 429]. For instance, in November 1993, shortly after paroxetine was approved for depression, GlaxoSmithKline convened an advisory board meeting at the Ritz Carlton Hotel in Palm Beach, Florida (including first class flight and $2500 to $5000 for attending the weekend meeting). The company invited ten advisory board members, including several DSM-IV work group members (Drs James Ballenger, David Dunner, Robert Hirschfeld and Michael Liebowitz), and the meeting was chaired by Dr Charles Nemeroff, then head of the psychiatry department at Emory University and presumably psychiatry's best paid key opinion leader (see also chapter Conflicts of Interest). The aim of the meeting was to help GlaxoSmithKline's marketing team to increase and expand the use of paroxetine, that is, to exploit the anxiety disorder market [30]. Later, this group (and similar others) would author various papers and consensus statements on the detection and treatment of both SAD and GAD, often supported by unrestricted grants from industry and published in industry-sponsored journal supplements. Many researchers rightly argue that this kind of academia–industry partnership is pharmaceutical marketing disguised as "independent" expert opinion [29, 376, 405, 406, 458, 459].

GlaxoSmithKline was of course not alone in the branding and commercialisation of anxiety disorders. Other companies also adopted this profitable disease marketing model and sought to increase their antidepressant sales by directing their promotional efforts towards anxiety disorder diagnoses. Roche, for instance, also invested in the marketing of social anxiety disorder by supporting a patient advocacy group and by funding a large conference on social anxiety disorder. These actions were part of a larger marketing strategy to popularise its antidepressant moclobemide as a treatment for social anxiety disorder [385]. Pfizer, in turn, was highly successful in marketing post-traumatic stress disorder (PTSD), for which condition its drug sertraline (Zoloft) gained regulatory approval in late 1999. Koerner briefly summarised this marketing campaign and its outcome as follows:

> "The company funded the creation of the PTSD Alliance, a group that is staffed by employees of Pfizer's New York public-relations firm, the Chandler Chicco Agency, and operates out of the firm's offices. The Alliance connects journalists with PTSD experts such as Jerilyn Ross, president and CEO of the Anxiety Disorders Association of America, a group that is heavily subsidized by Pfizer as well as GlaxoSmithKline, Eli Lilly, and other drug-industry titans. In the months following the launch of Pfizer's campaign, media mentions of PTSD skyrocketed. Just weeks after the Alliance's founding in 2000, for example, the New York Times ran a story citing Pfizer-supplied statistics on childhood PTSD, according to which 1 in 6 minors who experience the sudden death of a close friend or relative will develop the disorder. Other stories highlighted studies promoted by the alliance according to which 1 in 13 Americans will suffer from PTSD at some point in their lives". [429]

Other examples of economically successful disease-branding campaigns include the marketing of premenstrual dysphoric disorder by Eli Lilly to expand the patent of its SSRI fluoxetine [456, 460] and the marketing of bipolar disorder by various manufacturers of atypical antipsychotics to expand the market for this best-selling class of psychiatric drugs [67, 414].

Is Depression a Public Health Crisis?

As I have shown above, until the 1970s, depression was considered a severe but rare disorder. It was further assumed that, in general, it has a good prognosis even when left untreated. Depression experts of the time consistently emphasised that most people with depression would recover spontaneously and remain well [63, 132, 399]. This wide-held position changed dramatically between the 1970s and 1980s. Since then, depression has apparently become a "global crisis" [397]. The common view in psychiatry and clinical psychology nowadays is that depression is very common, severe, chronic or highly recurrent, and the leading cause of disability [77, 461]. For instance, a highly cited paper (725 citations as of June 2021), very typical of the mainstream description of depression nowadays, begins like this: "Mood disorders are among the most common and debilitating psychiatric disorders. The most common mood disorder is depression, which is the number-one cause of disability worldwide". Later, the authors assert that depressive disorders "recur at high rates, and most patients experience multiple episodes. These disorders are often chronic, and even minimal symptoms are associated with increased risk for subsequent episodes and considerable functional impairment". The authors also claim "Suicide is a major concern: About 15% of individuals with mood disorders will commit suicide (depression accounts for about 50% of all suicides)" [462].

By contrast, other authors challenged this alarming depiction of depression and maintain that the prevalence of clinical depression has been massively exaggerated [9, 25, 63, 414, 434, 448, 453]. For instance, according to Mulder, "the depression epidemic is an artifact related to the DSM criteria. As with most DSM diagnoses, the criteria for depression focus on well-delineated and manifest symptoms. All persons who report enough symptoms are counted as having a mental disorder, regardless of context or circumstances. Since most depressive symptoms are common—consider sadness, tiredness, apathy, insomnia, lowered concentration, and appetite changes—then depression will be reported as a widespread medical illness" [410]. Who is right then? And how accurate is the prevailing modern portrayal of depression as a serious chronic medical condition of epidemic proportions? In the following, I will examine each prominent claim carefully one by one.

Is depression typically severe? According to the Global Burden of Disease Study, only 11% of depression episodes were rated severe [116]. An analysis of nationwide insurance claims data from Germany likewise showed that of 35 million depression diagnoses made in 2017, only 11% fell under the category of a severe depression episode [463]. A large epidemiological study in Italian primary care practices showed that only 6% of all depression diagnoses were rated severe [464]. According to the UK primary care database, among adults aged 20–64 with a first depression diagnosis, merely 4% were rated severe [115], whereas in older adults aged 65–100, the proportion was 5% [465]. In Switzerland, federal data from 2008/2009 revealed that severe depression episodes accounted for 9% of all registered depression diagnoses [466]. Some epidemiological studies in the general population that did not account for context, including comorbid or underlying somatic medical conditions (e.g. cancer or endocrine disorders) produced somewhat higher (inflated) estimates, but even in these surveys only a minority of depression episodes qualified as severe or serious. For example, according to the WHO World Mental Health Survey, the proportion of severe/serious depression was 34% in developed countries [467], and according to the US National Comorbidity Survey Replication the proportion was 30% [468]. We can thus safely conclude that depression is typically not severe. In fact, most studies clearly indicate that severe forms of depression are rare and account for only about 10% of all depression diagnoses.

Is depression often chronic or highly recurrent? Major depression is an ill-defined, overinclusive, and heterogeneous diagnostic category comprising both mild, transient disorders and severe, more persistent disorders [4, 6, 7]. Community-based epidemiological studies have consistently shown that about half of all people with depression have a single episode with stable recovery and no recurrences long-term; about a third experience recurrences, of which most have one to three recurrences over the long-term; and 10–15% of people have chronic depression [190, 469–471]. In primary care samples, persistent severe depression is also a rare exception [472–474]. For instance, according to a large study conducted in 30 randomly selected Australian family practices, only 9% of patients with depression had chronically severe symptoms [472]. Highly recurrent and chronic depression is more frequently observed in samples of psychiatric inpatients, because people with severe and persistent psychopathology are more likely to be hospitalised [70, 475–477]. By consequence, the rate of highly recurrent and chronic depression is considerably overestimated in inpatient samples due to selection bias and not representative of the "typical" depression episode observed in community and primary care samples. We can thus safely conclude that in the general population, depression is typically not highly recurrent or chronic. In fact, half of all people with depression experience a single episode and, fortunately, only a small minority have chronic or highly recurrent depression.

Does untreated mild or subthreshold depression progress into severe depression? For sure a minority of people with mild/minor depression may develop more severe forms of depression over time, but research consistently shows that a much larger proportion of people fully recover from mild episodes and remain well independent of treatment received [472–474, 478, 479]. In patients with loss-related uncomplicated depression (i.e., brief reactive episodes without suicidality, psychotic symptoms, psychomotor retardation, and intense feelings of worthlessness) the rate of depression recurrence is not higher than the incidence rate in the general population with no baseline depression [480–482]. In addition, there is very little, if any, evidence that antidepressant treatment would improve the long-term outcome of depression, especially in mild-to-moderate episodes [190, 214, 219, 263, 264, 471, 483]. Let me detail some of these studies.

For instance, two pragmatic clinical trials (one randomised and the other non-randomised) compared the effectiveness of watchful waiting to antidepressant treatment in primary care patients with non-severe depression and found no meaningful difference at the 12-month follow-up [263, 264]. In a large naturalistic primary care study from Quebec, Canada, patients with mild baseline depression who received no adequate depression treatment had the same one-year outcome as patients who received antidepressants and/or psychotherapy [176]. According to a large international prospective observational study, primary care patients with undetected and untreated depression (mostly milder forms of depression) had, by tendency, even the better one-year outcome than patients diagnosed with depression and treated with antidepressants or sedatives, even after controlling for baseline severity [484]. Consistent with these results, in a prospective 30-year community cohort study, we found that antidepressant treatment in people with mostly mild to moderate depression was associated with a poorer long-term outcome, even after controlling for baseline severity [220]. Thus, there is neither robust evidence that mild/minor depression typically progresses to severe depression, nor that antidepressant treatment would improve the long-term outcome in mild/minor depression.

Is depression a leading contributor to the global burden of disease? The WHO now ranks depression the number 1 cause of disability burden [485], whereas according to the Global Burden of Disease Study, it is ranked number 3 cause after low back pain and headache disorders [486]. These estimates are, understandably, not without critics and should not been accepted at face value, as they are based on diagnostic concepts, epidemiologic characteristics (or parameters), data sources, and statistical models that are contested [65, 410, 487]. Among others, the burden of disease estimate, typically expressed as disability-adjusted life years (DALY), depends on the disability weights attributed to different levels of disorder severity, the rate of these levels of severity, the average duration of the disorder, and the estimated global prevalence of the disorder. Prevalence rates and average episode duration are estimated based on the best available epidemiological evidence. However, epidemiological studies may considerably overestimate the prevalence rates of clinical depression and other mental disorders, as these are based on semi-structured interviews (often conducted by lay people) that merely assess the presence of symptoms but largely ignore origin, context and/or meaning [65, 410, 488, 489]. For example, grief/despair after a critical life event is in most cases a normal emotional reaction, not a mental disorder (although it frequently meets diagnostic criteria). Most people will spontaneously recover after some time and thus should not be diagnosed with major depression.

Perhaps the most controversial (and least objective) part in the burden of disease estimates are the disability weights. In the Global Burden of Disease Study, the disability weights were determined by asking lay people from various countries how healthy they consider hypothetical cases with a particular health state based on "brief lay descriptions that focused on the major functional effects and symptoms associated with each health state" [490]. Even a modest change in the disability weight can have major impact on the global burden of disease estimate. So, how appropriate are these disability weights? Let's have a critical look.

The disability weights can range from 0 (no loss of health) to 1 (loss equivalent to death) [490]. The disability weight for mild depression was 0.16, for moderate depression 0.41, and for severe depression 0.66. In comparison, blindness had a disability weight of 0.19 and severe heart failure had a disability weight of 0.18, thus both just slightly above the disability attributed to mild depression. Tuberculosis with HIV infection had a disability weight of 0.41, identical to moderate depression. Both metastatic cancer and severe dementia had a disability weight of 0.45, which is just slightly above moderate depression but markedly below severe depression. Both AIDS without antiretroviral treatment and severe Parkinson's disease had a disability weight of 0.58, thus rated less disabling than severe depression. If we consider that according to double-blind randomised trials, 35–40% of patients with moderate to severe depression experience substantial clinical improvements (i.e. at least 50% symptom reduction) within 8 weeks while treated with an inert placebo pill [192], to me it is incomprehensible how the disability weight of moderate depression (0.41) could be on a similar level as tuberculosis with HIV infection (0.41), metastatic cancer (0.45), or severe dementia (0.45), which do not respond to placebo treatment and, contrary to moderate depression, never remit spontaneously. I do not contest that depression can be very severe and debilitating in some cases but declaring it sweepingly the leading cause of disability is, in my view and that of many other experts, certainly debatable [65, 410, 448, 487, 491].

Do 15% of people with depression die by suicide? The figure of 15% as cited by Hollon and colleagues [462] and many others has been accepted and propagated for many years by prominent psychiatrists and in various psychiatric textbooks. It was first reported by Guze and Robins in 1970 [492] based on their review of 17 studies of psychiatric inpatients with mostly severe (melancholic) depression. As frequently observed, large effects and spectacular findings are uncritically appraised in biomedical and psychological research, but quite often they eventually turn out to be false, unsubstantiated, or massively exaggerated [50, 493–496]. In 1997, Blair-West and colleagues conclusively demonstrated that it is mathematically impossible that 15% of people with depression die by suicide, otherwise population suicide rates would be much higher given the high prevalence of depression [497]. Based on their calculations, the suicide rate in depression would be 3.5% rather than 15%. Moreover, it has been shown that the suicide risk is strongly related to gender. While in men with depression the lifetime suicide risk was estimated to be 7%, in women with depression it was only 1% [498].

To authors familiar with the scientific literature it should thus have been evidently clear that the lifetime suicide risk of 15% derived from psychiatric inpatients as reported by Guze and Robins [492] was a massive overestimation of the true suicide risk in the broader population of people with depression [499], especially in women [498]. Even worse, it was shown back in 1998 that the statistical model applied by Guze and Robins was flawed. Based on an adequate statistical model, Inskip and colleagues [500] recalculated the lifetime suicide risk and derived a rate of 6% for inpatients with depression, thus less than half of the initial, erroneous estimate reported by Guze and Robins [492]. Comprehensive analyses later confirmed the much lower suicide risk in depression. For instance, Bostwick and Pankratz calculated a life-time suicide risk of 8.6% for inpatients ever hospitalised for suicidality (includes various diagnoses other than depression), 4.0% for affective disorder inpatients, and 2.2% for affective disorder outpatients [499]. Thus, while depression can be a serious and devastating disorder, the popular notion that 15% of people with depression will die by suicide is massively exaggerated and evidently wrong.

In conclusion, in the general population, severe forms of depression are fortunately rare [116]. Most people reporting depressive symptoms have mild or minor depression, which generally has a good prognosis [472, 478, 479]. It has further been shown that chronic or highly recurrent depression affects only a small minority [190, 471]. Depression undeniably is associated with an increased suicide mortality [501], but the lifetime suicide risk in depression is about 2–4% rather than the often quoted but erroneous figure of 15% [497, 499]. Moreover, while the suicide risk is substantially increased in men with depression, it is much less increased in women with depression [498]. It is therefore essential to differentiate between serious, debilitating depression and the much more frequent non-serious, milder forms of depression, which, unfortunately, are subsumed under the same diagnostic label [3, 6, 7, 410, 481]. To be clear, we must acknowledge that severe depression can be a chronic, devastating, and life-threatening disorder, but we must not generalise from these rare manifestations to the broader population of people with depression. Portraying depression based on its most serious form is misleading and misinforms public health policy, which may result in misallocation of limited healthcare resources and consequently both overtreatment (of mild depression) and undertreatment (of severe depression) [410, 414, 491]. I will discuss the misallocation of healthcare resources in the section "Bottom Line: a Public Health Analysis". But before I want to write about the biological revolution in psychiatry and the marketing of both depression as a brain disorder and its alleged chemical cure, the antidepressants.

Biological Reductionism

The Biological Revolution in Psychiatry

As briefly mentioned above, the 1970s and 1980s experienced a strong revival of biological psychiatry and the demise of psychoanalysis and psychosocial models, especially in the US. With the publication of the DSM-III in 1980, which corroborated the biomedical model of mental disorders, and the introduction of new drug classes (e.g. the atypical antipsychotics, SSRIs), a new psychiatric era began. Dr. Andrew Scull cynically summarised the biological revolution as follows:

> "Psychoanalysts were rapidly defenestrated, chucked out of their hold over academic departments of psychiatry and replaced by laboratory-based neuroscientists and psychopharmacologists. Psychoanalytic institutes found themselves bereft of recruits and forced to abandon their policy of admitting only the medically qualified. The very term 'neurosis' was expunged from the official nomenclature of mental disorder, along with the hypothetical Freudian aetiologies for various mental disorders. The 'surface' manifestations of mental diseases that the psychoanalysts had long dismissed as merely the symptoms of the underlying psychodynamic disorders of the personality became instead scientific markers, the very elements that defined different forms of mental disorder. And the control of such symptoms, preferably by chemical means, became the new Holy Grail of the profession". [394]

The biological revolution helped to establish psychiatry as a reputable and truly medical specialty [30, 63, 393]. Arisen from the neurosciences and generously supported by the pharmaceutical industry, biological psychiatry framed mental disorders as brain disorders and asserted to be finally equipped with "magic bullets", that is, drugs that cure the neurobiological abnormalities underlying mental disorders. This was also the main tenet of psychiatry professor Dr. Nancy Andreasen's influential book *The broken brain: The biological revolution in psychiatry*, published in 1984. In her book, Dr. Andreasen confidently announced that "these diseases are caused principally by biological factors and most of these reside in the brain". And she also had a clear advice on how we should treat mental disorders: "The best way to treat these biological abnormalities ... is to correct the underlying physical abnormality, usually through the use of somatic therapy" [502]. Soon this narrow and reductionistic view dominated almost the entire field of psychiatry [393]. For instance, among the 627 papers presented in the new research sessions at the annual meeting of the APA in 1992, 86% were biomedically oriented (mostly neurobiology, genetics, and psychopharmacology) [391].

Not much has changed since then. To this day, the biomedical model is still dominating in psychiatry, in both research and practice [392, 503, 504]. A clear indicator that contemporary academic psychiatry is often narrowly (and simplistically) reduced to neurobiology and psychopharmacology is the content of its top-tier journals. *Molecular Psychiatry*, *Translational Psychiatry*, and *Biological Psychiatry* publish exclusively biological research, and they have some of the highest journal impact factors, meaning their articles are among the most cited in the field. And if you look at other leading psychiatry journals, for instance the *American Journal of Psychiatry*, *JAMA Psychiatry*, and the *British Journal of Psychiatry*, you will easily recognise that the majority of published studies are about neurobiology, genetics, and drug treatment. There are few notable exceptions of top-tier journals with a more diverse content, including *Lancet Psychiatry* and *World Psychiatry*. Nevertheless, contemporary psychiatric research is largely (not exclusively) centred on the putative (neuro)biological causes of mental disorders and on drug treatments that are assumed to reverse neurobiological abnormalities. And with respect to practice, it is well established that drugs are the mainstay of mental healthcare and often the sole treatment provided [392, 477, 505].

But there are two major caveats. First, the scientific foundation of this neurobiological model of mental disorders is anything but cogent and reliable [395, 396, 506], and second, the new miracle drugs touted as "magic bullets", especially the new-generation antidepressants and atypical antipsychotics, proved neither curative nor highly effective [13, 80, 198, 507, 508]. In fact, most bio-psychiatric messages were (and still are) hyperbolic, poorly substantiated, and ill-founded [393, 396, 506, 509]. Meta-scientific studies have repeatedly shown that most biological research findings in psychiatry, especially neuroimaging and molecular genetic studies, do not replicate, are highly inconsistent, methodological artefacts, false-positive chance findings, or massively exaggerated [493, 510–520].

You may wonder what's wrong with centring research efforts on the neurosciences? Well, in short, neurobiological reductionism is likely a major driver of overprescribing and medicalisation [26, 394, 399]. And waiting for new scientific discoveries in the neurobiology of mental disorders is likely also the wrong strategy to improve public mental health and clinical practice [392, 396, 521]. To some authors these shortcomings (and negative consequences) of the bio-psychiatric paradigm are evidently clear. "Today one is hard-pressed to find anyone knowledgeable who believes that the so-called biological revolution of the 1980s made good on most or even any of its therapeutic and scientific promises. Criticism of the enterprise has escalated sharply in recent decades. It is now increasingly clear to the general public that it overreached, overpromised, overdiagnosed, overmedicated, and compromised its principles", wrote Dr. Anne Harrington, a professor of the history of science, in her book *Mind fixers: Psychiatry's troubled search for the biology of mental illness* [393].

Although the steep rise of biological psychiatry was heralded as a great scientific progress, the narrow focus on isolated neurobiological causes put psychiatry in a reactionary position in the late twentieth century. "During the second half of the 20th century, the approach to disease causation of major parts of psychiatry was out of step with the rest of medicine and medical epidemiology. Instead of multicausal models, the rising and soon to be dominant field of biological psychiatry pursued monocausal models for their major disorders" noted eminent psychiatry professor Dr. Kendler [522]. That is, while the rest of medicine turned towards complex multicausal models, allowing for environmental and social factors in the aetiology of physical health conditions, psychiatry, concerned with mental health conditions, largely ignored environmental and social factors and instead focused narrowly on simplistic and reductionistic monocausal neurobiological models. Many experts are still convinced that the neurosciences will ultimately reveal the pathogenesis (i.e. emergence, progression and maintenance) of mental disorders [523, 524], but others contend that this mission can impossibly succeed in view of the complex multifactorial nature of psychological problems that are so fundamentally embedded in unique individual biography, social environment, and culture [395, 521].

For instance, in a critical commentary published in the *New England Journal of Medicine*, Drs. Gardner and Kleinman, both psychiatrists, recently noted,

"Something has gone wrong in contemporary academic and clinical psychiatry. Checklist-style amalgamations of symptoms have taken the place of thoughtful diagnosis, and trial-and-error 'medication management' has taken over practice to an alarming degree. We are facing the stark limitations of biologic treatments, while finding less and less time to work with patients on difficult problems. Ironically, although these limitations are widely recognized by experts in the field, the prevailing message to the public and the rest of medicine remains that the solution to psychological problems involves matching the 'right' diagnosis with the 'right' medication. Consequently, psychiatric diagnoses and medications proliferate under the banner of scientific medicine, though there is no comprehensive biologic understanding of either the causes or the treatments of psychiatric disorders". [392]

That modern psychiatry is too narrowly focused on its descriptive symptom-based diagnoses, the search of putative neurobiological causes, and finding a chemical cure for whatever psychological problem, is not a recent insight. It was repeatedly stressed over decades by many mental health experts. For instance, it was already noted in 1993 by Dr. Carl Cohen, a US professor of psychiatry, who wrote a critical article about the "biomedicalization of psychiatry" [391]. And it was again emphasised in 2005 by Dr. Steven Sharfstein, then-president of the APA, who wrote "There is widespread concern of the over-medicalization of mental disorders and the overuse of medications. Financial incentives and managed care have contributed to the notion of a 'quick fix' by taking a pill and reducing the emphasis on psychotherapy and psychosocial treatments … We must examine the fact that as a profession, we have allowed the biopsychosocial model to become the bio-bio-bio model. In a time of economic constraint, a 'pill and an appointment' has dominated treatment" [525].

These justified concerns were later endorsed by various other psychiatrists. One of those is Dr. Joanna Moncrieff, professor of psychiatry at the University College London, who wrote a poignant critique of the reductionistic biomedical model in her influential book *The myth of the chemical cure* [80]. Another is Dr. Mark Sedler, professor of psychiatry, who wrote in 2016 in the journal *Medicine Health Care and Philosophy*, "As I have witnessed these much heralded changes over the course of my professional life—during which I was Chair of the Stony Brook University Department of Psychiatry and Behavioral Sciences for 18 years—I have observed that psychiatric training and practice have been given over almost exclusively to rendering diagnoses according to the DSM and prescribing drugs for virtually every complaint" [505]. And very recently a report by the World Health Organization emphasised:

> "The predominant focus of care in many contexts continues to be on diagnosis, medication and symptom reduction. Critical social determinants that impact on people's mental health such as violence, discrimination, poverty, exclusion, isolation, job insecurity or unemployment, lack of access to housing, social safety nets, and health services, are often overlooked or excluded from mental health concepts and practice. This leads to an over-diagnosis of human distress and over-reliance on psychotropic drugs to the detriment of psychosocial interventions—a phenomenon which has been well documented, particularly in high-income countries". [526]

But back in the late 1980s, these were distinct voices of the future and at that time few dared to question the triumph of the biological revolution, including the anticipated neuroscientific foundation and the hoped-for pharmacological cure of mental disorders. So let's look a bit closer at how this narrow focus on neurobiology and psychopharmacology came about.

The NIMH Mission

Perhaps the single most influential actor in the biological revolution, following changes in health policy (closing of large psychiatric hospitals), political pressure (antipsychiatry movement), and developments within the APA (disempowerment of psychoanalysts), was the NIMH [93, 391, 393, 396]. In 1990, initiated by Dr. Lewis Judd, the then-director of the NIMH, US Congress declared the 1990s the "Decade of the Brain" and this also sent the NIMH on an ambitious mission that would, so it was claimed, finally discover the neurobiological causes of mental disorders.

According to Dr. Alan Leshner, Judd's deputy at NIMH and later chief execute of the American Association for the Advancement of Science, "[Judd] was obsessed with educating the public and the profession … that mental illnesses were biological illnesses, that schizophrenia and depression were diseases of the brain" [527]. Within the NIMH and among many (perhaps most) academic psychiatrists, this idea quickly became an axiom, a general principle accepted as true without requiring proof.

"Mental illnesses are real, diagnosable, treatable brain disorders" wrote Dr. Steven Hyman, then-director of the NIMH in 1998 in the *American Journal of Psychiatry* [528]. In 2005, the new director of the NIMH, Dr. Thomas Insel, backed this bold claim and stressed again that mental disorders are brain disorders [523]. He also called for an integration of the clinical neurosciences into the discipline of psychiatry. According to Insel, "One of the fundamental insights emerging from contemporary neuroscience is that mental illnesses are brain disorders … While genomics will be important for revealing risk, and cellular neuroscience should provide targets for novel treatments for these disorders, it is most likely that the tools of systems neuroscience will yield the biomarkers needed to revolutionize psychiatric diagnosis and treatment" [523]. So he was basically advocating that all you need to diagnose and treat mental disorders is an understanding of neurobiology. That's also clear proof that various leaders in the field prefer a reductionistic biomedical model of mental disorders to an eclectic bio-psycho-social model [529]. Alas, up to this day, we are still waiting for these scientific breakthroughs and revolutionary treatments (and we will possibly wait forever if biological reductionism prevails). As a matter of fact, anno 2021, there are still no reliable biomarkers of mental disorders, no laboratory diagnostic tests, and no revolutionary treatments that are superior to the first psychiatric drug classes from the 1950s and 1960s (i.e. typical antipsychotics, lithium, tricyclic antidepressants, and benzodiazepines). But back to the ambitious and overly optimistic Dr. Insel and the NIMH.

In 2015, Dr. Insel succeeded in promulgating his reductionistic conviction in the prestigious journal *Science* with an article titled "Brain disorders? Precisely" [530]. However, just as his predecessors, Drs Hyman and Judd, and the many academic psychiatrists endorsing this view, he did not offer any convincing explanations as to what he means by ascribing complex psychological problems to brain disorders. Neither did he provide a clear rational for this claim except for citing various studies showing correlations between neurobiological measures and psychiatric symptoms, often by comparing patients with mental disorders to healthy controls. I will turn to this methodological issue in more detail later.

In 2010, under the leadership of Dr. Insel, the NIMH announced its Research Domain Criteria (RDoC) project, a "framework for research on pathophysiology, especially for genomics and neuroscience, which ultimately will inform future classification schemes" [531]. For many years now, the majority of NIMH grants have been awarded to neurobiological research programs. As stressed by Dr. Allen Frances, "NIMH was at the center of the neuroscience enthusiasm, dubbing the 1990s the 'decade of the brain' and betting the house on a narrow biological agenda to replace what previously had been a more balanced portfolio of research into not only the basic sciences, but also into treatments and health services. In effect, NIMH turned itself into a 'brain institute' rather than an 'institute of mental health'" [532]. But this move was apparently not radical enough for the NIMH leadership. In 2014, the NIMH even decided to stop funding clinical trials that do not include measures of neurobiology or genetics [533], which Markowitz and Friedman recently summarised in the title of a critical commentary as "NIMH's straight and neural path: The road to killing clinical psychiatric research" [534].

In result, "over the past half century, biologic research has come to largely replace all other forms of psychiatric research—psychosocial, cultural, public health, and community—which have thus been marginalized in spite of the useful knowledge these fields provide for everyday care of patients and prevention of mental illness. Similarly, psychotherapy, an essential and multifaceted tool that mobilizes the unique power of the clinician–patient relationship, has been increasingly neglected in psychiatric training and practice", wrote Gardner and Kleinman in 2019 [392]. Obviously (and sadly), Dr Sharfstein was proven right: psychiatry not only "allowed" but forced "the biopsychosocial model to become the bio-bio-bio model" [525]. But still many leaders in academic psychiatry have a different opinion and demand even more reliance on the neurosciences and psychopharmacology. You think I'm exaggerating? Well here are a few examples.

In 2008, a large group of influential UK psychiatrists wrote an article in the *British Journal of Psychiatry* titled "Wake-up call for British psychiatry" where they expressed grave concern about the increased provision of psychosocial interventions at community mental health services:

> "Evidence-based psychological and social interventions are extremely important in managing psychiatric illness. Nevertheless, the accompanying downgrading of medical aspects of care has resulted in services that often are better suited to offering non-specific psychosocial support, rather than thorough, broad-based diagnostic assessment leading to specific treatments to optimise well-being and functioning. In part, these changes have been politically driven, but they could not have occurred without the collusion, or at least the acquiescence, of psychiatrists. This creeping devaluation of medicine disadvantages patients and is very damaging to both the standing and the understanding of psychiatry in the minds of the public, fellow professionals and the medical students who will be responsible for the specialty's future". [535]

In a similar article from 2009 with the admonitory title "Why psychiatry can't afford to be neurophobic", also published in the *British Journal of Psychiatry*, psychiatry professor Dr. Bullmore (who is half-time employed at Oxford University and half-time at GlaxoSmithKline, of which major pharmaceutical company he also is a shareholder), urged the readers, "If psychiatry aspires to be a progressive modern medicine of the mind, it should be fully engaged with the science of the brain" [536]. Just two more examples. In 2009, a group of very distinguished US psychiatry professors, including the then-president of the APA, claimed "Psychiatry is grounded in clinical neuroscience. Its core mission, now and in the future, is best served within this context because advances in assessment, treatment, and prevention of brain disorders are likely to originate from studies of etiology and pathophysiology based in clinical and translational neuroscience" [524]. Finally, in 2015 another group of US psychiatry professors again asserted "The diseases that we treat are diseases of the brain. The question that we need to address is not *whether* we integrate neuroscience alongside our other rich traditions but *how* we work as a field to overcome the barriers that currently limit us" (emphasis in original) [537].

You may wonder how valid is the "mental disorders are brain disorders" notion that has dominated psychiatric research and practice for the last three decades and that has so pervasively shaped professionals' and the public's conception of mental disorders [25, 504, 538–542]. Thus, let us have a critical look.

Putting the "Mental Disorders are Brain Disorders" Notion to the Test

To avoid any misunderstandings, I first like to emphasise that biological factors are certainly involved in the occurrence and experience of mental disorders, sometimes also causally. For instance, there is strong empirical evidence that some prescription drugs can cause depression [543, 544], and it is well established that activating antidepressant agents (e.g. SSRIs) can cause agitation, anxiety, and panic [309, 310, 545]. That's clear proof that mental disorders, and psychological problems in general, can have biological causes. Thus, by no means I advocate for a radical position that mental disorders are exclusively psychosocial (or environmental) in origin. But saying that biological factors are involved (sometimes causally) in mental disorders and claiming that mental disorders are brain disorders are two different things.

The mind undoubtedly requires brain functions. Without brain activity, there would be no consciousness and, consequently, no mental states. Accordingly, emotions, thoughts, and behaviours necessarily are implemented in neural systems and thus correlate with brain activity. But this does not imply that a change in emotions, thoughts, and behaviours is necessarily caused by a physiological alteration in the brain. Association does not imply causation. Moreover, even if an alteration in brain function would be the proximate cause, it still doesn't follow that this equates to a brain disorder. To prove that depression is a brain disorder, you need to define that brain disorder in terms of neurophysiological abnormality and then you demonstrate that this specific brain disorder causes depression. You can't conclude that depression is a brain disorder simply because mental states correlate with brain activity.

When psychiatrists claim that mental disorders are brain disorders, their implicit assumption is that mental disorders are caused by an abnormality (or pathology) in the brain, be it structural or functional. The claim further purports that by understanding the brain we would eventually be able to explain the emergence and manifestation of mental disorders and to develop highly effective (perhaps even curative) biological treatments (like antibiotics for various infectious diseases or insulin for type I diabetes). As stressed by Dr. Friedman, "The doubling down on basic neuroscience research seems to reflect the premise that if we can unravel the function of the brain, we will have a definitive understanding of the mind and the causes of major psychiatric disorders" [503]. However, it is almost impossible to deduce (or explain) complex psychological problems, including emotion, motivation, and behaviour, from brain measures alone [395]. No enumeration of alterations in brain function or structure will ever be able to fully capture (and explain) what it means to have depression (or any other mental disorder). Put differently, "emotions are implemented in neural systems, but not reducible to them" [396].

Imagine, for example, a 45-year-old woman who developed intense despair, profound sadness, loss of interest and pleasure, negative thoughts about the future, indecisiveness, sleep problems, fatigue, and lack of appetite after she found out that her husband had a long-time secret love affair with a younger woman for whom he eventually left her. When these symptoms last longer than two weeks they fulfil the diagnostic criteria of a major depression episode and hence would indicate that she has a brain disorder (according to the mental-disorders-are-brain-disorders proponents). But how likely is it that this succession of events ("my husband cheated on me for years and then left me for his young lover which caused me severe distress and mental suffering") is neurologically recorded in a way that it can be assessed with, or deduced from, brain measures? How could this individual experience and the ensuing symptoms (based on unique biography, individual personality, subjective appraisal of events, social context, and culture) possibly be reduced to altered brain function or structure? To put it in a nutshell: it's neither possible nor sensible.

According to Miller, "there can be no comprehensive neurobiological account of emotion, because emotion refers to something psychological. What we can aim for is a neurobiological account of what the brain and the periphery are doing in emotion. Surely that goal is intriguing and valuable, but it could not be a full account of emotion, which is a psychological construct" [396]. Köhne and van Os expressed similar concerns: "The point here is that the 'representation' of mental processes in terms of biomarkers is not only reductionist, poor and insufficient but also not relevant enough for the understanding of mental processes" [521]. And, finally, why should we conceive of this particular depression episode as the result of a disordered brain, that is, a biomedical condition? As aptly stated by Dr. Friedman, "More fundamentally, the fact that all feelings, thoughts and behavior require brain activity to happen does not mean that the only or best way to change—or understand—them is with medicine" [503].

The prevailing view in academic psychiatry is that complex psychological problems (mental disorders) are caused by brain dysfunction [523, 524], but neurobiological alterations could also be the effect of mental states or merely realisations thereof [395, 396]. To return to our example from above, assume that before our woman was left by her cheating husband, she had been a sporty person. But after the breakup she became physically inactive for several weeks, ate unhealthy food, drank a lot of alcohol to numb her mental pain and started to use sleeping pills to fall asleep. So her acute mental state a few weeks after the onset of the depression symptoms certainly correlates with brain measures, but this association is not necessarily causal. The neurobiological alterations could also be the result of the lifestyle changes (i.e. unhealthy diet, physical inactivity, medication and alcohol use; [520]) and it is even possible that they are the effect of being depressed [395, 396]. Such a nuanced view gets completely lost when mental disorders are uncritically ascribed to undefined and yet to be demonstrated brain disorders.

In addition, neurobiological alterations are not inherently abnormal. They could reflect an adaptive process, also referred to as neuroplasticity [546, 547]. A specific change in brain structure or function under specific circumstances (here being depressed) first needs to be established as dysfunctional or pathological before it can be referred to as disordered.

That is, a change or difference in neurobiological measures is not per se abnormal, just as a temporary change in heart rate or hormone secretion in an acutely stressful situation is not necessarily pathological. Deep feelings of love are also associated with the secretion of various hormones, including but not limited to oxytocin [548, 549]. Does this indicate that love is an endocrine disorder?

Until now psychiatrists were not able to clearly define what kind of alterations in brain structure or function they consider disordered in relation to mental states. Perhaps they expect us to trust them that any change in a brain measure is pathological simply because it correlates with depression (or any other mental state). But that would be utterly unscientific and a very poor argument. Fever, for example, correlates with viral infections. In that case, however, fever is not the pathogen (i.e. the cause), it is merely an immune reaction. It is the viral infection that causes fever. Likewise, an increased or decreased activity in a certain brain region could very well be a normal neurophysiological reaction to feeling despair/distress, or any other cause, for example, lifestyle changes such as physical inactivity or substance abuse [520].

In sum, altered brain function or structure could be a symptom (or consequence) of psychological problems rather than a cause [396]. It could also be a spurious correlation due to uncontrolled confounders, including physical inactivity, medication use, and substance abuse [520]. For instance, a large international study showed that the minimal difference in hippocampus volume in patients with depression relative to healthy controls (1.2% reduction on average) was only apparent in patients with years of chronic/recurrent depression but was not observed in patients diagnosed with a first depression episode [550]. So in this case the brain alteration is most likely a consequence of persistent depression symptoms (e.g. hopelessness and anhedonia) and concomitant lifestyle factors (including physical inactivity and long-term medication use), but not the cause of depression (see also Moncrieff [551]). Arguing that altered brain measures in depression are indicative of depression being a brain disorder is akin to defining an infectious disease as a disorder of elevated body temperature (i.e. fever). It's simply poor reasoning.

Then why would a bit more or less of neuronal activity or a slight alteration in brain structure while someone is feeling depressed or anxious demonstrate that depression or anxiety are brain disorders? To the best of my knowledge, neither Dr. Hyman nor Dr. Insel or any other proponent of biological reductionism in psychiatry was able to convincingly answer that crucial question. But still the unsubstantiated and ill-founded notion that mental disorders are brain disorders has attracted massive media attention and many academic supporters proclaim it confidently as if it was an established fact rather than an unproven (some might say dodgy) hypothesis [506]. As summarised by Dr. Gardner,

> "Some critics [of neurobiological reductionism] contend, for example, that biological changes in depressed people are simply evidence of biological differences, not of a biologically caused depression. Others contend that changes in biochemistry can be a *result* of depressed symptoms (sadness, hopelessness) rather than a cause. Depression researchers declare these questions insignificant, contending that biological differences signify defect or illness—that depression is ultimately biologically based. The question of cause(s) is made mute, since the biological phenomenon is 'the problem'" (emphasis in original). [25]

As a case in point for biological reductionism and poor scientific reasoning in psychiatry serves a "mega-analysis" by Hoogman and colleagues on sub-cortical brain volume differences between children with ADHD and children without ADHD [552]. The study was published in the top-tier journal *Lancet Psychiatry* and reported that children with ADHD had, on average, marginally smaller volumes in a few brain areas (all effect sizes $d \leq 0.19$). I will give you some basic statistical background information in order to facilitate the interpretation of these findings. The differences in sub-cortical brain volumes were indeed so small that even in the area where the biggest group difference was found, the amygdala (effect size $d = 0.19$), the overlap between children with and without ADHD was 92% (in most other regions the overlap was about 95%). For the sake of simplicity, let's just focus on the amygdala, the region with the largest effect. With an average between-group difference of $d = 0.19$, the probability that a randomly chosen child with ADHD has a smaller sub-cortical brain volume than a randomly chosen child without ADHD would be just 55%. An identical average volume between groups with and without

ADHD would result in 50% probability, that is, a fifty-fifty chance akin to a coin toss. So you see how small this between-group difference of $d = 0.19$ in the amygdala actually is. Moreover, an effect size of $d = 0.19$ also means that 42% of children with ADHD, that is close to half, have a *larger* volume in this brain area than the average child without ADHD. So you see how substantial the within-group variability is. In other words, many children with ADHD have anything but a reduced amygdala volume. Various have indeed a relatively large amygdala volume compared to children without ADHD. Amygdala volume thus very poorly discriminates between children with and without ADHD.

Finally, and perhaps most importantly, this small association between ADHD diagnosis and reduced sub-cortical brain volume by no means implies causality. The association could be explained by various unmeasured factors (referred to as confounders). For example, being the youngest in class is associated with an increased probability of being diagnosed with ADHD and likely indicates that the youngest children in class are physically (and mentally) simply less developed relative to the older children in class [553]. Nonetheless, the uncertainty of a causal relationship, the huge effect variability and the utterly low levels of determinedness and predictability did not prevent Hoogman and colleagues from boldly concluding "the data from our highly powered analysis confirm that patients with ADHD do have altered brains and therefore that ADHD is a disorder of the brain" [552]. Sounds persuasive? How about that: on average, smaller people have a lower income [554], therefore, poverty is a disorder of body height. Sounds ridiculous? Yes, indeed, but it's the same logic as that applied by Hoogman and colleagues.

Fortunately, several authors noticed this shocking misinterpretation of the data and challenged the authors. Dehue and colleagues noted that "Hoogman and colleagues only found average differences with small effect sizes. This finding implies considerable overlap between groups and large within-group variation. Consequently, there is no point in conveying that a child with ADHD has a brain disorder. Moreover, brain scans can only differ and never tell which characteristics should count as a disorder … For instance, the youngest children in the classroom appear to have the highest probability to receive the diagnosis because their brains are possibly less developed, which can hardly justify the conclusion of a brain disorder" [555]. Batstra and colleagues wrote that "such small effect sizes mean that approximately 95% of the two groups overlap, and are usually interpreted as negligible or very small differences ... Within-group variation is always large and between-group differences are small and do not apply to many individuals diagnosed with ADHD. Furthermore, associations do not necessarily imply causality ... Biological differences do not automatically imply abnormality or pathology" [556].

Finally, as detailed in a revealing article by neuroimaging experts Drs Weinberger and Radulescu titled "Finding the elusive psychiatric 'lesion' with 21st-century neuroanatomy: A note of caution", neuroimaging findings are very susceptible to various biases [520]. MRI and other techniques do not provide a direct measure of brain structure. They capture only physical-chemical signals, and such signals can be influenced by a vast array of non-structural factors, including, but not restricted to, psychiatric drug use, differences in body weight, alcohol use, smoking, exercise, pain, and cortisol levels. In psychiatric neuroimaging studies, patients with a diagnosed mental disorder (e.g. major depression or ADHD as in the example above) are typically compared to healthy controls only matched for sex and broad age bands. The confounding factors thus vary systematically between the two groups as patients with the diagnosis are more likely to smoke, to drink more alcohol, to use medication, to weigh more, to have higher stress levels and to exercise less than healthy controls without the diagnosis. Any difference between patients and healthy controls could thus exclusively result from these confounding factors (which are rarely statistically controlled for). Although researchers generally assume that differences in the brain scans between patients and controls are due to biological abnormalities underlying mental disorders, they are probably better explained by systematic between-group differences in these confounding factors. Therefore, Weinberger and Radulescu conclude "the evidence that findings are neurobiologically meaningful is inconclusive and may represent artifacts or epiphenomena of uncertain value" [520].

Unfortunately, until such critical comments and expert opinion pieces are published, the damage has already been done, and the flawed message has been disseminated widely through academic media departments and the newspapers. For instance, shortly after the publication of the Hoogman and colleagues study and their unfounded interpretation/

conclusion, the *Daily Telegraph* headlined: "ADHD is result of brain disorder, not bad parenting", and in the article the journalist wrote: "The scientists behind the study say their findings prove for the first time that the condition has a physical cause" [506]. This fundamentally flawed statement couldn't be farther from the truth. Because it's so outrageous, I reiterate: the authors didn't demonstrate that ADHD is caused by a brain abnormality, they merely found a marginally small association between an ADHD diagnosis and average brain volume in a few areas based on a poorly controlled, observational, cross-sectional study.

Every researcher (and science journalist) should know that such poor evidence doesn't prove causation. This catastrophic misinformation of the public is not predominantly the result of bad journalisms, but first and foremost due to flawed reasoning, misconception, and very poor science communication by the study authors. That such an erroneous interpretation/conclusion passes peer review further demonstrates that all too many academics are all too eager to disseminate such unfounded and misleading bio-reductionistic messages. By consequence, we don't need to wonder that many patients hold unsubstantiated or unproven bio-causal beliefs (e.g. "my depression is due to a chemical imbalance") when even leading academics disseminate such erroneous claims. Moreover, the media commonly don't pick up corrections as those detailed above. Neither do they cover subsequent replication studies that fail to confirm the reported association. In psychiatry, about three-fourth of the sensationalist study results published in leading medical journals covered by newspapers were actually disconfirmed by subsequent meta-analyses. But the media rarely inform the public about these disconfirmations, so what sticks in the public mind are the initial erroneous reports [506, 557]. This also happened with the chemical imbalance theory of depression [558], which I will discuss in detail below.

The Failure of the Biological Revolution

Though many mental health researchers and practitioners certainly oppose biological reductionism; the dominant view in academic psychiatry is that mental disorders are brain disorders and that progress in the neurosciences will eventually reveal the true causes of mental disorders and, consequently, the long promised pharmacological cure for psychological suffering [523, 524, 536, 537]. Such calls have repeatedly been made since the 1980s by many leading psychiatrists, but these promises are still unfulfilled and as detailed above, they are largely unsubstantiated, unrealistic, or even downright invalid [392, 395, 506, 521]. As summarised by Dr Miller,

> "The headlong rush in recent decades to construe a host of psychological events as being biological events or being reducible to them is, at best, premature. This construal is rampant in scholarly and public spheres, it is indefensible based on available theory and data, and it is at least very suspect on logical grounds. That is, the scientific basis for it is far from adequate, and it can be argued that it could never be adequate. The problem extends well beyond psychopathology, although that is a domain with particularly high stakes, because the misconstrual is doing severe damage to clinical science, clinical practice, and public policy, including federal research-funding and health-care-policy priorities in the biobehavioral sciences, with consequences for fostering mental health and preventing and treating mental illness". [396]

So what do we know about the neurobiology of depression and other common mental disorders? The damning verdict is, almost nothing. And which progress has been made in mental healthcare based on over 30 years of extensive neurobiological research? Again, the damning verdict is, almost none. That is, the biological causes of depression and other common mental disorders remain unknown, no reliable biomarkers of disease states have been detected, no biological diagnostic tests have been developed, and treatment outcomes are not better than about 60 years ago when the first major drug classes (i.e. antipsychotics, antidepressants, and benzodiazepines) were introduced. Dr. Ross Baldessarini, professor of psychiatry at Harvard Medical School, wrote in 2014, "As increasingly technically sophisticated and detailed information is developed in such fields as neuroimaging and neurogenetics, we are repeatedly reminded that almost all major mental disorders remain fundamentally idiopathic. Most lack not only known etiologies but also even a coherent pathophysiology" [559]. In 2019, Drs Gardner and Kleinman noted, "Biologic psychiatry has thus far failed to produce a comprehensive theoretical model of any major psychiatric disorder, any tests that can be used in a clinic to diagnose clearly defined major psychiatric disorders, or any guiding principle for somatic treatments to replace the empirical use of medications". And in the year 2020, the editors of the top-tier journal *Lancet Psychiatry* had to admit that "no other [medical] specialty lacks the basic biological knowledge underlying its most common disease states the way psychiatry does" [560].

An obvious but inconvenient explanation for this lack of knowledge would be that mental disorders are not really brain disorders [395]. As a matter of fact, the great promises of the biological revolution in psychiatry, overoptimistically reiterated for decades in scientific journals and the media, remain largely (or entirely) unfulfilled [393, 395, 506, 561], and yet, as stressed by Dr Kleinman, "academic psychiatry and the funders of research still proceed as if the great breakthrough is just around the corner" [540]. Some argue that this is not true and routinely refer to the recently developed pharmacogenetic tests, which are heavily promoted to physicians as efficient tools that allow for genetically informed individualised psychiatric drug treatment (i.e. choosing the best drug based on a patient's genetic makeup). However, the advocates of pharmacogenetic tests likewise massively overpromised [249]. The benefits of these tests remain uncertain and, with respect to the pharmacotherapy of depression, it is debatable whether pharmacogenetic decision support improves the outcome of antidepressant treatment [562–564].

Even Dr. Thomas Insel, former director of the NIMH and a fervent promotor of neurobiological reductionism, recently admitted in an interview,

> "I spent 13 years at NIMH really pushing on the neuroscience and genetics of mental disorders, and when I look back on that I realize that while I think I succeeded at getting lots of really cool papers published by cool scientists at fairly large costs—I think $20 billion—I don't think we moved the needle in reducing suicide, reducing hospitalizations, improving recovery for the tens of millions of people who have mental illnesses. I hold myself accountable for that". [565]

Here I agree with Dr Insel for once. It is well established that the enormous investments in the neurosciences and genetics of mental disorders, accompanied by a massive increase in drug treatments, have, to this day, not improved the burden of mental disorders [539, 566–570]. If anything, it appears that the long-term outcome of severe mental disorders, including gap in life expectancy, years lived with disability, and permanent sick leave, have even worsened over the last decades [399, 571–574]. Further reason for concern lies in the fact that low- and middle-income countries, which have few mental health services and low treatment rates [575], have the same prevalence of common mental disorders as high-income countries that provide much more mental healthcare [576]. It simply doesn't add up.

Compared to the enormous progress medicine has made in many other fields (e.g. treatment of infectious diseases and cardiovascular diseases), the lack of advancement in psychiatry, both in research and practice, is staggering and calls for reform [390, 392, 577]. Yet the claim that mental disorders are brain disorders and that the neurosciences would eventually lead to major breakthroughs in the prevention, diagnosis, and treatment of mental disorders is fiercely upheld by many leaders in the field. This raises legitimate questions. "But does this not seem, after more than 30 years of failure, more akin to a religious or, albeit culturally influenced, persistent strong belief than one based on scientific grounds? Just where is the rational justification for ploughing the same furrow again and again?" asked Dr. Kingdon [561]. I fully agree with him.

Contemporary psychiatry is in crisis, and according to various authors, an even greater (and more reductionistic) emphasis on psychopharmacology and the neurosciences are part of the problem rather than solutions [147, 390, 392, 399, 503, 539, 561]. This was aptly stated by the UN Special Rapporteur on Human Rights, Dr. Dainius Puras, himself a trained psychiatrist. In a report to the UN he demanded no less than a revolution in mental healthcare. According to Dr. Puras, "Mental health policies and services are in crisis—not a crisis of chemical imbalances, but of power imbalances. We need bold political commitments, urgent policy responses and immediate remedial action … There is now unequivocal evidence of the failures of a system that relies too heavily on the biomedical model of mental health services, including the front-line and excessive use of psychotropic medicines, and yet these models persist" [578]. Thus, instead of advancing the field and helping patients, biological reductionism has presumably thwarted progress in the field and it may be harmful to patients [396, 539]. As summarised by Drs Dumas-Mallet and Gonon,

> "Most experts in the field of psychiatry recognize that neuroscience advances have yet to be translated into clinical practice. The main message delivered to laypeople, however, is that mental disorders are brain diseases cured by scientifically designed medications. Here we describe how this misleading message is generated. We summarize the academic studies describing how biomedical observations are often misrepresented in the scientific literature through various forms of data embellishment, publication biases favoring initial and positive studies, improper interpretations, and exaggerated conclusions. These misrepresentations also affect biological psychiatry and are spread through mass media documents. Exacerbated competition, hyperspecialization, and the need to obtain funding for research projects might drive scientists to misrepresent their findings … These misrepresentations affect the care of patients. Indeed, studies show that a neuro-essentialist conceptualization of mental disorders negatively affects several aspects of stigmatization, reduces the chances of patients' healing, and overshadows psychotherapeutic and social approaches that have been found effective in alleviating mental suffering. Public information about mental health should avoid these reporting biases and give equal consideration to the biological, psychological, and social aspects of mental health". [506]

Marketing and Promotion of Antidepressants

Antidepressants and other prescription drugs are often promoted, both directly and indirectly, via disease awareness campaigns [27, 29, 399, 427]. As detailed above, a main objective of the Defeat Depression Campaign during the 1990s was to teach GPs and the public to recognise depression [425]. However, perhaps the most salient message was that GPs and patients should recognise the value of drug treatment and embrace high-dose antidepressant use as long-term therapy. Thus, according to Medawar, "[the campaign] emphasised the need for radically different standards of treatment. Fears of dependence [from antidepressants] were misconceived and resulted from misunderstanding. In future, there should be more prescribing for depression and at higher dosages than before, and serious consideration should be given to continuing treatment indefinitely" [132].

D/ART also strongly advocated for more depression treatment, both pharmacological and psychological, but with a stronger emphasis on the former. According to the campaign leaders, "With pharmaceutical company support, APA also has sponsored a series of training sessions for primary care physicians. Particular emphases for nonmedical mental health providers have been on biological and pharmacological treatments; for medical specialists, diagnoses and a full range of treatment techniques have been emphasized" [424]. Although D/ART also mentioned that psychological therapies are effective, its assessment was biased towards pharmacological treatments and clearly overstated their benefits [448]. Unsurprisingly, Eli Lilly, which was just about to launch the marketing of fluoxetine (Prozac), financially supported the printing and distribution of eight million D/ART brochures which, among other things, explained the particular merits of serotonergic drugs in the treatment of depression [9].

The Defeat Depression Campaign and D/ART certainly helped to destigmatise clinical depression, to increase awareness of this potentially serious disorder, and to improve access to treatment. It is important to acknowledge these merits of the programs, but unfortunately that's just half the story. By now it's increasingly clear that these two campaigns and the many other programs they influenced also contributed significantly to the pharmaceuticalisation of human distress (despondency, sadness, unhappiness) and subsequent mass-prescribing of antidepressants not only for severe depression (where antidepressant treatment is indicated), but also for mild/minor depression and many forms of normal emotional reactions to stressful events and problems of everyday life (where antidepressant treatment is ineffective or even harmful) [9, 30, 132, 384, 448].

Various consumer organisations and patient advocacy groups have strongly endorsed the reductionistic view that depression is a brain disorder best treated with antidepressants [399]. According to Dr. Gardner, "Uninformed consumers view single cause research finding as 'knowledge' that all types of depression are illnesses, and that depression means the brain is sick and requires psychopharmaceutical treatment. In turn, pharmaceutical companies overestimate their findings, claiming that antidepressants simply work. These glossings are well-packaged for sound-bite promotional consumer information: depression is an illness, antidepressants work" [25]. Consumer organisations and patient advocacy groups are very valuable to pharmaceutical companies as their credibility and sincerity as the patient voice helps the industry to promote their drugs more efficiently. Unsurprisingly, many consumer/patient organisations are financially strongly supported by the pharmaceutical industry, in particular by companies that have costly, patented drugs on the market [579–582].

These industry payments to consumer/patient organisations are problematic for two main reasons. First, they are rarely fully and transparently declared [580, 583], and second, industry-funded groups generally support the sponsor's commercial interest in highly controversial issues [579]. These often-undeclared industry payments thus pose a serious conflict of interest and undermine the organisations' credibility and autonomy. As emphasised by Parker and colleagues, "Selective industry funding of groups where active product marketing opportunities exist might skew the patient group sector's activity towards pharmaceutical industry interests and allow industry to exert proxy influence over advocacy and subsequent health policy" [584].

A case in point is the National Alliance on Mental Illness (NAMI), one of the leading non-profit advocacy groups for mental disorders in the US. NAMI collaborates closely not only with both APA and NIMH, but also with the pharmaceutical industry. During the 1990s and 2000s, NAMI received most of its funding from the pharmaceutical industry [399, 585]. But the industry pays for service rendered, and not for altruistic reasons. In accordance, NAMI received mostly donations from the manufacturers of the drugs it promoted. NAMI also supported the industry in its lobbying efforts and pushed controversial legislation that benefitted the industry, it confidently asserted that depression and other psychiatric conditions are brain disorders, proffered the chemical imbalance theory of depression, promoted the use of SSRIs, opposed the regulatory safety warning on treatment-emergent suicidality, and downplayed the evidence that antidepressants increase the suicide risk in children and adolescents [399, 586]. NAMI is of course no exception. Other consumer/patient organisations were also exploited (or corrupted) by pharmaceutical companies seeking to expand their drug markets and to promote their products. One of these advocacy groups is the Anxiety Disorders Association of America (ADAA). As internal documents from Forest Laboratories (maker of escitalopram; Lexapro) stated, "Marketing opportunities with ADAA will increase when Lexapro labeling expands to include anxiety disorders. At that time, Forest can take advantage of opportunities to disseminate important brand information to their members" [29].

After the introduction of the SSRIs and spurred by aggressive pharmaceutical marketing (including advertising to both consumers and prescribers), neurobiological explanations of depression and antidepressants as corrective (curative) treatments became dominant themes in the mainstream literature and were widely adopted by lay people and consumers [25, 558, 587]. But what's the issue with marketing depression in order to promote antidepressant treatment? You may legitimately argue that there is certainly nothing wrong with informing people about a serious health condition and helping them to get treatment. In principle yes, if marketing would only reach those who really need treatment and who likely benefit from it. But in practice it seems that those people predominantly influenced by marketing campaigns are not those most in need of treatment. Often marketing addresses those people who don't benefit from treatment, for a main objective of marketing is to expand markets and to create consumers. Marketing thus also leads to unnecessary (harmful) use of medicines, that is, overtreatment [374, 387, 455]. Let's look a bit closer at this issue.

There is compelling scientific evidence that drug advertising and disease marketing leads to pharmaceutical overuse and overprescribing [427, 430, 588, 589]. Marketing messages persuade healthy people that they might be ill (see example of depression screening instruments above) and thus prompt consumers to ask their doctors for a treatment that is not indicated (and potentially harmful) for them. In a revealing experiment, Kravitz and colleagues showed that people meeting diagnostic criteria for adjustment disorder (a condition for which antidepressants are not indicated) were prescribed antidepressants at an alarmingly high rate by primary care physicians when they requested a brand-specific or general antidepressant. While only 10% of people not making a request were prescribed an antidepressant, 39% and 55% of people requesting a general antidepressant and a specific brand, respectively, received an antidepressant prescription [590].

"Direct marketing to consumers also leads to increased demand for medications and inflates expectations about the benefits of medications. As a profession, we need to be concerned about advertising and the impact it has on the over-medicalization of our field", warned Dr. Sharfstein, then-president of the APA, in 2005 [525]. Fluoxetine, for example, was intensively advertised by its manufacturer Eli Lilly and soon heralded as a new miracle drug for depression in various popular magazines and newspapers [9, 132]. For instance, on December 18, 1989, fluoxetine made it on the cover of the *New York Magazine*, with a title announcing "Bye, Bye Blues. A new wonder drug for depression" and on March 26, 1990, the *Newsweek* cover proclaimed "Prozac: A breakthrough drug for depression" [399]. It has long been noted with concern that the popular media tends to inadequately promote the benefits of new medical interventions, often parroting uncritical commercial material provided by pharmaceutical companies or quoting experts on industry payroll (i.e. key opinion leaders) [429, 558, 591].

Clarke and Gawley [538] examined the media portrayal of depression from 1980 to 2005 in high-circulating magazines published in Canada or the United States (e.g. *Vogue*, *Newsweek*, *Time Magazine*, *Reader's Digest*, and *The New Republic*). While in the 1980s, only 38% of all articles on depression had a narrow biomedical focus, this proportion increased to 53% in the 1990s and further to 66% in the early 2000s. The proportion of articles endorsing medical interventions as the preferred treatment (usually antidepressants) also steeply increased from 50% in the 1980s to 92% in the 1990s and 88% in the early 2000s. When drugs were depicted in stories of depression, they were portrayed as positive in 38% of articles from the 1980s, in 45% of articles from the 1990s, and in 73% of articles from the early 2000s. Most importantly, "In the 1980s depression was described in a multitude of ways, some seemingly casual descriptions of lifestyles and behaviors clearly within the range of the normal; others were more narrowly medical. Often there were contradictory and multi-faceted understandings of depression presented within the same article. There was no clear or unanimous definition of depression that was repeated from story to story", wrote Clarke and Gawley [538]. "By contrast the definition of depression in the 1990s and beyond almost entirely relied on different aspects of biology, biochemistry, genetics and other biomedical explanations from the human biological sciences". In consequence, the same articles also frequently promoted antidepressants as remedies that would rectify an (inherited) chemical imbalance in the brain.

But lay media are not the only culprits. There are also many mental health professionals who massively exaggerate the alleged benefits of antidepressants and other drug classes [16, 79, 592, 593]. Dr. Peter Kramer, a prominent professor of psychiatry, went even one step further in his bestseller *Listening to Prozac*. In this book, Kramer claimed that fluoxetine (Prozac) could not only cure depression, it could also enhance people's personalities, making them better than well. Kramer called this new opportunity "cosmetic psychopharmacology" and described it as follows: "Prozac seemed to give social confidence to the habitually timid, to make the sensitive brash, to lend the introvert the social skills of a salesman" [594]. His praising of the almost magical powers of fluoxetine was so astonishing that an independent commission in France investigated the possibility that Kramer had been hired by Eli Lilly (manufacturer of fluoxetine) to write this book; however, the investigation concluded that he was not [393]. In any case, *Listening to Prozac* was a priceless marketing vehicle for fluoxetine and the new class of the SSRIs.

The Chemical Imbalance Theory of Depression

Pharmaceutical companies have spent billions US$ in the marketing of antidepressants, but perhaps the single most influential marketing move of the pharmaceutical industry was to establish the unsubstantiated (some say erroneous or flawed) notion that depression is caused by a chemical imbalance (neurotransmitter deficiency) that can be rectified with antidepressants [26, 595]. However, it is important to stress that the chemical imbalance theory (or monoamine theory), even though heavily promoted by the manufacturers of antidepressants, was not invented by the pharmaceutical industry. In fact, it was developed by academic psychiatrists. The chemical imbalance theory became such a dominating paradigm in psychiatry, in both research and practice, that it inaugurated the modern antidepressant era [93]. According to Dr. Mulinari, "monoamine theories could be invoked to increase the scientific credentials of psychiatry's subject matter: Its drugs, diseases, and explanations, in this way, finally allow psychiatry to place itself at the heart of the biomedical thought collective" [596]. Most psychiatrists and GPs eagerly endorsed some form of a chemical imbalance theory of depression [597, 598], and the theory helped to spur the biological revolution in psychiatry by providing impetus to neurobiological and psychopharmacological research [93]. In short, "For nearly 50 years the monoamine hypothesis has been the leading theory about the neuropathologic processes that underlie depression", noted Baumeister and colleagues in 2003 [599]. So let's have a closer look at this influential theory.

The chemical imbalance theory has its roots in the late 1950s and early 1960s, when antidepressants' main mechanism of action was discovered, that is, blocking the absorption of the monoamines, especially norepinephrine and serotonin, and thus increasing the concentration of these neurotransmitters in the brain [1, 93, 599]. In 1965, the US psychiatrist Dr. Joseph Schildkraut formulated his famous hypothesis of affective disorders in the *American Journal of Psychiatry*, which "proposes that some, if not all, depressions are associated with an absolute or relative deficiency of catecholamines, particularly norepinephrine, available at central adrenergic receptor sites. Elation, conversely, may be associated with an excess of such amines" (catecholamines are a specific subgroup of monoamines) [600].

In 1967, in an article in the *British Journal of Psychiatry*, his European colleague Dr. Alec Coppen agreed that depression was caused by a depletion of monoamine levels in the brain, but contrary to Dr. Schildkraut, he believed that serotonin, not norepinephrine, was the main neurotransmitter in the pathophysiology of depression [601]. The basic argument advanced by both Schildkraut and Coppen largely rested on selected reports that drugs that deplete norepinephrine or serotonin, respectively, can cause depression (in particular the drug reserpine), whereas drugs that enhance the availability of these neurotransmitters would cure depression (that is, MAOIs and tricyclic antidepressants). However, in his original paper, Schildkraut also acknowledged that his theory is "undoubtedly, at best, a reductionistic oversimplification of a very complex biological state" [600] and Coppen likewise stated that his work was "inevitably influenced by the reviewer's own interests and prejudices" [601]. So there clearly was reason to be cautious about the monoamine (chemical imbalance) theory.

In the early 1970s the NIMH launched an extremely large and costly research program to test the monoamine (chemical imbalance) theories [596]. The NIMH "Program on the Psychobiology of Depression" [602, 603] included key researchers such as Drs James Maas, Martin Katz, Joseph Mendels, Stephen Koslow, Eli Robins, Gerald Klerman, John Davis, George Winokur, Paula Clayton and Robert Spitzer, in short, the who's who in US academic psychiatry. The project ultimately extended over 18 years and the aim was no less than to achieve "a complete biological evaluation of the depressive disorders". As we all know (to this day there is no biological understanding of depression), the NIMH Program on the Psychobiology of Depression failed to achieve this ambitious goal, but "in a sense it was still a successful enterprise since it provided a major scientific, methodological, financial, and institutional momentum to biological research in US psychiatry" [596].

Arguably that money could have been saved. Various findings already available at the time Schildkraut and Coppen had written their seminal articles should have led them (and other researchers) to call the monoamine theory into question [93, 599]. First, it was known that antidepressants increase serotonin and/or norepinephrine concentration almost instantly, whereas the clinical effect only occurs after at least two to three weeks of continuous treatment. Second, cocaine, a drug that also increases norepinephrine levels, was shown to have no antidepressant effects. And third, it was questionable whether reserpine, which depletes both norepinephrine and serotonin, really causes depression, as a double-blind placebo-controlled trial published in 1955 in fact showed that it lowers depression symptoms.

It has further been demonstrated that both Schildkraut and Coppen cherry-picked findings that supported their theory while they ignored conflicting evidence certainly known to them [596]. Thus, from the beginning the theoretical foundation of the chemical imbalance theory was shaky and dubious. It is also important to stress that one main argument of Schildkraut and Coppen, that is, the efficacy of antidepressants, is an *ex juvantibus* argumentation, that is, reasoning backwards to make assumptions about disease causation based on the observed effect of treatment. This is a problematic logic and a poor scientific argument, for as Lacasse and Leo aptly state, "the fact that aspirin cures headaches does not prove that headaches are due to low levels of aspirin in the brain" [26]. Despite these arguments, are you still convinced that the chemical imbalance theory has strong empirical support? Okay, here we go.

Perhaps the most convincing counterargument to the chemical imbalance theory of depression is the limited efficacy of antidepressants, because if a monoamine deficiency, in particular a lack of serotonin, was the cause of depression in most, if not all, people affected according to Coppen [601], then the average treatment effect of SSRIs would certainly not be that small and of dubious practical relevance [20, 26]. Moreover, antidepressants' serotonergic activity is not associated with efficacy [604]. That is, drugs with a potent serotonergic action are no better than drugs with a weak or no serotonergic action. Neither do SSRIs (which all have a relatively potent serotonergic action) demonstrate a dose–response relationship, meaning that low doses that moderately increase serotonin levels are just as effective as high doses that strongly increase serotonin levels [268]. So again, there is absolutely no evidence that increased serotonin levels yield better treatment outcomes. As observed by Dr. Kirsch, "Some antidepressants increase serotonin levels, some decrease it, and some have no effect at all on serotonin. Nevertheless, they all show the same therapeutic benefit" [605]. By now it is also well established that reserpine (which lowers both serotonin and norepinephrine levels) does not cause depression [599]. Other substances that deplete serotonin and/or norepinephrine don't lower mood in healthy people either [606]. Finally, there is no direct proof that people with depression lack serotonin or that serotonin levels correlate with depression severity [26, 595]. Taken together, these various lines of evidence clearly indicate that a chemical imbalance (and specifically a lack of serotonin) is not the cause of depression.

Despite a lack of robust evidence (and many conflicting findings), the chemical imbalance theory, in particular the serotonin hypothesis of depression, was aggressively marketed by the manufacturers of the SSRIs to both the public and prescribers during the 1990s and early 2000s [1, 93]. Lacasse and Leo [26] show that many direct-to-consumer drug advertisements included the notion of a serotonin deficiency in depression and that the SSRIs could correct this chemical imbalance. For instance, an advertisement for citalopram from 2005 states, "Celexa helps to restore the brain's chemical balance by increasing the supply of a chemical messenger in the brain called serotonin. Although the brain chemistry of depression is not fully understood, there does exist a growing body of evidence to support the view that people with depression have an imbalance of the brain's neurotransmitters". Anxiety disorders were explained in the same way, and an advertisement for paroxetine from 2001 asserts "Chronic anxiety can be overwhelming. But it can also be overcome … Paxil, the most prescribed medication of its kind for generalized anxiety, works to correct the chemical imbalance believed to cause the disorder" [26].

Zetterqvist and Mulinari [607] examined antidepressant advertisements printed in the *Swedish Medical Journal* from 1994 through 2003. They found that 12 of 124 (10%) unique antidepressant advertisements, or 62 of 722 (9%) total antidepressant advertisements, professed some form of an unevidenced chemical imbalance theory. Relatedly, Mulinari [608] analysed information provided on the Swedish website Fass.se, one of the world's most visited medicine information sites through which the pharmaceutical industry is allowed to disseminate regulator-approved medicines information to the general public. Many drug information materials from the manufacturers posted on Fass.se contained a statement that depression is caused by a neurotransmitter deficiency that can be rectified with SSRIs, even though according to drug regulators, this is a wrongful claim, for such a neurotransmitter deficiency has never been scientifically established.

Advertising the chemical imbalance theory to both consumers and doctors was undeniably a great commercial success for the pharmaceutical industry. Endorsing a neurogenetic aetiology of depression is associated with a greater acceptance and perceived utility of antidepressants [541, 609]. While there is certainly nothing wrong with that per se, the downside is that the endorsement of a chemical imbalance notion may propel patients into believing that their depression is a chronic brain disease that necessarily requires (long-term) antidepressant treatment [610, 611]. That is, patients who are convinced that they have a chemical imbalance fear that they cannot live without drugs and thus may continue antidepressant use unnecessarily [612, 613], which puts their health at risk due to the adverse long-term effects of the drugs [307, 614, 615]. Research also indicates that the belief that a chemical imbalance is the cause of one's depression lowers the perceived efficacy of psychotherapy and worsens the outcome of non-pharmacological treatments [616–618].

Finally, there is mounting evidence that neurogenetic causal explanations, including chemical imbalance attributions, may increase the stigmatisation of people with depression and other mental disorders [542, 619, 620]. Although neurogenetic explanations may reduce blame, they also induce pessimism (e.g. "it's a chronic disorder") and reinforce the perception that people with mental disorders are unpredictable and dangerous [621, 622]. On balance, it is thus reasonable to conclude that the chemical imbalance theory has mostly benefitted the pharmaceutical industry, but presumably did a disservice to patients and the general public. As stressed by Miller, "If depression is just a chemical imbalance, and if drugs are the only way that a chemical imbalance can be addressed (two separate faulty assumptions), it is no wonder we have a dysfunctional mental health system" [396].

There is little doubt nowadays that the chemical imbalance theory of depression was aggressively promoted by the pharmaceutical industry as a marketing vehicle to sell evermore antidepressants [1, 26, 595, 623, 624]. However, it was also strongly endorsed by academic psychiatry and taught to both psychiatric trainees, GPs, and to patients [522, 597, 598]. Dr. Kendler, a leading professor of psychiatry, recently remembered in an article, "Although the original articles proposing these theories were couched in qualifications, as a psychiatry resident in the late 1970s, I was taught these theories as monocausal explanations … Decades later, I would commonly see patients who would say some version of 'my psychiatrist said I have a chemical imbalance in my brain' and then proceed to summarize one or more of these theories" [522]. Although most experts in psychiatry and psychopharmacology now agree that this theory is unsubstantiated or disconfirmed [26, 595, 597, 624], the general public, antidepressant users, and many prescribers remain largely unaware. Roughly 70–90% of the general public (including antidepressant users) believe that depression is caused by a chemical imbalance [541, 609, 625]. What's even worse, in a recent survey of GPs in the UK, 77% of physicians agreed that a chemical imbalance is a cause of depression, and in total 23% even strongly agreed [369]. So the chemical imbalance myth is undeniably well and alive.

Paradoxically, what I now increasingly observe are attempts made by eminent psychiatrists to discharge psychiatry from any fault in the widespread dissemination of this flawed (or unsubstantiated) theory. In particular, one vocal psychiatry professor, Dr. Ronald Pies, was very active in this endeavour. For instance, in 2011, Dr. Pies wrote "The 'chemical imbalance' trope has been tossed around a great deal by opponents of psychiatry, who mendaciously attribute the phrase to psychiatrists themselves ... In truth, the 'chemical imbalance' notion was always a kind of urban legend—never a theory seriously propounded by well-informed psychiatrists" [624]. Based on the historical accounts detailed above, it is evidently clear that Dr. Pies is factually wrong. But more on this below. Quite ironically, it was the same Dr. Pies who, in 1992, articulated a chemical imbalance theory of self-injurious behaviour with onset in childhood or adolescence in an article published in the *American Journal of Psychiatry*. In this piece he mused that "two principal neurotransmitter abnormalities" were responsible for youth-onset of self-injurious behaviour, specifically "a primary dopamine deficiency which, over time, may lead to secondary dopamine receptor hypersensitivity and/or a dysregulation of serotonergic systems". Based on this, he argued that "treatment with either dopamine agonists or antagonists may be helpful, depending on the point of 'transition' between primary dopamine deficiency and dopamine receptor hypersensitivity. Serotonergic agents (e.g., fluoxetine, clomipramine) are also helpful in this type, particularly in patients with 'obsessive spectrum' symptoms such as trichotillomania [compulsive hair pulling]" [626].

Lacasse and Leo [627] cite various prominent psychiatrists who publicly stated that depression is caused by a chemical imbalance that can be corrected with antidepressants, including, for example, Dr. Richard Harding in 2001 (then-president of the American Psychiatric Association and someone most would consider a "well-informed psychiatrist"). Even the American Psychiatric Association, in a patient information leaflet from 2005, claimed that "Antidepressants may be prescribed to correct imbalances in the levels of chemicals in the brain". Perhaps even more concerning than this unsubstantiated claim is the fact that this patient information leaflet was confidently titled "Let's Talk Facts About Depression". As I'll detail below, this is pharmaceutical marketing rather than telling facts. This leaflet is of course no exception. Educational materials framed in such misleading ways were very common during the 1990s and 2000s. For instance, in an "Education program for primary care physicians" financially supported by various pharmaceutical companies, Dr. Steven Cole and colleagues wrote "The physician should stress that depression is a highly treatable medical illness caused by a chemical imbalance" [628]. Are there still doubts that Dr Pies is willfully blind to the seminal role his psychiatric colleagues played in the widespread dissemination of the chemical imbalance theory? If so, I'd like to add a few other examples.

Among the vocal leaders who firmly endorsed the chemical imbalance theory of depression was also prominent US psychiatry professor and industry's most precious key opinion leader Dr. Charles Nemeroff, who claimed confidently in 2007, "There is truly a real deficiency of serotonin in depressed patients" [627]. Contrary to Dr. Pies, Nemeroff at least does not deny that the chemical imbalance theory was propounded by "well-informed psychiatrists" like him, for in an article from 2020 on the "pathophysiology and optimal treatment of depression" he frankly admitted that "If I were writing this review 20 years ago, I would have related a tidy story about how three monoamine systems in the brain—serotonin, norepinephrine, and dopamine—are the major players in the pathophysiology of depression". He went on to write that "In those years, clinicians discussed patient symptoms as being a picture of a 'dopaminergic' depression, with severe anhedonia and psychomotor retardation, or a 'serotonergic' depression, with sleep disturbance and reduced libido" [597].

Although the chemical imbalance theory of depression is now less frequently endorsed by psychiatrists in public, it anything but disappeared. For instance, in 2015, Dr. Ulrich Hegerl, a professor of psychiatry and president of the German Depression Support Charity ("Stiftung Deutsche Depressionshilfe"), spoke at a large patient conference on depression in Leipzig, Germany. In his keynote address, he stated that "everything we say or do involves brain functions. Same with depression. Hormones in the brain can get out of balance. Perhaps you heard of serotonin". He then went on to explain that drugs can correct such a chemical imbalance in the brain, asserting that antidepressants "do not only resolve symptoms, they also target the illness at its core" [translated from German] [629]. Of note, Dr. Hegerl is also a member of the advisory boards and speakers bureaus of several pharmaceutical companies (see for instance the conflict of interest statement in this article of Hegerl from 2016 [630]).

Finally, as a last example I want to mention the Austrian Depression Report [631], an authoritative governmental document written by leading Austrian depression researchers. In a chapter on the explanatory models of depression, Drs Christoph Kraus, Rupert Lanzenberger, and Siegfried Kasper (the latter two are both professors of psychiatry at the Medical University Vienna) claim that "It is considered established that depression involves changes in structure and function of several brain regions, especially in the limbic system." The authors then assert that "One of the most important pathophysiological mechanisms in depression is depicted by the 'monoamine-hypothesis'. That hypothesis states that an imbalance in the neurotransmitter system serotonin, norepinephrine and dopamine is crucially involved in the emergence of depression. By now this hypothesis is scientifically well established by numerous molecular imaging studies such as positron emission tomography (PET)" [translated from German].

A few things warrant consideration. Perhaps the reader is interested to learn that there are no scientifically established neurobiological alterations in depression. Two comprehensive meta-analyses found no significant association between depression and specific brain functions [516,

632], whereas structural differences are inconsistent across studies, very small on average, and not specifically related to depression [597, 633, 634]. In a highly cited study by Schmaal and colleagues [550], the largest study on structural brain alterations in depression conducted to date, the differences in cortical gray matter volume between adults with depression and healthy controls were marginally small (all effect sizes $d < 0.15$), indicating that people with depression have gray matter volumes ranging from very small to very large and that their average volume is almost indistinguishable from non-depressed people. Moreover, such minor effect sizes could easily be methodological artifacts of neuroimaging measures due to uncontrolled confounding factors such as medication use, general health status, and lifestyle factors [520].

It is also interesting that the few studies cited by Kraus and colleagues in support of the chemical imbalance theory by design cannot demonstrate that a neurotransmitter deficiency is causally involved in the emergence of depression, since the study participants first underwent neuroimaging when they already were depressed. Temporality is an essential premise of cause–effect relationships and refers to the necessity for a cause to precede an effect in time [635, 636]. Thus, to establish that a chemical imbalance causes depression one needs to show that the chemical imbalance (the cause) precedes the depression episode (the effect) in time. It is thus impossible to demonstrate temporality when people first undergo neuroimaging when they are already depressed. Therefore, and at the risk of repeating myself, association does not imply causation. You certainly get the message by now. If only some vocal biological psychiatrists would pay more attention this this crucial distinction. Finally, as we detail in a recent umbrella review of the serotonin hypothesis of depression, such neuroimaging studies are seriously underpowered (and hence at risk of biased effect estimates) and confounded by previous antidepressant use, which leads to physiological changes in the serotonergic system [637]. Pooled over all available studies, there is no robust and consistent association between depression and the serotonergic system. If anything, and considering the major limitations detailed above, these studies hint at an *increased* serotonin concentration or activity in depression. This finding is in conflict with the serotonin hypothesis, as this notion claims that the concentration or activity of serotonin is *reduced* in depression [637].

Bottom Line: A Public Health Analysis

Since the 1980s, mental health organisations like the NIMH, APA, and RCP quite understandably called for more antidepressant use in what they perceived of as an epidemic of untreated depression. There is per se nothing wrong with that and their intentions were certainly honest, in so far as serious clinical depression was indeed undertreated in the 1960s and 1970s [93]. During the 1990s, the pharmaceutical industry aggressively advertised SSRIs to both consumers and doctors, often misleadingly as curative drugs that correct a chemical imbalance [26, 607]. Drug companies also financially supported various depression awareness campaigns and patient advocacy groups which further promoted antidepressant use directly and indirectly by altering the perception and recognition of depression [27, 30]. According to Dr Mulder, "Those with incentives, particularly financial ones, have elevated rates of major depression because it serves their interests. These incentives are particularly powerful for drug companies to improve their sales and profits. Drug companies attempt to expand their market for depression as for all medical illnesses, and they sponsor depression awareness campaigns, medical education, depression carer meetings, and conferences" [410]. Meanwhile, the popular media fuelled the perceived need for antidepressants by proffering the chemical imbalance notion and other reductionistic biomedical concepts of depression, and by cherishing the idea that we are amidst a depression crisis of epidemic proportions [25, 538].

Even today, some people with severe and debilitating depression who could benefit from treatment (pharmacological and/or psychological) do not receive adequate mental healthcare [105]. However, the problem with the relentless marketing of both depression and antidepressants is that it not only attracted people in need of treatment but many more people with mild/minor depression and normal emotional reactions to common problems of daily life, that is, the so-called worried well [414, 447]. The consequence is an alarming disbalance in contemporary mental healthcare provision. Some people with severe (melancholic) depression who clearly need medical treatment and other forms of professional support (including social, legal and vocational support) don't receive help while a much larger group of people with mild and subthreshold depression who don't necessarily need treatment consume the majority of mental healthcare resources, especially antidepressants [105, 410, 414].

There is now compelling evidence that depression is overdefined and overdetected in primary care [3, 5]. The promotion of the chemical imbalance theory and other pharmaceutical marketing strategies caused many people to attribute psychosocial problems to faulty brain chemistry requiring (long-term) antidepressant treatment [610, 611]. These factors have undoubtedly contributed to overdiagnosis and overtreatment. Olfson et al. [105] found that among people treated for depression (mostly with antidepressants), only 30% screened positive for depression and only 22% had serious psychological distress. Moreover, patients with non-serious distress were more likely to be treated with antidepressants than patients with serious distress (89% vs. 81%). Likewise, Mojtabai [117] showed that only 38% of people with clinician-identified depression met the liberal diagnostic criteria for major depression. Among those with subthreshold depression, 74% were prescribed psychiatric medication (mostly antidepressants). Finally, a comprehensive meta-analysis provided clear evidence that depression is overdetected (or misdiagnosed) and, consequently, overtreated in primary care [450].

Since the 1990s, treatment rates of depression and anxiety have increased substantially while population prevalence rates remained largely constant [566, 568, 638]. It is also well established that depression and anxiety are mostly diagnosed and treated by GPs and that antidepressants are the preferred (and often sole) treatment modality [105, 439, 575, 639]. People with severe disorders are more likely to seek treatment but given that only a small minority of people has serious psychological distress, according to Olfson and colleagues, "the absolute increase in outpatient mental health service use was almost completely the result of growth in outpatient mental health service use by individuals with less serious or no psychological distress" [477]. Likewise, the WHO World Mental Health Survey Consortium emphasised that "Due to the high prevalence of mild and subthreshold cases, the number of those who received treatment far exceeds the number of untreated serious cases in every country". The surveys further showed that "either the majority or a near majority of people in treatment in each country are either noncases or mild cases" [640]. These findings confirm that doctors indeed mostly treat the worried well [414, 447] and that "unmet need for treatment among serious cases is not merely a matter of limited treatment resources but that misallocation of treatment resources is also involved" [640].

These disparities in healthcare provision grew considerably during the 1990s, most likely due to the broadening of the diagnostic criteria for depression, overdetection fuelled by depression and anxiety disorder awareness campaigns, and aggressive promotion of antidepressant treatment by pharmaceutical companies, psychiatric associations, and patient organisations alike. Mojtabai [106] found that, in the US, the rate of antidepressant treatment increased more than fourfold between the early 1990s and the early 2000s, but antidepressant use increased significantly more in the group of less severely ill individuals than in individuals with severe psychopathology (which were often socio-economically disadvantaged). He thus concluded, "Sociodemographic disparities in antidepressant treatment persisted over the last decade in the US, lending support to concerns about undertreatment among traditionally underserved groups, whereas the greater increase in the rate of antidepressant treatment in the less severely ill group lends support to concerns about antidepressant overtreatment in this population" [106]. This trend continued unaltered from 2004/2005 to 2014/2015, as shown in a recent analysis by Olfson and colleagues. "The recent increase in outpatient mental health service use occurred during a period of decline in serious psychological distress. Adults with less serious psychological distress accounted for most of the absolute increase in outpatient mental health service use" [477].

In conclusion, today the typical primary care patient treated for depression has a mild/minor disorder, and not a severe/serious disorder. By consequence, the majority of antidepressants are prescribed to people with mild and subthreshold disorders. This provides clear evidence for the misallocation of limited healthcare resources. Put differently, a large group of people with mild and transient depression (and/or anxiety) is evidently overdiagnosed and overtreated, while a small group of people with severe disorders remains undetected and undertreated. Undertreatment and overtreatment thus co-exist, and "in light of these findings, it is important to strengthen efforts to align depression care with each patient's clinical needs" [105]. But while overtreatment is steadily growing, undertreatment is fortunately on the decline. Given that most forms of depression (and anxiety) are mild or subthreshold and that most antidepressants are prescribed to this group of patients [105, 115, 116, 477], the bottom line is that overtreatment affects a much larger portion of the population than undertreatment. As argued by Dr. Marcia Angell, people with minor ailments (which constitute the majority of healthcare users) may suffer more from overtreatment and its associated risks, especially adverse drug effects, than from undertreatment [458]. Or, as Dr. Vilhelmsson put it, "For the sake of public health, arguments for increased diagnosis must therefore be related to a possible danger of medicalizing social problems and life crises. By including people with mild problems in estimates of mental illness, we risk losing support for treating those people who have legitimate disorders" [491].

4

Flaws in Antidepressant Research

Before I scrutinise the design, conduct, and reporting of antidepressant trials it is worthwhile to briefly outline under which medico-scientific framework healthcare services are assessed and provided nowadays. Contemporary healthcare is devoted to evidence-based medicine, a new approach to clinical decision making that developed in the early 1990s [641]. According to the founders of this paradigm, "Evidence based medicine is the conscientious, explicit, and judicious use of current best evidence in making decisions about the care of individual patients. The practice of evidence based medicine means integrating individual clinical expertise with the best available external clinical evidence from systematic research" [642]. To determine what the best clinical evidence is, the new approach established a hierarchy of scientific evidence. High-quality evidence is provided by double-blind randomised controlled trials, low-quality by observational studies (i.e. case-control and cohort studies), and very low-quality by any other evidence (i.e. case reports, animal research, in-vitro research, and expert opinion). However, the quality of evidence from observational studies can be upgraded when effect estimates are very large, when a dose–response relationship can be demonstrated, or when all relevant confounders (e.g. treatment selection) can be excluded. By

M. P. Hengartner, *Evidence-biased Antidepressant Prescription*,
https://doi.org/10.1007/978-3-030-82587-4_4

contrast, the quality of evidence from both randomised controlled trials and observational studies needs to be downgraded when the studies have serious limitations (e.g. unblinding of participants and/or clinical investigators), when the effect estimates are inconsistent across studies, when the effect estimate is indirect (e.g. due to unrepresentative samples or surrogate outcomes), when there is imprecision in effect estimates, or when reporting or publication bias is likely [641, 643]. By this means a systematic assessment of observational studies can obtain a high evidence grade, whereas a synthesis of randomised controlled trials can yield a low or very low evidence grade.

A large and well-controlled double-blind randomised clinical trial certainly provides the strongest evidence to evaluate efficacy and safety/tolerability of medical interventions, that is, the balance between benefits and harms in a large group of patients. Randomised means that patients are randomly assigned to treatment conditions (e.g. new drug vs. active comparator or placebo) to avoid that treatments are differently assigned to patients based on specific characteristics, which could produce incomparable treatment groups and thus biased efficacy estimates (e.g. when those with less severe illness are assigned to the new drug and those with more severe illness to the comparator drug). Double-blind means that neither the patients nor the clinical investigators ought to know which treatment a patient receives, as this could also bias the outcome due to treatment expectations. When a particular drug has been tested in several trials, as is mostly the case, a systematic review and meta-analysis of all available studies then provides the best evidence of efficacy and safety/tolerability, for results of individual studies could differ due to sampling variability. Depression, for example, is a very heterogeneous condition, and depending on treatment setting (e.g. urban psychiatric hospital vs. rural primary care practice), samples of patients with depression may differ substantially from study to study with respect to age, sex, ethnicity, socio-economic background, illness severity, symptomatology, medical comorbidity, and functional impairment. Differences in sample composition could thus affect treatment effects of antidepressants (i.e. efficacy and safety estimates).

In sum, evidence-based medicine attempts to provide the best healthcare according to the most reliable scientific evidence. To that end, it incorporates not only the quality of individual studies but also considers the strength of evidence based on assessments of all available studies to determine whether a specific treatment is safe and effective in a specific patient population. These systematic reviews of clinical trials are the foundation of treatment guidelines and inform clinical decision making in modern healthcare. Put differently, evidence-based medicine replaced so-called eminence-based medicine, that is, treatment decisions based on unsystematic, uncontrolled observations and physiological reasoning. According to Drs Djulbegovic and Guyatt, "The basis for the first EBM [evidence-based medicine] epistemological principle is that not all evidence is created equal, and that the practice of medicine should be based on the best available evidence. The second principle endorses the philosophical view that the pursuit of truth is best accomplished by evaluating the totality of the evidence, and not selecting evidence that favours a particular claim" [641]. Arguably, the most important and best resource for the practice of evidence-based medicine is Cochrane, an international non-profit organisation that produces systematic reviews and meta-analyses of medical interventions to inform clinical decision making. According to the Cochrane website, "Our vision is a world of improved health where decisions about health and health care are informed by high-quality, relevant and up-to-date synthesized research evidence. Our mission is to promote evidence-informed health decision-making by producing high-quality, relevant, accessible systematic reviews and other synthesized research evidence" [644].

The Corruption of Evidence-Based Medicine

It comes without saying that evidence-based medicine was a great achievement that improved healthcare in various medical conditions and therapeutic domains. However, in some sense, the movement became a victim of its own success. Various doctors seem to ignore (or simply are unaware) that medical research is fallible and subject to falsification and correction. Research findings in support of a medical intervention remain valid temporarily and never provide a clear confirmation that will necessarily stand the test of time. Medicine is a probabilistic, not an exact science. We cannot be certain about best medical practice, and quite often the scientific evidence allows for nothing more than a wild guess, that is, a treatment decision with huge uncertainty [383]. The history of medicine is replete with examples of new (breakthrough) interventions that quickly became established best medical practice (or standard of care) and later turned out to be in error [645]. Again and again medicine had to fundamentally change its "best" practice due to new results from methodologically superior clinical trials showing that the standard of care was ineffective or that its harms exceeded its benefits, a phenomenon now commonly termed "medical reversal" [646, 647]. Contending that a medical intervention clearly works for most patients because it became standard medical practice (an argument often made to defend the widespread prescription of psychiatric drugs) is thus utterly naïve and misinformed. Best medical practice may eventually turn out to be bad medical practice. I give an example.

During the 1980s, it was accepted best medical practice to treat patients who had suffered myocardial infarction with antiarrhythmic drugs in the conviction that this intervention would reduce mortality. But in 1989, the first placebo-controlled trial that examined mortality as treatment outcome showed that antiarrhythmic drugs accounted for an excess of deaths from major adverse cardiac events and also for higher all-cause mortality [648]. That is, antiarrhythmic drugs were not beneficial in this patient population, they were harmful. Instead of reducing mortality, they actually increased mortality! According to Dr. Jeremy Howick, an expert in evidence-based medicine from the University of Oxford, "Given the widespread use of the drugs, it has been estimated that tens of thousands of people were killed by the drugs each year" [649].

But how come antiarrhythmic drugs were even approved for the treatment of patients with myocardial infarction? Put simply, the pharmaceutical companies seeking marketing approval for these drugs made sure that they did not need to establish effectiveness based on mortality (even though, ironically, the aim of antiarrhythmic drugs was precisely to reduce mortality). Instead, the companies managed to claim effectiveness based on a surrogate outcome, namely ventricular extra beats, a common type of cardiac arrhythmia [649]. This example illustrates nicely how surrogate outcomes can mislead and give a false impression of treatment benefits when in fact a drug is harmful. It also demonstrates that drug regulators may erroneously approve drugs as safe and effective when they don't require the pharmaceutical industry to study the right treatment outcomes.

So there can be no doubt that medical research is fallible. And because medical research is fallible and evidence-based medicine became so influential, it was soon corrupted by the biomedical industry [29, 376, 377, 650]. The pharmaceutical and medical device industry had quickly realised that by managing (or dominating) the scientific literature with study results that support their commercial interests, they could exert a significant influence over healthcare policy and clinical practice [649, 651, 652]. This led to a myriad of serious flaws that threaten (or undermine) the validity of evidence-based medicine. More to the point, given the inherent hierarchy of scientific evidence, with the synthesis of clinical trials on top, the industry was able to co-opt evidence-based medicine and turn this movement into an efficient marketing tool to boost its profits. The companies did so by sponsoring thousands of clinical trials, often systematically biased and selectively reported, that were then eligible for the systematic reviews and meta-analyses that guide clinical practice [377, 653]. How is this possible? Let me briefly explain.

Given that original research is expensive, most biomedical research, especially drug trials, are sponsored by the pharmaceutical industry [654–656]. The typical drug trial is thus sponsored by the pharmaceutical company that seeks regulatory marketing approval for a treatment indication (premarketing/preapproval trials) or increased market share in approved indications (postmarketing/postapproval trials). These trials are designed by the sponsoring company with input from industry advisors and conducted by contract-research organisations. These firms organise a network of study sites, which may number in dozens across the globe, designate the clinical investigators and implement the trial protocol at those sites. During the trial, the contract-research organisations monitor the study sites and send report forms to the sponsoring company. Once the trial is completed, the sponsoring company conducts the data analysis and evaluates and interprets the results. If the results are not too unfavourable to the sponsor's drug, the company will publish the results (or selected parts thereof). For it the company hires a medical communication firm that produces several manuscript drafts based on instructions from the marketing department of the sponsoring company. When the company is satisfied with the manuscript, the marketing department selects key opinion leaders, often senior researchers from prestigious academic departments who serve on the company's advisory board and/or speaker's bureau, to be listed as "authors" on the publication. At this final stage, the academic researchers comment on the manuscript, make some edits, and lend the study the badge of scientific excellence and academic independence. However, the sponsoring company almost always has the final say on the manuscript to be submitted for publication and it owns the data. That is, the trial data are property of the sponsor and the eminent researchers from the prestigious universities listed as "authors" on the publication hardly ever have full access to the raw data. They only know the data and results the company was willing to show them, and often they only give intellectual inputs but don't write a single sentence, let alone an entire paragraph of the manuscript. Most articles are thus not written by the academic "authors" listed on the publication; they are largely ghostwritten, that is, drafted by industry employees and medical communication firms that are not declared as authors on the paper's by-line [29, 428, 459, 657, 658].

As detailed by Matheson, "Through a patchwork of diminutions, aggrandizements, omissions, euphemisms, fudges, and misnomers, academics are positioned as masters, and proprietors as their worthy aides. The company is placed in the shop window—but nobody is told it owns the shop … The language of corporate 'sponsorship' and academic 'investigators' and superficial arrangements of trial committees suggest that companies merely provide finance and that independent academic institutions are in true command, while the actual role of commerce in instigation, analysis, framing, writing, and data ownership is politely shepherded into the margins by diverse attributional tricks—and that is how medicine likes it." [659]. So the pharmaceutical company gets its commercially tailored research article, senior academics and medical institutions get reputation and credits, and the journals get impact points and revenues. According to Matheson, "each party benefits in its own way. Companies get the elixir of endorsement on which advocacy marketing depends; academics reap the rewards of authorial status and generally feel that they deserve top billing; journals sell reprints; and culturally, I believe, academic medicine and its journals crave the sense that the research scene remains in their hands" [659]. Put differently, evidence-based medicine has been corrupted by the pharmaceutical industry, and academic medicine eagerly cooperated to advance its own agenda [377]. The interests least served by this commercial research enterprise are often those of both patients and the public [29, 459, 650, 660].

There is of course an inherent financial conflict of interest in industry-sponsored drug trials, for being critical towards the efficacy of its own drug and fully transparent (or honest) about adverse effects and safety issues undermines the company's commercial interest. As a result, industry-sponsored trials often have systematic methodological biases so that the sponsor's drug appears more effective, better tolerated and safer than it really is [29, 62, 661]. Another pervasive bias is the selective reporting of treatment outcomes [61, 662]. Trials with unfavourable results are either not published or the prespecified primary outcomes are not fully reported in the published article when they are negative [89, 663, 664]. Of course, selective reporting affects not only efficacy outcomes but also safety and tolerability data [87, 664, 665]. Likewise, statistical analyses often deviate from the model prespecified in the study protocol (the analysis intended before the data was inspected), for instance, by using a different statistical model or by focusing on a different analysis population (i.e. including only a subset of participants in the analysis) [666]. A last form of scientific misconduct briefly mentioned here is spin, that is, the deliberate misrepresentation and misinterpretation of negative trial results [667]. A typical example of spin is reporting and interpreting a trial with non-significant primary outcome as if the intervention was unequivocally effective [668–670].

Together these issues systematically bias the benefit–harm ratio of medical interventions reported in the scientific literature, resulting in the overestimation of efficacy and underestimation of harms [29, 85, 89, 428, 459]. Perhaps you'll doubt that the situation is that bad and you are right to challenge these conclusions, given that they call into question the whole of modern medicine that we need (and want) to rely on when we seek healthcare. Perhaps you assume that most medical interventions are supported by strong evidence and thus argue that twisting and bending of the scientific evidence is only an issue for a small minority of interventions. If you think so, then you're mistaken. As a matter of fact, the scientific evidence supporting the effectiveness of contemporary medical treatments is generally poor. A substantial portion (presumably the majority) of the scientific literature on medical interventions is inconclusive and unreliable. But don't just take my word for it. Instead, let's have a quick look at two pertinent studies.

First, a recent systematic review showed that only 4% of contemporary medical interventions were supported by high-quality evidence. The quality of evidence was low or insufficient in 74% of surgical interventions, 82% of pharmacological interventions, and 86% of psychosocial interventions [671]. Second, according to a recent analysis of Cochrane reviews of medical interventions (mostly drug treatments), only 10% provided high-quality evidence for the effectiveness of treatments; 37% provided moderate-quality evidence, 31% low-quality evidence, and an alarming 22% very low-quality evidence [672]. I reiterate: about half of medical interventions (53%) are "supported" by low or very low quality evidence. That's not reassuring…

Another common view is that with the accumulating number of trials for a specific treatment, the scientific evidence on its benefits and harms will improve. However, this is not true either. On average, Cochrane reviews updated with new trial results did not provide improved quality of evidence. By tendency, it was rather the other way round. After inclusion of new trial results, the quality of evidence was downgraded in 58% of reviews and upgraded in 42% of reviews, but of the latter only a very small minority achieved a high-quality rating [672]. The evidence base for the effectiveness of antidepressants in depression is no exception to the rule. According to the most recent systematic reviews, the quality of evidence is in general low to very low, and this applies to both adult clinical trials [13, 141] and paediatric clinical trials [292, 294].

What does the low quality and unreliability (i.e. poor credibility) of the scientific evidence for medical interventions imply? A brilliant study by Heres and colleagues impressively demonstrated what the consequences are. They examined the comparative efficacy of popular antipsychotic drugs in the treatment of schizophrenia or schizoaffective disorder [673]. For the sake of simplicity, let's call them drug A, B, and C. Logic dictates that if in head-to-head trials A beats B, and B beats C, then A must also beat C. By consequence, if the evidence is reliable, then A would be the most effective drug, B the second best, and C the least effective. However, the "reality" looks different. The scientific literature shows that when the manufacturer of A sponsors the trial, then A beats both B and C. If, however, the manufacturer of B sponsors the trial, then B beats both A and C, and, you certainly sense what's coming, if the manufacturer of C sponsors the trial, then C beats both A and B. So ultimately the scientific evidence provides no clue as to which drug is best in the treatment of schizophrenia or schizoaffective disorder. The confusing and conflicting evidence on the comparative efficacy of antipsychotics is thus basically meaningless.

Based on this study it is obvious that pharmaceutical companies can quite easily get the results they want (i.e. the results that present their own product in the most favourable light relative to competitors). And given that there is little reason to assume that the trial results from one company are more (or less) credible than the findings from the other companies, it follows that the industry-sponsored studies on the comparative efficacy of antipsychotics, and by extension all other drugs, are neither trustworthy nor reliable. I deliberately wrote "by extension", because the disturbing findings from Heres and colleagues [673] were later replicated in a much larger study examining head-to-head trials in general medicine [674]. The authors of the latter study concluded from the data that "The literature of head-to-head RCTs [randomised controlled trials] is dominated by the industry. Industry-sponsored comparative assessments systematically yield favorable results for the sponsors, even more so when noninferiority designs are involved" [674]. These studies thus clearly indicate that pharmaceutical companies have the capabilities (or possibilities) to create the "scientific evidence" that best suits their commercial interests. In the following sections I will detail how sponsors get (or at least try to get) the results they want. To that end, I will outline methodological biases in clinical trials and then provide an account of reporting biases.

Methodological Biases

Why is the quality (and credibility) of evidence for the effectiveness of most medical interventions so dismayingly poor? In my view the two main reasons are the serious methodological limitations of most clinical trials and the lenient criteria for drug approval adopted by regulatory agencies. Scientists at the European Medicines Agency (EMA) evaluated 111 successive applications submitted from September 1997 to May 2001 to their agency [169]. In 49% of applications, the EMA objected the quality of long-term safety data, in 42% they noted a lack of adequate randomised controlled trials, in 38% they objected the robustness of methodology, in 33% they criticised the selected patient population, in 29% the choice of outcomes, in 18% the insufficient long-term follow-up data, in 17% the inadequate duration of treatment, and so on. However, the only major methodological limitation that was independently related to the agency's decision to approve or reject an application was the lack of adequate randomised controlled trials [169]. The other limitations did not seem to influence their decision to approve or reject a new drug application, including quality of long-term safety data, robustness of methodology, the selected patient population, choice of outcomes, and duration of treatment. Given that this analysis dates a few years back, perhaps standards have improved? Unfortunately, this is not the case.

The results of a recent analysis indicate that, overall, the methodological quality of clinical trials conducted for regulatory approval of new drug applications has arguably even decreased in more recent years. Zhang and colleagues examined the methodological characteristics of pivotal trials supporting new treatments approved by the FDA [675]. While in 1995–1997 altogether 94% and 79% of trials were randomised and double-blind, respectively, in 2015–2017 these rates dropped to 82% and 68%. Moreover, in 1995–1997 altogether 44% of pivotal trials had a clinical outcome (e.g. cardio-vascular events), but in 2015–2017 only 23% had so, while the rate of the less stringent surrogate outcomes (e.g. cholesterol levels) increased from 48% in 1995–1997 to 59% in 2015–2017. Likewise, the rate of active comparators decreased from 44% in 1995–1997 to 29% in 2015–2017, while the rate of uncontrolled trials (i.e. neither active nor placebo comparator) increased from 9% in 1995–1997 to 18% in 2015–2017. The only positive development was an increase in both median sample size (277 patients in 1995–1997 vs. 467 in 2015–2017) and median trial duration (11 weeks in 1995–1997 vs. 24 weeks in 2015–2017). As recently summarised by Drs Kesselheim and Avorn, both highly respected professors of medicine at Harvard Medical School,

> "In recent years, under steady pressure from the pharmaceutical industry and the patient groups it funds, the FDA has progressively lowered its standards of effectiveness and safety required for drug approvals. New drugs are now more likely to be supported by fewer studies and less adequate clinical trial designs than in the past. Worse, more than half of new drugs are now approved based on what's called surrogate endpoints—changes in the body measured by lab tests that may not reflect clinical benefit—rather than requiring that the drug affect how a person feels, functions or survives". [676]

You may rightly object that the main issue detailed above is the use of surrogate outcomes and uncontrolled trial designs. Thus, all should be fine if researchers and regulatory agencies would adhere to clinical outcomes assessed in randomised controlled trials, shouldn't it? Unfortunately, this is not true. The double-blind randomised controlled trial is widely considered as the gold standard to determine efficacy as well as tolerability and safety of medical interventions, for it has good internal validity (refers to the degree of confidence that the causal relationship being tested is trustworthy and not influenced by other factors). However, due to narrowly defined (unrepresentative) patient populations, extensive monitoring and short treatment duration, all of which considerably deviate from routine practice, the external validity of most clinical trials is poor (refers to the extent to which results from a study can be generalised to other situations or patient populations). Many double-blind randomised controlled trials also have other serious methodological limitations, implying that their results are systematically biased and no meaningful conclusions can be drawn from the data, even when objective clinical outcomes are assessed [29, 62, 84, 661, 677, 678]. A list of common methodological limitations is provided in Table 4.1.

Most clinical trials are of very short duration and sample size is modest [165, 675], making it impossible to determine sustained treatment benefits and to detect rare adverse drug reactions [679]. Small sample size also implies low statistical power, which reduces the chance to find a true treatment effect but also produces both inflated treatment effects and false-positive results [680, 681]. Most trials have extensive exclusion criteria and preselect those patients assumed to respond best to the medication, especially younger male patients without comorbid (concomitant) medical conditions [682]. Many placebo-controlled trials are inadequately blinded (or blinding is not ascertained), meaning that investigators and patients may correctly identify whether they receive the active drug or inert placebo [683]. This is an important issue, for unblinding is associated with stronger effects on subjective outcomes like quality of life or mental health ratings [684, 685]. When a new drug is compared to another active drug, often an inferior comparator drug is chosen, the

Table 4.1 Common methodological limitations in double-blind randomised controlled trials

Problem	Examples
Inadequate samples	Unrepresentative patient population due to restrictive selection criteria; sample size too small
Inadequate trial duration	Only acute treatment trials; no long-term trials and post-treatment follow-up
Poor comparators	Only placebo control; inferior active comparator; too high or too low dosed comparator drug
Inadequate randomisation	Inadequate generation of randomised sequence; Treatment allocation not concealed
Unblinding of both participants and investigators	Unblinding due to lack of side effects in placebo group; unblinding due to drug-specific side effects in active controlled trials
Poor outcomes	No clinical outcomes; only subjective outcome measures; only surrogate outcomes
Inadequate harm assessment	No reporting of severe adverse events and discontinuation due to adverse events; only reporting of common adverse events; unsystematic and unstructured harm assessment; inconsistent coding of adverse events; no grouping of adverse events

dose of the comparator drug is too high (so that the sponsor's drug appears safer and better tolerated) or too low (so that the sponsor's drug appears more effective) [62, 84].

Contrary to efficacy outcomes, adverse events are typically assessed in an unsystematic and unstructured way by simply asking patients whether they experienced any unwelcome medical events since the last study visit [686]. In trial publications, often only the most common adverse events are reported, while no information on severe adverse events and discontinuation due to adverse events is given at all [687]. A specific adverse event is sometimes coded with different (and inadequate) terms which leads to misrepresentation and underestimation of its true prevalence rate [688]. Adverse events are rarely grouped by anatomic or physiological system, which further limits the detection of harm signals and significant adverse drug effects [689]. Due to unsystematic assessment, inadequate recording and poor reporting, common adverse drug effects can be systematically underestimated and, occasionally, missed altogether [29, 87, 687]. Finally, the identification of rare but serious adverse drug reactions is almost impossible in clinical trials, even when they have more than 1000 participants [690], a sample size unusually large in general medicine and especially in psychiatry [165, 675]. For these various reasons, Healy and Mangin also referred to clinical trials as "the gold standard way to miss adverse events" [691].

In sum, trial protocols, especially industry-sponsored trials, are typically designed in a way that they produce the best possible outcome for the sponsor's drug. These strategies compromise not only the internal validity of a trial, but also (and perhaps in particular) its external validity. The biases that they create are often systematic, that is, in favour of the sponsor's drug, resulting in overestimation of benefits and underestimation of harms. A main consequence of these various limitations is that it can be difficult (some might say impossible) to determine whether a drug shown to be safe and effective in a clinical trial also works in real-world routine practice. That is, generalisations of clinical trial results outside the narrowly defined study population may be invalid and the sustainability of treatment effects beyond the acute treatment phase is often uncertain [679, 692]. It follows that various drugs approved by drug regulators as safe and effective were in fact neither safe nor truly effective outside the restricted and tightly controlled experimental setting [171, 173, 376, 458]. Therefore, when a new drug is introduced into the market, "the amount of information on benefits and risks, especially long term, is relatively small, and often based on highly selected populations with respect to age, comorbidities, use of concomitant medications, and other factors" [690].

I will now revisit these issues in more detail as they pertain specifically to antidepressant trials. I will guide you through these trial characteristics step by step. I'll start with limitations relevant to efficacy estimates and then turn to limitations relevant to safety/tolerability estimates.

Methodological Biases Distorting Efficacy Estimates

Antidepressant trials have myriads of (serious) methodological limitations [14, 102, 144, 693–695]. The first crucial aspect is the size and composition of the study sample. The average sample size in antidepressant trials is just about 224 participants [141], which is small but sufficiently large to reliably detect a minimally important treatment effect. But are the effects measured in these samples generalisable? So let's look at the selection of trial participants. Ideally, the study sample is representative of the broader patient population that will use the investigated drug in clinical practice, for it makes little sense to demonstrate efficacy and safety in a narrowly defined study population that is very untypical of the average patient being prescribed the drug in real-world routine practice. Unfortunately, this is exactly the case in antidepressant trials.

Trial participants are carefully preselected by applying very restrictive selection criteria. Most trials enrol psychiatric outpatients or people from the community recruited through advertisements, but neither psychiatric inpatients (those with mostly severe clinical depression) nor primary care patients (the largest group of antidepressant users). In addition, antidepressant trials commonly exclude participants with depression severity below or above a certain cutoff, participants with bipolar and psychotic features, participants with substance abuse or dependence, participants with acute suicidal ideation, as well as participants with comorbid (concomitant) mental disorders and general medical conditions [144, 188].

As you may easily recognise, these stringent selection criteria result in very narrowly defined and unrepresentative patient populations. Several studies have consistently shown that between 78% and 88% of patients who seek treatment in primary care and psychiatric outpatient clinics would be excluded from antidepressant trials due to these restrictive selection criteria [696–698]. Given that patients treated in psychiatric hospitals (inpatient clinics) very frequently have comorbid mental and general medical conditions and often are acutely suicidal, almost all psychiatric inpatients would arguably be excluded from a typical placebo-controlled antidepressant efficacy trial.

Another alarming finding is that selection criteria in antidepressant trials have become yet more restrictive over time, thus trial participants are even less representative in more recent studies [188]. While on average 84% of treatment-seeking patients would be excluded from antidepressant trials published between 1995 and 2009, this rate grew to 91% based on selection criteria applied in trials published from 2010 to 2014 [697]. Finally, it appears that these restrictive inclusion and exclusion criteria introduce a systematic bias. According to results of the STAR*D study, patients typically excluded from efficacy trials have a poorer treatment outcome than the unrepresentative participants preferably selected into these studies (response rates were 39% vs. 52% and remission rates 25% vs. 34%) [696]. In another analysis it was shown that the large group of patients with depression typically excluded from antidepressant trials due to restrictive selection criteria are more chronically ill [699], a patient group often unresponsive to antidepressants and thus commonly referred to as "treatment resistant" [227, 700].

A very common, almost universal, design feature in antidepressant trials is the so-called placebo run-in phase (also referred to as placebo washout) [166, 194]. The placebo run-in phase puts all participants on placebo before randomisation and typically lasts about a week. It serves two main purposes. First, many participants enrolled in antidepressant trials are already on an antidepressant and thus need to be withdrawn from this drug before they can be randomised to either the investigational drug, an active comparator, or placebo. Second, participants who improve significantly in the placebo run-in phase are typically excluded from the trial. By consequence, placebo run-in (washout) phases likely induce a systematic bias in favour of the drug. In an older meta-analysis, the effect size for active drug against placebo was 0.50 in trials with placebo run-in and 0.41 in trials without placebo run-in, but this difference was statistically not significant [701]. However, this study was based on a small set of studies, thus lacking statistical power. In addition, as can be seen from the surprisingly high effect sizes (0.50 and 0.41, respectively), the dataset was unrepresentative, for the average treatment effect size in antidepressant trials is considerably lower (about 0.3) [17, 57, 141]. In a subsequent analysis based on a much larger and representative dataset, the effect sizes in trials with and without placebo run-in were 0.31 and 0.22, respectively, and this difference was statistically significant [13]. It is thus reasonable to conclude that placebo run-in (washout) results in inflated efficacy estimates.

Another common but problematic design feature in antidepressant trials is the permission of rescue medication, that is, sedative-hypnotic drugs such as benzodiazepines. Between 30% and 40% of antidepressant trials, including the influential STAR*D study, allowed the comedication with sedative-hypnotic drugs [141, 191]. However, these figures are most likely grave underestimates of the true rate, for use of comedication is often not reported in trial publications. According to Walsh and colleagues, only 60% of antidepressant trial reports stated explicitly whether comedication was permitted or not, and in these trials the rate of comedication was 84% [166]. Likewise, Dr Healy noted that comedication with sedative-hypnotic drugs (typically benzodiazepines) was a standard design feature in SSRI premarketing trials [9]. This certainly confounds the effects of the investigational drug. But then, why would antidepressant trial protocols permit the use of other psychotropic drugs when their main objective is to evaluate the efficacy of a specific psychotropic drug? The answer is simple and straightforward. Many antidepressants, especially the activating agents, frequently cause insomnia, nervousness, and agitation, which can be alleviated with sedative-hypnotics.

So comedication is permitted in many, likely even most, antidepressant trials. The fundamental question now is how many participants in a trial eventually received this rescue medication. If the rate is high, then the issue is serious, given that a doctor's decision to additionally prescribe a sedative-hypnotic drug is certainly non-random. The few data available indeed indicate that the majority of participants randomised to activating antidepressants are co-medicated with sedative-hypnotic drugs, whereas participants randomised to sedating antidepressants less often receive comedication [241]. This comes as no surprise, for the whole idea of permitting comedication with sedative-hypnotics was to mitigate the common side effects of activating antidepressants [9]. This design feature thus clearly compromises the internal validity of many antidepressant trials, for sedative-hypnotics not only alleviate antidepressant side effects, thus inflating tolerability/safety estimates, in fact they also treat depression, for anxiety, insomnia, and agitation are also common depression symptoms [1, 702]. That is, the treatment effects of antidepressants and sedative-hypnotics are necessarily confounded, but it is not clear whether this bias is systematic, since patients in the placebo group may also benefit from comedication.

It is well established in general medicine that unblinding of investigators or outcome assessors, also referred to as observer bias, produces exaggerated efficacy estimates in subjective outcome measures [685, 703–706]. Given that ratings of depression severity, and by consequence their transformation into response and remission rates, are inherently subjective (i.e. not based on objective clinical tests), unblinding is a serious issue in antidepressant trials [707]. This is particularly true since antidepressants, to varying degree, can cause marked side effects that are detectable by the clinical investigators who make the outcome assessments. This unblinding issue is well known for decades (but still largely ignored) and calls into question the integrity of the double-blind procedure in antidepressant trials.

Back in 1967, Dr Leyburn wrote in the *Lancet* "Patients who come into the consulting-room for assessment, perhaps for the sixth time and rather bored with the whole thing, but with their mouths so dry that one can hear their tongues scraping and clicking about in their mouths, are likely to be taking, say, amitriptyline, rather than the placebo" [400]. In 1993, Fisher and Greenberg likewise wrote that the double-blind procedure is deficient in placebo-controlled antidepressant trials [708], a conclusion also drawn by Even and colleagues in 2000 [707]. According to the latter authors, "This raises troublesome questions. For example, have all antidepressants consistently demonstrated their efficacy? Would the defects in design of therapeutic trials have smoothed out differences in strength of the available antidepressants? Might truly blind trials enable us to discriminate between efficacious and inefficacious antidepressants?" [707].

Because there are only very few truly double-blind antidepressant trials, and because unblinding is rarely ascertained in psychiatric drug trials [683, 684], we won't be able to answer these fundamental questions. But we know that unblinding is mostly due to the detection of side effects and the drugs' psychotropic effects, especially sedation and activation [400, 707, 708]. We can further assume that, due to treatment expectations, unblinding will result in more favourable outcome ratings in active treatment groups. To establish an association between unblinding and inflated efficacy estimates, we need to answer the following questions. How often is the blind broken in antidepressant trials? And how strongly are efficacy estimates affected by unblinding?

A few studies have examined how reliable clinical investigators can identify treatment allocation in trials of older antidepressants (tricyclics and MAOIs) for various indications and found that investigators (outcome assessors) were able to correctly guess the active drugs in about 80–90% of cases, and patients in roughly 70–80% of cases [707, 708]. Even less studies assessed the integrity of the double-blind in trials of new-generation antidepressants. A rare exception is the Depression Hypericum Trial, a 8-week three-arm trial that compared the efficacy of hypericum perforatum (St John's Wort) and sertraline against placebo [151]. If patients and clinicians were effectively blinded, stochastics (probability theory) dictates that, by chance, rates of correct guesses should be 33% in each group. However, at the end of 8 weeks, the proportion of patients guessing their treatment correctly was 55% for sertraline, 29% for hypericum, and 31% for placebo, a difference that was statistically significant. The probability of clinicians correctly guessing treatment allocation was 66% for sertraline, 29% for hypericum, and 36% for placebo, again a statistically significant difference. The findings from the Depression Hypericum Trial thus demonstrate that many clinicians, and to a lesser extent also patients, were able to correctly guess sertraline treatment, but not hypericum and placebo treatment.

According to Baethge and colleagues, only 1.8% of antidepressant trials provide an assessment of blinding [684]. Pooled across trials in schizophrenia and affective disorders, 58% and 70% of patients and investigators, respectively, correctly guessed active treatment. Finally, in a recent trial of sertraline against placebo in primary care (PANDA study), 46% of participants on sertraline thought they were taking the active drug compared to 19% of participants on placebo [152]. Thus, 81% of placebo-recipients correctly guessed that they were on placebo, demonstrating that the blind was broken in a substantial portion of participants. The literature reviewed so far thus clearly indicates that unblinding is a serious issue in antidepressant trials. I will now detail if this methodological limitation biases the trial results systematically.

As in general medicine, unblinding most likely also inflates efficacy estimates in antidepressant trials. According to Baethge and colleagues, correct guessing of treatment assignment in schizophrenia and affective disorder trials was correlated with higher treatment effect sizes [684]. Khan and colleagues examined all sorts of depression treatments, including antidepressants and psychotherapy, and found that unblinded trials produced larger treatment effects (relative to placebo) than blinded trials for any treatment modality, but most pronounced in combination therapy (i.e. antidepressants and psychotherapy combined) [709]. Given that most antidepressants can cause marked side effects, an effectively blinded trial is basically impossible when inert placebo pills are used in the control group. A few tricyclic trials therefore used active placebos, that is, placebos that cause side effects comparable to some of the tricyclic side effects (especially dry mouth). A meta-analysis of these active placebo-controlled trials produced a pooled effect size much smaller than that typically found in trials with inert placebos [710]. Thus, taken together, these findings strongly indicate that unblinding introduces a systematic bias in favour of antidepressants, thus producing inflated efficacy estimates [18].

A last issue that warrants scrutiny is the handling of study dropouts (i.e. participants who discontinue treatment prematurely and thus terminate the trial). It is well known that when information on an outcome variable is missing, this may lead to a significant distortion of results when missing values are not adequately addressed [161, 711]. Even in short-term antidepressant trials of 8 weeks duration, the dropout rate is roughly 30% [163, 175]. That is, almost a third of participants stops the treatment prematurely and thus their outcome at the end of the trial is unknown. This is problematic, since a loss of 20% or more can cause biased efficacy estimates and limits the generalisability of results [144]. In clinical trials, the intention to treat (ITT) analysis is standard practice now [712]. It requires that all participants randomised to treatment must be analysed, and not only those participants that completed the trial (referred to as per protocol or completer analysis). ITT increases the external validity of trial results, for in real-world routine practice it is common that patients discontinue treatment prematurely. But since the treatment outcome of study dropouts is unknown, these data must be imputed.

The most common statistical method in ITT analyses is the Last Observation Carried Forward (LOCF), which "is a data imputation process used in longitudinal repeated-measures clinical trials in which the last obtained data entry is substituted for any subsequent missing data, in an attempt to minimize the problem of dropout-associated missing data" [163]. For instance, if a participant stops a 8-week antidepressant trial prematurely at week 2 (let's say due to side effects) with a Hamilton depression score of 20 points, this last measure (observation) will be projected (carried forward) to be his/her 8-week treatment outcome. LOCF became the preferred method during the 1990s and was applied in about 80–90% of all antidepressant trials in the late 1990s and early 2000s [712]. That is, the efficacy of most new-generation antidepressants (especially SSRIs and SNRIs) was evaluated with LOCF method. More recently, however, the rate of LOCF fell to about 50% as it was increasingly replaced by more adequate methods [712]. But what's the issue with LOCF?

The LOCF method has serious limitations if the timing and reason of dropout differs between treatment groups, for it assumes that a given depression score at time of discontinuation would remain unchanged until the end of the trial [144]. This is of course a false assumption, for spontaneous remission and regression towards the mean (extremely high scores are often inflated due to random error and thus decline over time when repeatedly measured) will result in a reduction of average depression scores independent of treatment [177]. If patients on placebo drop out earlier due to a felt lack of efficacy than patients on active drug, it's very likely that they discontinue with higher depression scores, even though many would have improved considerably until the end of the trial had they continued participation. The timing of dropout is seldom reported in antidepressant trials, but it's well established that participants receiving placebo more often discontinue treatment due to lack of efficacy than participants receiving antidepressants [367]. LOCF thus likely introduces systematic bias in favour of active treatment and thus inflates efficacy estimates [163, 695].

This assumption has been empirically confirmed. Siddiqui and colleagues [161] compared LOCF to the Mixed-Effect Model Repeated Measure (MMRM) model, a newer, more accurate method that predicts missing outcome scores based on all available data, including symptom trajectories from other participants (i.e., the average decline of scores over time for participants with similar scores). They ran a simulation study and an analysis based on phase III trials submitted to the FDA as part of a new drug application. First, "The simulation studies demonstrate that LOCF analysis can lead to substantial biases in estimators of treatment effects and can greatly inflate Type I error rates of the statistical tests, whereas MMRM analysis on the available data leads to estimators with comparatively small bias". A Type I error indicates that an estimated effect reached statistical significance when there likely is no true effect [48, 713]. Second, "analysis of 48 clinical trial datasets obtained from 25 New Drug Applications (NDA) submissions of neurological and psychiatric drug products, MMRM analysis appears to be a superior approach in controlling Type I error rates and minimizing biases, as compared to LOCF" [161]. That is, the widespread application of LOCF in antidepressant trials during the 1990s and early 2000s has most likely resulted in various false-positive results, meaning that in some trials efficacy estimates became statistically significant even though true treatment effectiveness was uncertain.

Methodological Biases Distorting Safety/Tolerability Estimates

Safety refers to the adverse effects of a drug (also termed harms or side effects), whereas tolerability represents the degree to which adverse effects can be tolerated by patients. Per convention, adverse effects occurring in at least 10% of people are considered "very common", those affecting 1% to 10% "common", those affecting 0.1% to 1% "uncommon", those affecting 0.01% to 0.1% "rare", and those affecting less than 0.01% "very rare". The average sample size in antidepressant trials is 224 and most trials last merely 6–8 weeks [141]. As detailed above, this is sufficient to measure short-term efficacy of a drug, but insufficient to reliably detect even common adverse effects and to establish long-term safety [679, 692]. As detailed by Berlin and colleagues [690], with a sample size of 1000 participants there is a 82% chance to statistically detect an adverse drug effect that increases a harm event from 5% baseline risk to 10% during treatment (common adverse effect). Thus, even with such a large sample size rarely seen in antidepressant trials, there is a 18% chance to miss a common adverse drug effect. If a drug increases an adverse event rate from 1% to 2% (also falling into the rubric of common adverse effects), then with a sample size of 1000 there is only a small chance of 17% to statistically detect it. In that case, it would require a sample size of 5000 participants to detect it with a probability of 80%. When a drug increases the risk of an adverse event from 0.1% to 0.2% (uncommon adverse effect), then with a sample size of 1000 there is a meagre 5% chance to detect it, with a sample of 5000 participants the chance would be 7%, with a sample of 10,000 it would be 17%, and only with a sample of 50,000 it would be 79%. Thus, even if we pool the results from 10 trials with a sample size of 224 each, the resulting total sample size of 2240 participants will not generate enough statistical power to detect uncommon, let alone rare and very rare, adverse drug effects.

But even a large trial with a sample size of say 1000 participants won't guarantee that common adverse drug effects are statistically detected, for inadequate assessment and analysis of adverse events is a serious issue in randomised controlled trials [29, 686, 688, 689, 691, 714]. In most antidepressant trials, adverse event assessments fully rely on spontaneous patient reports prompted through open-ended questions, that is, unstructured and unsystematic assessments. This can lead to a considerable underestimation of both frequency and severity of side effects, especially when patients are not comfortable discussing sensitive adverse events such as sexual dysfunction [29, 275, 335, 691].

The pharmaceutical companies seeking regulatory approval for their SSRI drugs already observed in the phase I trials (the first small, uncontrolled trials conducted in humans as part of a new drug application) that over 50% of healthy volunteers developed sexual dysfunction after SSRI exposure [334]. The companies realised this was a serious tolerability/safety issue, and therefore sexual dysfunction was avoided (or concealed) as much as possible in subsequent trials. That is, systematic assessment of sexual dysfunction did deliberately not take place in phase II and III trials (unlike phase I trials that are conducted in small samples of healthy volunteers to assess drug safety and dosing, phase II and III trials are conducted in larger clinical samples with the specific condition the drug is supposed to treat, and assess efficacy, safety, and tolerability). When sexual dysfunction was spontaneously reported by patients, it was commonly ascribed to the underlying condition, that is, the depressive disorder. And sometimes, clinical investigators were even instructed by the trial sponsor not to enquire about sexual dysfunction [9]. The unsystematic assessment and inadequate recording of adverse events thus allowed the companies to profess sexual dysfunction rates of less than 5% in phase II and III trials. A rate of less than 5% for sexual dysfunction was also the figure given in the initial SSRI drug labels [334]. How seriously did these official rates underestimate the true prevalence of treatment-emergent sexual dysfunction with antidepressants? Let's have a look.

In the pivotal premarketing placebo-controlled clinical trials of fluoxetine, treatment-emergent sexual dysfunction was recorded in merely 1.9% of participants receiving fluoxetine, but in postmarketing (postapproval) trials, based on systematic assessment with questionnaires, rates as high as 75% were reported. With respect to SSRIs as a class, spontaneous reports of sexual dysfunction produced rates of 2% to 7%, but these rates rose to 55% when systematically enquired via questionnaires [275]. Finally, according to a recent meta-analysis focusing exclusively on clinical trials with a systematic assessment of sexual dysfunction, the rates are even higher for various SSRI drugs, being around 70% to 80% for fluoxetine, paroxetine, citalopram, sertraline, and venlafaxine (the latter is an SNRI), but only about 12% in placebo groups [336].

Treatment-emergent suicidality was also evident right from the beginning when the first SSRIs were clinically tested in humans. The new onset (occurrence) of suicidal ideation and behaviour on fluoxetine was also a main reason why the German drug regulators first refused to approve Eli Lilly's new drug application [9]. It was also quite clear that treatment-emergent suicidality was linked to fluoxetine's activation syndrome, that is, disinhibition, agitation, anxiety, nervousness, and akathisia. For Eli Lilly it was thus prerequisite to eliminate these side effects in antidepressant trials, which is why it (and other companies seeking approval for SSRIs and other activating antidepressants) by default permitted the comedication with sedative-hypnotic drugs. The companies further obfuscated the risk of treatment-emergent suicidality by systematically misrecording suicidal events [9, 29, 322, 323, 715]. For instance, suicidal events occurring in the lead-in phase (i.e. before randomisation) were counted as events in the placebo group, suicidal events leading to treatment discontinuation were not listed as adverse events, and discontinuation due to suicidality was often miscoded as discontinuation due to lack of efficacy. Some suicides and suicide attempts were not coded as serious adverse events but simply as study dropouts, and events clearly described as suicidal ideation or behaviour on case report forms were misrepresented by coding them as "emotional lability" or "worsening depression". Together these unethical and fraudulent practices led to a systematic underestimation of the risk of treatment-emergent suicidality in antidepressant trials. Although the drug regulators spotted most of these deceptions in the new drug applications for the SSRIs and SNRIs, they led the pharmaceutical companies get away with it and granted approval [9, 715, 716].

Finally, adverse events are inconsistently coded, commonly divided into multiple subcategories, and rarely grouped by anatomic or physiological system [29, 688, 689]. That is, the very same adverse event is frequently coded with different terms (e.g. akathisia interchangeably as agitation, nervousness, or restlessness), while events belonging to the same syndrome are commonly coded with different subcategories (e.g.

sexual dysfunction specifically as abnormal ejaculation, reduced libido, impotence, or anorgasmia). These methodological limitations impede the detection of harm signals. Imagine a clinical trial where 100 people were randomised to an antidepressant and 100 to placebo. In the antidepressant group, 9 patients developed akathisia, whereas in the placebo group there was only 1 such adverse event. According to a Chi-square test, this difference is statistically significant ($p < 0.05$) and would suggest that the antidepressant causes akathisia. However, if the 9 akathisia events are coded as nervousness in 3 cases, agitation in 3 cases, and restlessness in 3 cases, none of these adverse events would significantly differ from placebo and thus it would appear that the antidepressant does not cause akathisia or any of these coded adverse events. An important harm signal would thus go unnoticed. To account for this, lumping techniques were developed (i.e. grouping by anatomic or physiological system), but they are rarely used. It is therefore difficult or almost impossible to statistically detect adverse drug effects in modestly sized short-term trials when they are not very common. Along with the unsystematic assessment of adverse events detailed above (i.e. spontaneous self-reports), these biases corroborate (or amplify) the systematic underestimation of antidepressants' harm potential.

Although statistical analyses often lack the power (due to small sample sizes and low event rates) to reliably detect differences between treatment groups in subcategorised adverse event rates, such tests are frequently performed [686]. By consequence, these tests don't demonstrate statistically significant between-group differences even when the rate is considerably larger in one treatment group (e.g. 6% vs. 2%) [714, 717]. What's worse is that these statistically non-significant differences are often erroneously interpreted as no difference [718], even though researchers should know that "absence of evidence is not evidence of absence" [719]. Just because a difference in adverse event rates is statistically not significant does not indicate that there is no difference. It simply means that the sample was not large enough to draw reliable (or conclusive) statistical inferences from the data.

As detailed above, comedication with sedative-hypnotic drugs may bias the efficacy estimates of antidepressants. However, permitting the use of sedative-hypnotics in antidepressant trials has another important implication. Since insomnia, agitation, and anxiety can also be symptoms of depression and withdrawal symptoms in participants who were on antidepressants before being randomised to placebo, sedative-hypnotics are also frequently used in placebo groups [241]. This may inflate the rate of specific adverse events in the placebo group, for sedative-hypnotics also have side effects, for example drowsiness and dizziness [720]. On the other hand, comedication may also mitigate some depression symptoms in the placebo group, for example insomnia and agitation. Therefore, the use of sedative-hypnotics will not necessarily change the rate of any adverse event. But since tolerability of an antidepressant is determined by comparing the rate of treatment discontinuation due to adverse events in the antidepressant group to that recorded in the placebo group, the use of sedative-hypnotics may bias this group difference. In any case, comedication certainly lowers the incidence rate of specific antidepressant side effects such as insomnia, agitation, nervousness, and anxiety, for these symptoms are effectively alleviated through the administration of sedative-hypnotics [9, 720, 721].

The narrow selection of younger participants without complicated illness and comorbid medical conditions is a standard feature of clinical trial protocols [682]. I already discussed that this may inflate the real-world effectiveness of antidepressants. It may, however, also bias safety estimates. Serious adverse drug reactions are more common in older people with various chronic medical conditions, often in interaction with other prescription drugs [722, 723]. Depression is very common in older people with comorbid chronic medical conditions [724] and antidepressant use by consequence is highest in this vulnerable patient population [725]. The patients most likely to be prescribed antidepressants in real-world practice are thus exactly those people at highest risk of adverse drug reactions. The safety and tolerability of antidepressants in these vulnerable patients is largely unknown though, since clinical trials preferably select younger patients without comorbid chronic medical conditions. However, given that frail patients (i.e. old adults with various chronic medical conditions on multiple medications) are more susceptible to adverse drug effects, the safety of antidepressants is certainly poorer in this high-risk population than in the patients typically included in antidepressant trials [300].

Discontinuation Trials, Placebo Response, and Other Issues

As you might remember, I did not discuss the evidence from antidepressant discontinuation trials for relapse prevention (assumed to assess long-term prophylactic effects) in the section on the long-term efficacy of antidepressants in depression. This is due to serious methodological limitations and systematic biases in these trials, which is why they are presented here.

In relapse-prevention (discontinuation) trials, participants are first treated open-label with an antidepressant (commonly for about 3–6 months), but it is important to note that many participants were already taking antidepressants (sometimes for years) before entering the actual treatment trial. Participants who by the end of the open-label acute treatment phase stably improved on the investigational drug (mostly defined as being in remission) enter the double-blind placebo-controlled maintenance phase. At the beginning of this second phase, participants are randomly assigned either to remain on the drug or to have the antidepressant rapidly discontinued (in most studies abruptly) and replaced by an inert placebo pill. Double-blind means that both patients and clinical investigators ought not to know whether someone was put on placebo or whether active treatment was continued. The blinded placebo-controlled trial phase commonly lasts about 6–12 months; there are only a few small trials for older drugs that lasted 24 months or longer [726]. The primary outcome in these trials is the resurgence of clinically relevant depression symptoms (defined as relapse), which is commonly based on a cut-off score on a depression rating scale such as the HDRS [726–728]. The main finding from discontinuation trials is that over an average observation period of 12 months, about 20% of participants maintained on antidepressant compared to 40% of those switched to placebo experience a relapse, yielding a rate ratio of 2 and a number needed to treat of 5 [214].

These figures are so impressive that some leading psychiatric academics consider antidepressants "one of the most effective of all drugs" [22]. However, as I previously noted about this subject, "as researchers, we should not be seduced into believing that a drug is highly effective simply because a specific trial protocol has consistently produced impressive treatment effects, as these effects could be the result of a flawed trial protocol" [214]. And in the case of relapse-prevention (discontinuation) trials, there is indeed compelling scientific evidence that the protocol is seriously flawed and the results thus inconclusive, probably even misleading [9, 12, 214, 215, 228, 230, 235, 237]. Let me explain.

First, only patients who remitted during the acute treatment period (which is typically a minority of all patients) are randomised to either continued antidepressant use or abrupt discontinuation. The results of the randomised maintenance phase thus apply only to a particular subgroup of patients with a good short-term treatment outcome, but not to those who experience spontaneous recovery or those with a poor response to acute treatment. Second, the outcome in the double-blind randomised maintenance phase is merely a re-assessment of the unblinded acute-phase outcome (i.e. sustained response is assessed in acute treatment responders). Third, because participants were already treated open-label (unblinded) in the acute phase, they may instantly recognise when they are randomised to placebo and abruptly taken off the active drug. Various participants (and by consequence the investigators) are thus most likely unblinded. These three serious limitations systematically bias the results in favour of maintenance therapy and thus lead to inflated efficacy estimates [12, 215, 230, 234, 729].

Most important, however, is the fact that the outcome in relapse-prevention (discontinuation) trials is confounded, since many (sometimes most) relapses in the placebo group occur shortly after discontinuation of the antidepressant and are thus most likely withdrawal reactions [214, 228, 235, 237, 239, 729, 730]. It is well established that abrupt discontinuation of antidepressants can cause withdrawal syndromes, both acute and protracted, that often mimic a depression relapse or that may trigger a depression relapse (e.g. due to stressful physical withdrawal symptoms) [238, 345, 347, 731–735]. As a result, relapse-prevention (discontinuation) trials cannot differentiate between a true relapse, that is the recurrence of a genuine depression episode, and the consequences of a neurophysiological adaptation to prolonged drug exposure (pharmacodynamic effect) causing severe mental and physical withdrawal symptoms after abrupt/rapid discontinuation (also referred to as oppositional tolerance) [217, 223, 351]. What may seem a benefit of continued antidepressant treatment (i.e. a long-term prophylactic effect) could very well be construed as an adverse treatment effect (i.e. iatrogenic harm) [214, 239]. Therefore, discontinuation trials cannot demonstrate that antidepressants truly prevent depression relapses [214, 228, 230, 235, 237, 238]. Whether continuing antidepressant use beyond the acute treatment phase relative to abrupt/rapid discontinuation prevents relapses or rather the occurrence of withdrawal reactions is still fiercely debated, but our recent analysis of relapse prevention (discontinuation) trials submitted to the FDA indicates that it is most likely the latter [239].

Various authors argued that the placebo response (i.e. observed improvements in placebo groups) has significantly increased in antidepressant trials over time and that this is a main reason for the modest/poor efficacy estimates of new-generation antidepressants [736–738]. The placebo response has indeed increased during the 1980s, mostly due to the broadening of the diagnostic criteria for depression (leading to the inclusion of many people with milder conditions) and changes in trial designs (with the advent of large multi-centre trials with longer duration and fixed dosing) [166, 192, 736]. But what about increased placebo response during the 1990s and 2000s? A comprehensive analysis based on published and unpublished trials by Furukawa and colleagues showed that since the early 1990s the placebo response remained largely constant [192]. By contrast, Khan and colleagues found evidence for increasing placebo response during the 1990s and 2000s, but they also showed that the average drug–placebo difference remained unchanged and that the rate of positive trials (i.e. statistically significant drug–placebo differences) has even increased, which argues against the hypothesis that an increasing placebo response prevents the demonstration of efficacy [739]. Moreover, when Furukawa and colleagues re-analysed the data by Khan and colleagues, they found no increase in the placebo response after controlling for changes in trial designs [740]. To further complicate matters, the most recent analysis even suggests that the placebo response slightly decreased from 2001 to 2015 [741]. In any case, there is no consistent evidence that the placebo response has increased since the mid-1990s and no evidence at all that a higher placebo response is associated with smaller efficacy estimates or a higher rate of negative trials.

Another popular argument is that the improvement seen in placebo groups (i.e. observed placebo response) is mostly due to the placebo effect [11, 742]. By contrast, others argued that the placebo effect in antidepressant trials is trivial or inexistent [743]. The truth most likely lies somewhere in between these extreme positions [144]. However, it is quite clear that most apparent improvements observed in placebo groups (and by consequence also in antidepressant groups) are due to spontaneous remission, regression to the mean, and unspecific treatment effects (e.g. regular contact with a physician, clinical management, and comedication with sedative-hypnotic drugs) [177]. As demonstrated in many other medical fields, what has often been misconstrued as a genuine placebo effect is much better explained by other factors [744, 745]. Thus, as I outlined elsewhere, "it follows that the placebo effect in antidepressant trials is largely (though not entirely) a methodological artefact, and that the symptom reduction seen in placebo recipients is mostly due to both regression to the mean and spontaneous remission" [177].

Last but not least, there is ongoing controversy about the most popular scale to assess depression in clinical trials, the Hamilton Depression Rating Scale 17-item version (HDRS-17) [746, 747]. Various authors suggested that the HDRS-17 has poor validity and may underestimate antidepressant efficacy, for the scale is not unidimensional and may capture antidepressant side effects (e.g. insomnia, gastrointestinal symptoms, agitation, sexual dysfunction) [748, 749]. However, thus far there is no convincing evidence that alternative scales that more specifically assess core depression symptoms, for instance the Bech scale (HDRS-6) or the Montgomery-Asberg Depression Rating Scale (MADRS), generate significantly higher efficacy estimates, especially in severe depression [17, 258]. With respect to patient-centred outcomes, that is, quality of life and social functioning, effect size estimates again do not differ meaningfully from the HDRS-17 effect size [750, 751]. Moreover, it is also important to stress that simply because antidepressants may aggravate some depression symptoms (e.g. sleep problems, psychomotor agitation, sexual dysfunction, loss of appetite), this by no means legitimates the exclusion of these symptoms in the assessment of depression [752]. Instead of removing such symptoms from a depression rating scale, one should rather wonder why we call a drug an antidepressant when in fact it worsens (or causes) various established depression symptoms [18, 753].

The quality of the depression ratings obtained through clinician-administered interviews (e.g. HDRS-17, MADRS) is another methodological limitation. An analysis of HDRS-17 assessments showed that "interviews were brief and cursory and the quality of interviews was below what would be expected in a clinical drug trial" [754]. Based on a small study, Kobak and colleagues suggested that antidepressants may fail to demonstrate efficacy due to these low-quality interviews [755]. However, the evidence is inconsistent, and a subsequent study by Khan and colleagues found the exact opposite [756]. According to their study, significant drug-placebo differences were only detected in trials where traditional semi-structured (low-quality) interviews were conducted, but not when a stringent (high-quality) interview technique was applied (i.e. structured interview guide with audiotaping and rater applied performance scale). It is thus debatable whether low-quality outcome ratings introduce systematic bias. But given that self-report instruments (quality of life, depression) produce comparable or even smaller effect sizes as the common clinician-administered rating scales (i.e. HDRS-17, MADRS), it is highly unlikely that lack of efficacy is due to low-quality interviews. Low-quality clinician outcome ratings may even inflate efficacy estimates, possibly due to unblinding of clinical investigators [18]. In this respect it is also important to note that patient self-reports of depression assessed with questionnaires such as the Beck Depression Inventory (BDI) produce significantly smaller effect sizes than clinician rating scales such as the HDRS-17 [147, 757, 758].

Selective Reporting and Spin

As I have outlined above, antidepressant trials are marred with methodological limitations, of which various seem to result in inflated efficacy estimates and underestimation of harms. Despite these systematic biases in the design and conduct of antidepressant trials, about half of all placebo-controlled trials failed to demonstrate efficacy [57, 175]. This is, however, not the impression a physician gets when he/she consults the scientific literature, where almost all trial publications report positive results [174]. How is this possible? How can the scientific literature paint such a false and misleading picture of the actual scientific evidence? The answer is as simple as it is shocking: the trial data are misrepresented and selectively reported. Before I go into detail on how the evidence on the efficacy and safety of antidepressants is systematically biased in the scientific literature, I will briefly outline how clinical trial results are misreported in general medicine.

The scientific evidence consistently shows that about 20–50% of clinical trials remain unpublished and trials with positive results are about 2 to 5 times more likely to get published. The primary outcome reported in the published article is discrepant to the pre-specified primary outcome in about 30–40% of all trial publications, and roughly 40–60% of all negative primary outcomes (i.e. pre-specified primary outcomes that failed to demonstrate efficacy) are not reported in trial publications (i.e. journal articles). Moreover, about 30–50% of all negative primary outcomes are misrepresented as positive in the published article [85, 86, 89, 90, 668, 759, 760]. In addition, safety outcomes and (serious) adverse events are inadequately described and massively underreported in the scientific literature [90, 677, 687, 761, 762]. According to a comprehensive analysis by Golder and colleagues, only 36% of all adverse events are reported in trial publications and 54% of all publications provide no information on adverse events at all [87]. The authors thus concluded "There is strong evidence that much of the information on adverse events remains unpublished and that the number and range of adverse events is higher in unpublished than in published versions of the same study" [87]. Even deaths, the most serious adverse events, are not reported in most trial publications [665, 763].

How do we know about these issues? By comparing the trial results reported in journal articles to other sources, including results posted on trial registries, reviews provided by the drug regulators, internal industry documents released through litigation, and clinical study reports available to some medical authorities and researchers. Clinical study reports are very comprehensive documents of many hundred (sometimes thousands) pages written by the trial sponsors. They come the closest to the raw data and regulatory agencies base their drug reviews on these extensive documents, for full raw data are property of the trial sponsors and not even regulators have access to them. The problem is that, with very few exceptions, clinical study reports are publicly unavailable. Pharmaceutical companies don't publish them and except for drug regulators and a few other health authorities (e.g. research ethics committees), it is very difficult or almost impossible to get access to them. The detailed results provided by the clinical study reports are thus rarely known to the public unless a pharmaceutical company is required to release them through litigation. Trial registries such as ClinicalTrial.gov are another important data source, albeit much less detailed and complete as the clinical study reports [665]. Since 2007, with a few exceptions, trial sponsors, including both industry and non-industry, are mandated to publish clinical trial results in a publicly accessible registry within one year of trial completion. Unfortunately, sponsors poorly comply with these legal requirements. According to a recent analysis, only 41% of trial results were reported within the 1-year deadline and 64% had results submitted at any time; 36% of trial results were thus not reported in the trial registry [764].

You may wonder how it could be that eminent medical academics selectively report outcomes, conceal (serious) adverse events, and if that doesn't help to create a positive message about the drug, prefer not to publish the trial? That is, why do so many leading academics (often professors of medicine) behave in such unscientific (and unethical) ways? Although there are certainly various reasons, including professional and personal interests, the two most important factors arguably are that, first, in most cases the authors don't analyse the data themselves, and second, they actually don't even write the articles [29, 459, 657, 659, 765–767]. The data from industry-sponsored trials are the property of the sponsor and analysed in-house by the company's own statisticians or else by a contract-research organisation. And most articles are ghostwritten, that is, they are largely (sometimes entirely) written by a medical communication firm hired by the company's marketing department, and not by the eminent medical academics listed as "authors".

The next question is, what to make of these findings? We can safely draw three main conclusions. First and foremost, the evidence is clear and compelling that the efficacy and safety of medical interventions is significantly overestimated in the scientific literature. Therefore, trial results reported in journal articles are arguably the least reliable and most incomplete source. Second, trial registries can provide valuable information, for they allow to evaluate whether publications fully report all prespecified trial outcomes. Sometimes registries also allow to access trial results that were not reported in journal articles, but results posted in trial registries are often incomplete or lacking altogether. Third, clinical study reports are certainly the most reliable and most comprehensive data source, but they are not publicly available and often inaccessible. And that's why evidence-based medicine largely fails, for the scientific literature (i.e. evidence from peer-reviewed journal articles) is the cornerstone of clinical decision making in modern healthcare. Respected medical authorities such as Cochrane who provide systematic reviews relevant to clinical decision making strongly rely on publications in scientific journals. When the evidence is unreliable and biased due to selective reporting, so are the overall assessments of efficacy and safety of medical interventions. This serious issue has not gone unnoticed, and several EBM experts called for a careful reevaluation of the E in EBM (Evidence-Based Medicine) [29, 377, 378, 650, 768]. According to Jefferson and Jorgensen,

> "So, should we ignore evidence from journal articles? If steps are not taken urgently to address the situation, then 'probably' would be our answer. By the law of Garbage In Garbage Out, whatever we produce in our reviews will be systematically assembled and synthesised garbage with a nice Cochrane logo on it. One major problem is our ignorance of the presence of garbage, as its invisibility makes its distortions credible and impossible to check. This is how some of us happily signed off a Cochrane review with findings which had been completely and invisibly subverted by reporting bias". [653]

Selective Reporting in Antidepressant Trials

The most extreme, though not necessarily the most pernicious, form of selective reporting is publication bias, meaning that trials with favourable results are published, often multiple times, whereas trials with unfavourable results will never see the day of light and thus remain unknown to physicians and the public. About a third of antidepressant trials for adult depression remain unpublished [57, 174]. And, of course, trial sponsors (mostly pharmaceutical companies) do not decide at random whether they publish a trial or not. They intentionally, and almost exclusively, publish trials with positive results [174], of which some are published multiple times as part of repeated pooled analyses [56, 769]. Let's start with a telling example.

The German Institute for Quality and Efficiency in Health Care (IQWiG) conducts health technology assessments to determine whether statutory health insurance should cover the costs of a new prescription drug. The health technology assessment report for Pfizer's reboxetine (the first selective norepinephrine reuptake inhibitor for depression) was impeded by Pfizer for not providing a complete list of all unpublished trials as requested by IQWiG [82]. The institute had received data from 3 published trials, but based on secondary publications reporting results for subsamples and other outcomes, IQWiG knew that the main efficacy results of many reboxetine trials were never published. Pfizer first refused to provide these data, but after long negotiations finally decided to cooperate and provided data for 10 unpublished short-term efficacy trials. Thus, according to IQWiG, Pfizer published only 3 of 13 efficacy trials (23%) of its antidepressant reboxetine and data on altogether 74% of trial participants remained unpublished. This is unethical on its own right, but the real scandal became only apparent when IQWiG compared the results of the published and unpublished trials. In the few published trials, reboxetine was superior to placebo and equally effective as SSRI comparator drugs. However, when IQWiG included the data from the many unpublished trials, reboxetine was no better than placebo and inferior to the SSRIs. Put differently, Pfizer did only publish a small subset of trials where reboxetine was superior to placebo and not inferior to SSRIs but tried to hide the majority of trials where its drug not only failed to beat placebo but also lost to the SSRIs. Based on the full data from all trials, the authors therefore concluded "Reboxetine is, overall, an ineffective and potentially harmful antidepressant. Published evidence is affected by publication bias, underlining the urgent need for mandatory publication of trial data" [82].

Unfortunately, reboxetine is no exception and Pfizer's selective reporting of favourable trial results is standard operating procedure in the pharmaceutical industry. A comprehensive analysis by Turner and colleagues showed that according to the scientific literature (i.e. journal articles), 94% of antidepressant trials for adult depression are positive. However, based on the FDA's evaluation of trial data submitted to them for marketing approval, only 51% of antidepressant trials are positive. How is this possible? In total 74 placebo-controlled efficacy trials were submitted by pharmaceutical companies to the FDA as part of a new drug application for 12 new antidepressant drugs eventually approved between 1982 and 2004. In total 38 trials were positive (51%), and all but one of these (97%) were published. But there were also 36 trials, that is about half of all trials submitted to the FDA, with questionable or negative results. And this is where it gets really dirty. Of the 12 trials with questionable results, 6 (50%) were not published and 6 (50%) were published as positive. You think it can't get worse than this? Well, it does. Among the 24 negative trials, only 3 (12%) were published as negative, whereas 5 (21%) were published as positive and 16 (67%) were not published. That's why in the scientific literature almost every antidepressant trial appears positive when in reality just about half truly are. Resulting from this selective reporting of antidepressant trials, the efficacy of new-generation antidepressants was inflated by 32% in the scientific literature [57].

But how can a pharmaceutical company publish a trial as positive when the results were negative (i.e. no significant drug-placebo difference on the primary efficacy outcome)? Unfortunately, this is quite easy as there are multiple ways how the drug manufacturers can cheat [29, 56, 57, 60, 459, 767]. For instance, a company can decide to publish the more favourable per protocol analysis instead of the more conservative (but more accurate) intention to treat analysis. They can also report the results for a study subsample from selected study sites instead of the full study population. Or else they can switch the primary outcome when a statistically significant effect could be demonstrated on a secondary outcome or a newly created outcome measure. The leading academics commonly listed as "authors" on these publications are perhaps not even aware of the extent of fraud they are indirectly supporting (and lending their badge of scientific excellence), for, as detailed above, in most cases they neither analysed the data nor did they actually write these articles [29, 78, 657].

That is, most antidepressant trials with negative results are distorted and presented as positive or else are simply not published [56, 57, 174]. But still many unpublished trials sooner or later appear in the scientific literature. They just rarely report the primary efficacy outcomes. The data from negative trials are often pooled to answer a different question by presenting data on a secondary outcome that do not reveal that the drug failed to beat placebo and are by and large positively framed (e.g. by focusing on selective safety outcomes) [174, 769]. This constant production of favourable publications is no longer research conducted in the spirit of advancing scientific knowledge but mere marketing. As bluntly stated by Spielmans and colleagues, "Such redundant publications add little to scientific understanding" [769]. It further indicates that the pharmaceutical industry actively (and efficiently) manages the scientific literature in order to advance its commercial interests (i.e. expanding markets and increasing prescription rates) [651, 658].

But selective reporting is not restricted to efficacy data. It equally affects safety data. Maund and colleagues compared the adverse events reported in clinical study reports of duloxetine trials for depression to those reported in the published journal articles for the same trials [83]. They found that in each trial, a median of 406 treatment-emergent adverse events were not reported in the journal articles. The total number of treatment-emergent adverse events reported in journal articles was less than half the number reported in the clinical study reports. Hughes and colleagues compared result summaries posted in a mandatory trial registry to the corresponding information provided in journal articles for the same trials. In 35 duloxetine trials, the trial registry listed a total of 11 deaths and 4 suicides; all (100%) were reported in the corresponding journal articles. However, of 40 suicidal events reported in the trial registry, only 33 (82.5%) were reported in the corresponding journal articles, and of 27 events of treatment-emergent psychiatric symptoms, only 21 (77.8%) were reported in journal articles. For the 7 sertraline trials listed in the trial registry, the situation was even worse. Of 11 deaths reported in the trial registry, none (0%) was reported in the journal articles. No suicides were reported in both trial registry and journal articles. But of 5 suicidal events and 11 treatment-emergent psychiatric symptoms listed in the trial registry, again none (0% each) was reported in the corresponding journal articles [763].

Wieseler and colleagues assessed a large sample of antidepressant trials for depression (including bupropion, duloxetine, mirtazapine, reboxetine and venlafaxine) and various non-psychiatric drug trials for other conditions (e.g. diabetes and asthma). They compared the completeness of safety data reported in the clinical study reports to the corresponding data published in journal articles. Mortality, adverse events, and serious adverse events were completely reported in 100%, 92%, and 88% of clinical study reports, but only in 30%, 21%, and 24% of journal articles [665]. So, just like in general medical interventions [87], there is clear evidence that safety outcomes are underreported in antidepressant trials. The main question now is whether this incomplete information introduces a systematic bias in favour of the drugs comparable to the inflated efficacy estimates detailed above [57].

De Vries and colleagues compared safety evaluations provided by the FDA to the data presented by the drug manufacturers in the corresponding journal articles [81]. The risk of discontinuation due to adverse events in antidepressant groups compared to placebo groups was similar for FDA evaluation and journal articles (in depression the risk is about 2 times higher with antidepressants compared to placebo), suggesting that tolerability is not subject to reporting bias. Likewise, according to the comprehensive analysis of reboxetine trials by IQWiG detailed above, the risk of adverse events was similar for published and unpublished data [82]. However, while in the few published trials the increased risk of adverse events did not reach statistical significance, in the much larger database of unpublished trials the same effect estimate was statistically highly significant (due to increased statistical power). Moreover, while the few published trials suggested that discontinuation due to adverse events was no more likely with reboxetine than with placebo (suggesting the drug is well tolerated), according to the unpublished data the risk was about 2.5 times higher with reboxetine (indicating that the drug is not well tolerated). When both published and unpublished data were pooled, the risk was about 2 times higher with reboxetine and the effect estimate was statistically highly significant. So according to these findings, selective reporting of antidepressant trials can indeed lead to distorted and exaggerated tolerability estimates.

There is also evidence that the underreporting of serious adverse events leads to systematically inflated safety estimates in antidepressant trials. According to De Vries and colleagues, there were discrepancies in the number of serious adverse events between the FDA evaluation and the corresponding journal articles in 43% of trials. In 78% of these discrepant cases, the published data (journal articles) led to a smaller or reversed drug–placebo difference and thus a systematically more favorable drug–placebo comparison [81]. Sharma and colleagues analysed the clinical study reports of 70 antidepressant trials (including duloxetine, fluoxetine, paroxetine, sertraline, and venlafaxine) obtained from European drug regulation agencies with a total of 18,526 patients. 16 deaths occurred in these trials, of which four deaths were misreported by the drug company, all systematically in favour of the antidepressant. For instance, "A patient receiving venlafaxine (trial 69) attempted suicide by strangulation without forewarning and died five days later in hospital. Although the suicide attempt occurred on day 21 out of the 56 days of randomised treatment, the death was called a post-study event as it occurred in hospital and treatment had been discontinued because of the suicide attempt" [323]. Moreover, of 62 suicide attempts, 27 events (44%) were misreported as "emotional lability" or "worsening depression" in the treatment-emergent adverse event tables, although in patient narratives or individual patient listings they were clearly identified as suicide attempts. Likewise, 32 of 63 suicidal ideation events (51%) were again misreported as "emotional lability" or "worsening depression". As detailed in the section "Methodological biases distorting safety/tolerability estimates", this misreporting and miscoding of suicidal events was a deliberate (and nefarious) tactic of the pharmaceutical companies to conceal the suicidality harm signal in antidepressant trials [9, 29].

The amount of selective reporting is even worse in paediatric antidepressant trials. The majority of these studies remain unpublished, and in the few that were published, the sponsoring pharmaceutical companies distorted and selectively reported the outcome data [29, 58, 290, 322,

770]. Not only were efficacy outcomes selectively reported, but harm outcomes as well. Especially treatment-emergent suicidality was systematically underreported and deliberately obfuscated on a large scale. The outcome data of antidepressant trials in children and adolescents was so terribly manipulated, misreported, and misrepresented that the Lancet Editors felt compelled to write an article titled "Depressing research", where they stated

> "It is hard to imagine the anguish experienced by the parents, relatives, and friends of a child who has taken his or her own life. That such an event could be precipitated by a supposedly beneficial drug is a catastrophe. The idea of that drug's use being based on the selective reporting of favourable research should be unimaginable ... The story of research into selective serotonin reuptake inhibitor (SSRI) use in childhood depression is one of confusion, manipulation, and institutional failure ... In a global medical culture where evidence-based practice is seen as the gold standard for care, these failings are a disaster. Meta-analysis of published data supports an increasing number of clinical decisions and guidelines, which in turn dictate the use of vast levels of health-care resources. This process is made entirely redundant if its results are so easily manipulated by those with potentially massive financial gains". [771]

Creating the Right Marketing Message for Antidepressants

A comprehensive analysis by Healy and Cattell [78] showed that a large number of articles on sertraline published between 1998 and 2000, including the vast majority of clinical trials from various therapeutic areas, were sponsored by Pfizer (manufacturer of sertraline) and written by a medical communication firm. The latter information was available to the authors due to an internal Pfizer document released through litigation, for on most publications the involvement of the medical communication firm was not disclosed (which is a violation of publication ethics). Most importantly, all ghostwritten trial publications were favourable to Pfizer's sertraline. The academics listed as authors on these articles had a large number of publications and the articles also appeared mostly in high-impact journals and had a high citation rate. By contrast, articles on sertraline not sponsored by Pfizer and not prepared by a medical communication firm often reported negative findings (mostly safety issues), were typically published in low-impact journals, and the authors had a relatively small publication output. Healy and Cattel thus concluded "The profile of the articles reported here suggests that the background of certain authors may have increased the possibility of the company's publications appearing in the most prestigious journals. Specific journals seem to have been targeted. The combination of distinguished journal, distinguished author, an efficient distribution system and sponsored platforms appears to have led to an impact on the therapeutics domain greatly in excess of 50% of the impact of the rest of the literature on sertraline" [78].

From a commercial perspective, selective reporting of favourable results in journal articles allegedly written by leading academics clearly pays off for the pharmaceutical companies. They can be published in top-tier journals and are massively disseminated due to their high citation rates. Indeed, positive antidepressant trials are much more cited than the very few published trials with negative results [81]. The reach and impact of positive trials is further increased through multiple publications of the same trial results [56, 769]. And to make sure that the right marketing message is firmly established in the scientific literature, namely antidepressants being effective (at least based on the published articles), the pharmaceutical companies also heavily produce meta-analyses that synthesise these selectively reported positive results over and over again. Between January 2007 and March 2014, that is in roughly 7 years, an incredible number of 185 meta-analyses of antidepressant trials for depression were published, of which 54 (29%) were authored by industry employees and altogether 147 (79%) of meta-analyses had some link to industry (sponsored by industry or authored by industry employees or academics with financial relationships to industry) [772].

Publishing an abundance of favourable efficacy data is one way to disseminate the right marketing message; ignoring safety issues is another way to make sure that medical organisations and prescribers receive only positive information about a drug. It is thus worthwhile contrasting the 185 meta-analyses on the efficacy of antidepressants published between

2007 and early 2014, most sponsored or otherwise supported by the pharmaceutical industry, with meta-analyses specifically focusing on important safety issues relevant to public health and clinical decision making. So what about treatment-emergent suicidality and withdrawal syndromes, two prominent topics discussed in detail in the chapter "Conflicts of interest in medicine" that were fiercely debated for decades (for critical overviews, see for example [351, 357, 715, 773])? Let's have a look.

The first case reports highlighting and discussing antidepressant withdrawal were published soon after the introduction of the first antidepressants in the early 1960s [774, 775], but it took almost 40 years until the first randomised controlled trial, sponsored by Eli Lilly, was published [735]. The first systematic review followed in 2015 [347] and the first meta-analysis in 2019 [345], both conducted by researchers without industry-ties. As regards treatment-emergent suicidality, this was first prominently discussed in the early 1990s after the introduction of fluoxetine [326, 776], followed by a meta-analysis conducted by Eli Lilly in 1991 attempting to settle any doubts [777]. Then there were a few non-industry sponsored meta-analyses in the early and mid-2000s (e.g. [327, 330, 778, 779]), including the comprehensive FDA-analysis that led to the suicidality safety warning (referred to as black box warning) in children and adolescents [321, 780]. Between 2007 and early 2014, however, to the best of my knowledge there was only one other meta-analysis, that is the FDA analysis that led to the expansion of the suicidality black box warning to also include young adults [324]. In sum, while 185 meta-analyses on the efficacy of antidepressants were published between January 2007 and March 2014, during the same period there was not one meta-analysis on withdrawal syndromes and only one meta-analysis on treatment-emergent suicidality. Even very common side effects such as treatment-emergent sexual dysfunction are rarely studied. As far as I am aware, there were only two meta-analyses of treatment-emergent sexual dysfunction published during the period 2007–2014, namely, a study by Serretti and Chiesa from 2009 [336] and another by Reichenpfader and colleagues from 2014 [781].

Spin is another pernicious issue in the reporting and interpretation of antidepressant trials. Spin is defined as "a specific reporting that fails to faithfully reflect the nature and range of findings and that could affect the impression that the results produce in readers, a way to distort science reporting without actually lying … Reporting results in a manuscript implies some choices about which data analyses are reported, how data are reported, how they should be interpreted, and what rhetoric is used. These choices, which can be legitimate in some contexts, in another context can create an inaccurate impression of the study results … It is almost impossible to determine whether spin is the consequence of a lack of understanding of methodologic principles, a parroting of common practices, a form of unconscious behavior, or an actual willingness to mislead the reader. However, spin, when it occurs, often favors the author's vested interest (financial, intellectual, academic, and so forth)" [667]. The most basic depiction of spin is the standard conclusion stated in almost every single positive antidepressant trial that the investigated drug was effective, safe, and well tolerated, even when efficacy estimates were marginally small, some adverse events considerably higher with antidepressants, and treatment discontinuation due to adverse events significantly increased compared to placebo. I will now provide two compelling examples of how spin manifests in antidepressant trials and how it contributes to the exaggeration of efficacy and minimisation of harms. I deliberately chose two governmentally sponsored trials to illustrate that spin is not exclusively an issue in industry-sponsored trials.

The Depression Hypericum Trial tested hypericum perforatum (St John's Wort) and sertraline against placebo [151]. Both active drugs failed to beat placebo on the primary efficacy outcome, the mean change in HDRS-17 total score from baseline to 8 weeks. The rates of full response at week 8 were 23.9% for hypericum, 24.8% for sertraline, and 31.9% for placebo, with no statistically significant between-group difference. In addition, there were five secondary efficacy outcomes (a self-report measure of depression, one measure of disability, one measure of global functioning, and two measures of general illness severity). Hypericum failed to separate from placebo on all of them and sertraline on four of them. That is, one weak but statistically significant difference was found between sertraline and placebo on one of the measures of general illness severity (the Clinical Global Impressions-Severity scale). Nevertheless, the results were quite clear and consistent overall. Both hypericum and sertraline failed to conclusively improve depression, disability, global functioning, and general psychopathology in comparison to placebo.

But still, the authors, oddly enough, concluded in the main text "According to available data, hypericum should not be substituted for standard clinical care of proven efficacy, including antidepressant medications and specific psychotherapies, for the treatment of major depression of moderate severity" [151]. This conclusion does not logically follow from the data. In this trial St John's Wort was indeed not effective, but so was sertraline, the "standard clinical care of proven efficacy". If the authors judge St John's Wort ineffective in this patient population (which they obviously did), then they must also conclude that sertraline is ineffective. Moreover, their conclusion did not logically follow from the broader scientific literature. Considering all studies, of which many were already available when the Depression Hypericum Trial was published, St John's Wort is just as effective as standard antidepressants and also superior to placebo, though, as with antidepressants in general, the effect size is small [203]. Thus, according to all available data, the only appropriate conclusion would be that standard antidepressants are no better than St John's Wort. If the authors, which had extensive financial ties to manufacturers of antidepressants, including shares in Pfizer (the manufacturer of sertraline), consider St John's Wort ineffective in major depression, then so are standard antidepressants like sertraline.

The second example is the TADS trial, a governmentally sponsored 12-week randomised treatment trial evaluating the efficacy of fluoxetine and cognitive-behavioural therapy (CBT) against placebo in adolescents with depression [782]. Although the study was sponsored by the NIMH, many authors had received research support and honoraria for serving as consultants and/or speakers for Eli Lilly, the manufacturer of fluoxetine. The study was also supported by an unrestricted educational grant from Eli Lilly. Two primary efficacy outcomes were prespecified; first, the continuous score on the Children's Depression Rating Scale-Revised, and second, response (much or very much improved) based on the Clinical Global Impressions scale. The two secondary efficacy outcomes were the Reynolds Adolescent Depression Scale and the Suicidal Ideation Questionnaire-Junior High School Version. Let us first look at the summary of the results as stated in the abstract, often the only part of a paper that busy clinicians have the time to read.

"Compared with placebo, the combination of fluoxetine with CBT was statistically significant (*P*=.001) on the Children's Depression Rating Scale-Revised. Compared with fluoxetine alone (*P*=.02) and CBT alone (*P*=.01), treatment of fluoxetine with CBT was superior. Fluoxetine alone is a superior treatment to CBT alone (*P*=.01). Rates of response for fluoxetine with CBT were 71.0% (95% confidence interval [CI], 62%–80%); fluoxetine alone, 60.6% (95% CI, 51%–70%); CBT alone, 43.2% (95% CI, 34%–52%); and placebo, 34.8% (95% CI, 26%–44%). On the Clinical Global Impressions improvement responder analysis, the 2 fluoxetine-containing conditions were statistically superior to CBT and to placebo. Clinically significant suicidal thinking, which was present in 29% of the sample at baseline, improved significantly in all 4 treatment groups. Fluoxetine with CBT showed the greatest reduction (*P*=.02). Seven (1.6%) of 439 patients attempted suicide; there were no completed suicides. Conclusion: The combination of fluoxetine with CBT offered the most favorable tradeoff between benefit and risk for adolescents with major depressive disorder". [782]

So the authors stressed that fluoxetine combined with cognitive-behavioural therapy (CBT) was more effective than placebo, fluoxetine alone, and CBT alone on the first primary outcome (Children's Depression Rating Scale-Revised). They also emphasised that fluoxetine alone was more effective than CBT alone on both primary outcomes and that fluoxetine (alone and in combination with CBT) was more effective than placebo on the second primary outcome (Clinical Global Impression scale). However, they did not mention that fluoxetine was not significantly better than placebo on the first primary outcome (Children's Depression Rating Scale-Revised). Neither did they state that fluoxetine failed to beat placebo on the two secondary efficacy outcomes, the Reynolds Adolescent Depression Scale and the Suicidal Ideation Questionnaire-Junior High School Version. Instead they mentioned that suicidal thinking significantly improved in all treatment groups and that fluoxetine with CBT showed the greatest reduction. You might rightly argue that the authors only mentioned statistically significant results, which is what clinicians are mostly interested in. Okay, fair enough. But in that case, why did the authors not mention that various adverse events were significantly more frequent in fluoxetine-treated patients compared to CBT and placebo? Let's look a bit closer at these safety data.

According to spontaneous adverse event reporting, there were significantly more treatment-emergent events of self-harm (including self-injurious and suicidal behaviours) in patients treated with fluoxetine compared to non-fluoxetine treated patients (including CBT alone and placebo). The rate of treatment-emergent self-harm was 10.2% in patients treated with fluoxetine compared to 4.9% in patients not treated with fluoxetine and the difference was statistically significant ($p < 0.05$). The rates of self-harm for fluoxetine alone was 11.9% as compared to 5.4% for placebo, but due to lack of statistical power, this difference was statistically not significant [782]. Moreover, rates of suicide attempts were 2.8% for fluoxetine treatment (with or without CBT) and 0.4% for non-fluoxetine treatment (CBT alone or placebo). The authors claimed that the numbers were too small for statistical comparison, but according to my own calculation the difference fell just short of statistical significance according to a two-tailed Fisher's exact test ($p = 0.064$) and are thus concerning in view of the significantly increased risk of treatment-emergent self-harm. In addition, 14.8% of patients treated with fluoxetine (with or without CBT) and 4.5% of patients not treated with fluoxetine (CBT alone or placebo) experienced a treatment-emergent psychiatric adverse event (mostly mood dysregulation and insomnia, which are known side-effects of fluoxetine). This difference is statistically highly significant according to a two-tailed Fisher's exact test ($p < 0.001$).

In sum, in the abstract, the TADS authors emphasised significant efficacy outcomes for fluoxetine (alone and in combination with CBT) but did not mention that fluoxetine alone failed to beat placebo on three of four efficacy outcomes (of which one was a primary outcome). Moreover, they did not mention that the rates of treatment-emergent self-harm and other psychiatric adverse events were significantly higher in patients treated with fluoxetine than in patients not treated with fluoxetine. Clinicians simply skimming the abstract may thus understandably gain the false impression that fluoxetine alone is both effective and safe in adolescents. This false impression was reinforced in the conclusions of the main text, where the authors claimed "The effectiveness outcomes were clear and the clinical implications straightforward … Fluoxetine alone was effective, but not as effective as fluoxetine with CBT" [782]. This statement is problematic, for there was no definite statistical evidence for the efficacy of fluoxetine against placebo on one of two primary outcomes. Conclusive statistical evidence of effectiveness would imply that fluoxetine was significantly better than placebo on both primary outcomes. Fluoxetine also failed to demonstrate efficacy on both secondary outcomes, that is, patient self-reported depression and suicidal thinking. Moreover, the data clearly indicate that fluoxetine treatment was associated with increased rates of self-harm and other psychiatric adverse events, which was not mentioned in the abstract and in the conclusions of the main text. Finally, and worthy of note, at the naturalistic 36-week follow-up reported in another publication, the response rates for fluoxetine combined with CBT, fluoxetine alone, and CBT alone did not differ (86%, 81% and 81%). That is, although CBT alone was less effective than fluoxetine (alone or in combination with CBT) in the acute placebo-controlled 12-week phase, at week 36 it was just as effective as medication, indicating that psychotherapy, quite understandably, takes a bit longer to work than medication. Moreover, at week 36 there were significantly more suicidal events in patients treated with fluoxetine alone (14.7%) as compared to combination therapy (8.4%) or CBT (6.3%) [783]. According to these long-term outcomes, fluoxetine alone seems not indicated in adolescents with major depression due to increased risk of self-harm.

Paroxetine Study 329

Nowhere else became the deleterious impact of selective reporting and spin coupled with aggressive off-label promotion (i.e. promotion for an unapproved condition) more evident than in antidepressant prescribing for paediatric depression [289, 771, 784]. A particularly revealing (and shocking) case in point is the study 329, a paroxetine trial in adolescents with depression sponsored by its manufacturer GlaxoSmithKline. Various books and articles had been written about this infamous, fraudulent trial that served as an infomercial to promote off-label paroxetine prescribing in youth [29, 322, 770, 785, 786]. The trial even has its own Wikipedia entry, https://en.wikipedia.org/wiki/Study_329. Before I will go into detail of why this study is a prime example of fraud in industry-sponsored antidepressant trials, it is important to stress that we would never have known the full extent of this scandal if GlaxoSmithKline had not been pressured to release internal documents and provide free access to the clinical study report (which comes close to the raw data) through litigation. The original article by Keller and colleagues on the 8-week acute phase results reported that paroxetine (93 participants), but not imipramine (95 participants), was significantly better than placebo (87 participants) on four of eight efficacy outcomes. Rates of withdrawal from the study because of adverse events were 9.7% for paroxetine, 31.5% for imipramine, and 6.9% for placebo. The article further reported 11 serious adverse events in the paroxetine group, 5 in the imipramine group, and 2 in the placebo group. 5 suicidal and self-injurious adverse events were reported for paroxetine, 3 for imipramine, and 1 for placebo. The authors concluded that "Paroxetine is generally well tolerated and effective for major depression in adolescents" [787].

The documents released through litigation, including the clinical study report, and a comprehensive re-analysis of the data by independent academics, tell of a completely different story [29, 322, 770, 785]. The Keller et al. article was largely ghostwritten by a medical communication firm in close collaboration with GlaxoSmithKline's marketing department. Most "authors" listed on the paper had financial relationships with GlaxoSmithKline (mostly honoraria for serving on advisory board and speakers' bureau), which were not declared in the published article. The two primary outcomes and the five secondary outcomes designated in the study protocol were all negative, that is, paroxetine failed to beat placebo on any of the prespecified efficacy outcomes. All four efficacy outcomes demonstrating statistical significance in the Keller et al. article were introduced post-hoc by GlaxoSmithKline after dredging the data (also referred to as p-hacking). The two prespecified primary outcomes that failed to demonstrate efficacy were reported in the article but presented as if they were secondary outcomes. Of the five prespecified secondary outcomes (which also failed to demonstrate efficacy), only two were reported in the article, the others were omitted. Thus, in short, paroxetine unequivocally failed to demonstrate efficacy. It is only through concealing prespecified outcomes and creating new ones post-hoc that GlaxoSmithKline could give a false impression of some questionable efficacy [322, 770, 785].

But GlaxoSmithKline also deceived on a large scale to present paroxetine as safe and "generally well tolerated" [787]. The comparator drug imipramine was dosed way too high, so that it caused a lot of side effects and discontinuation due to adverse events (the latter at an incredibly high rate of 31.5%) [29, 770]. As detailed above, overdosing a comparator drug is a common strategy so that the sponsor's drug looks safer and better tolerated in comparison [62, 84]. In addition, many adverse events were miscoded and misreported, including reasons for premature treatment discontinuation. Contrary to the rate of discontinuation due to adverse events of 9.7% for paroxetine reported by Keller et al., the independent re-analysis of the data by Le Noury et al. showed a rate of 15.0% for paroxetine [322], that is, about twice the rate for placebo (6.9%). According to the clinical study report, the rate of serious adverse events (mostly suicidal and self-injurious events) were 11.8% for paroxetine and 2.3% for placebo, a statistically significant difference [785]. Very concerning was also the misrepresentation of suicidal and self-injurious behaviours. These adverse events were mostly miscoded as "emotional lability" and some events listed in the appendix were not included. Contrary to 5, 3, and 1 events for paroxetine, imipramine, and placebo reported by Keller et al., the clinical study report stated 7, 3 and 1 events, and the re-analysis by Le Noury et al. found 11, 4, and 2 events [322]. That is, paroxetine use was related to a clear excess of suicidal and self-injurious behaviours. According to my own calculation, the rate was significantly higher with paroxetine compared to placebo based on the data given by both the clinical study report (7.5% vs. 1.1%) and Le Noury et al (11.8% vs. 2.3%). In this respect it's also important to mention the number of severe psychiatric adverse events (including but not limited to suicidal and self-injurious behaviours) reported in the re-analysis. Le Noury et al found 32 severe psychiatric adverse events for paroxetine (among 93 participants) compared to 4 for imipramine (among 95 participants) and 6 for placebo (among 87 participants), a difference that is clinically meaningful and statistically highly significant (my own calculation).

In conclusion, the ghostwritten report of study 329 by GlaxoSmithKline (i.e. Keller et al., 2001) stated that paroxetine was effective and generally well tolerated in adolescents with depression [787]. However, careful examination of the clinical study report and a comprehensive re-analysis of the raw data by independent academics showed that paroxetine was not only ineffective, but harmful [322, 785]. GlaxoSmithKline applied a variety of fraudulent and unethical strategies to misrepresent the efficacy and safety of paroxetine, including a comparator drug dosed way too high, selective reporting of efficacy outcomes, post-hoc creation of new outcomes, and both underreporting and miscoding of (severe/serious) adverse events. In addition, GlaxoSmithKline intentionally withheld data from a second paroxetine trial for adolescent depression that also failed to demonstrate efficacy and safety (study 377). This second trial was completed in 1998, that is, long before the results of study 329 were published in 2001. When pooled together, these two trials showed that paroxetine was completely ineffective and associated with a significantly increased rate of suicidal behaviour compared to placebo [58, 786]. To withhold the data of both trials from drug regulators (which would have immediately noted these issues), the company did not seek regulatory approval for paroxetine in adolescent depression [788].

In an internal GlaxoSmithKline document titled "Seroxat/Paxil Adolescent Depression: Position piece on the phase III clinical studies", the marketing department gave recommendations on how to deal with the two negative adolescent trials. "Effectively manage the dissemination of these data in order to minimize any potential negative commercial impact", the document states. And further, "It would be commercially unacceptable to include a statement that efficacy had not been demonstrated, as this would undermine the profile of paroxetine" [788]. So GlaxoSmithKline clearly knew that paroxetine should not be used in adolescents, but the company remained silent about lack of efficacy and increased risk of suicidal behaviour. Quite the contrary, the company exploited the distorted Keller et al. publication to aggressively promote off-label use of paroxetine for adolescent depression, knowing that it was neither effective nor safe [29, 322, 770, 785]. In a memorandum to its sales representatives, the company stated "This 'cutting edge,' landmark study is the first to compare efficacy of an SSRI and a TCA with placebo in the treatment of major depression in adolescents. *Paxil* demonstrates REMARKABLE Efficacy and Safety in the treatment of adolescent depression" [785]. This message was further disseminated at conferences and in the media by GlaxoSmithKline's key opinion leaders, influential academic psychiatrists on the company's payroll [29, 770].

Fortunately, in mid-2003, drug regulators issued a safety warning and stressed that paroxetine should not be used in children and adolescents due to treatment-emergent suicidality [789]. Based on their evaluation, the UK Committee on the Safety of Medicines (CSM) concluded that there is "a clear increase in suicidal behaviour versus placebo" [786]. As summarised by McGoey and Jackson,

> "It seems unarguable, then, that for five years, GSK [GlaxoSmithKline] deliberately failed to disclose clinical trial data which provided evidence that Seroxat should not be prescribed to under-18s. Given that, in 1999 alone, 32 000 prescriptions for Seroxat had been issued to children in the UK, it is clear that in the time-lag between the completion of the relevant clinical trials (1998) and the CSM's warning notices (2003), tens of thousands of under-18s were prescribed a drug that was unlikely to work, and which carried an unacceptable risk of a serious, indeed fatal, adverse reaction. We do not know how many, if any, under-18s actually committed suicide between 1998 and 2003 as a result of taking Seroxat, but given the large number of children involved, it is certainly possible that deaths occurred which could have been avoided by prompt disclosure of this information". [786]

Years later, in 2012, GlaxoSmithKline pleaded guilty and was fined US$3 billion by the US Department of Justice for large-scale healthcare fraud, including illegal promotion of paroxetine for unapproved adolescent depression, creating misleading journal articles making unsubstantiated and/or false representations or statements about safety and efficacy of paroxetine, and hiding paroxetine trials that had negative findings [790]. But what about the fraudulent publication of study 329 by Keller et al., which has in total 808 citations as of June 2021? You would certainly think that a scientific journal has the ethical and legal obligation to retract a fraudulent research article. Well, you err. Despite several requests and unequivocal evidence that the article misreports and misrepresents the efficacy and safety of paroxetine, including a legal conviction by the US Department of Justice, the *Journal of the American Academy of Child and Adolescent Psychiatry* who published the article, refuses to retract it [29, 770, 791]. In fact, the American Academy of Child and Adolescent Psychiatry, the owner of the journal, deliberately turns a blind eye to this nefarious study. As stated by Dr. Doshi, "No correction, no retraction, no apology, no comment" [791]. By consequence, the false and misleading findings of study 329 remain in the scientific literature and the article is still widely cited, not only as a prime example of scientific fraud, but also as "evidence" that paroxetine is effective and generally well tolerated in adolescents with major depression.

In sum, the efficacy and safety of antidepressants is systematically misrepresented in the scientific literature due to methodological biases, selective reporting, and spin. It is therefore almost impossible to evaluate the drugs' true treatment effects, especially in real-world routine care. The chapter has also shown that the pharmaceutical industry, psychiatric associations, and eminent academics play a major role in this pervasive distortion of the scientific evidence. This leads us directly to the next chapter, "Conflicts of interest in medicine".

5

Conflicts of Interest in Medicine

Multiple factors contribute to overprescribing of antidepressants (especially in mild and subthreshold depression), including the adoption of managed care plans, consumerism, the unsubstantiated public (and professional) belief that depression is caused by a chemical imbalance that can be fixed with a pill, physicians' time constraints, restricted access to or unavailability of non-pharmacological treatments, depression awareness campaigns, disease marketing and aggressive promotion of pharmaceuticals, an unevidenced (false) conviction that antidepressants work in mild and subthreshold depression, overestimation of antidepressants' benefits and underestimation of harms due to selective reporting of favourable trial results and systematic methodological biases in antidepressant trials, and physicians' overreliance on pharmacological treatments coupled with a reluctance to accept non-pharmacological treatments as effective and safe alternatives [9, 11, 13, 14, 25, 26, 57, 134, 188, 368, 369, 623, 792, 793]. These factors were discussed in detail in the chapters "The transformation of depression" and "Flaws in antidepressant research". In this chapter I will address a pernicious and pervasive problem that is closely related and often a driver of the factors detailed above: conflicts of interest in medicine.

M. P. Hengartner, *Evidence-biased Antidepressant Prescription*,
https://doi.org/10.1007/978-3-030-82587-4_5

In his fierce but legitimate critique of evidence-based medicine, leading medical researcher Dr. John Ioannidis, professor at Stanford University, stressed:

> "As EBM [evidence-based medicine] became more influential, it was also hijacked to serve agendas different from what it originally aimed for. Influential randomized trials are largely done by and for the benefit of the industry. Meta-analyses and guidelines have become a factory, mostly also serving vested interests. National and federal research funds are funneled almost exclusively to research with little relevance to health outcomes. We have supported the growth of principal investigators who excel primarily as managers absorbing more money. Diagnosis and prognosis research and efforts to individualize treatment have fueled recurrent spurious promises. Risk factor epidemiology has excelled in salami-sliced data-dredged articles with gift authorship and has become adept to dictating policy from spurious evidence. Under market pressure, clinical medicine has been transformed to finance-based medicine. In many places, medicine and health care are wasting societal resources and becoming a threat to human well-being". [377]

To be clear, this is not just some opinion of a dissenting academic; these are established facts, consistently supported by compelling scientific evidence [57, 149, 592, 674, 767, 772, 794–799]. "Moral arguments for transparency aside, there is little debate that relevant financial or other professional and intellectual interests can, and have, distorted medical research, education, guidelines, and practice", recently wrote the editor in chief of the *British Medical Journal* and the director of the Centre for Evidence-Based Medicine at the University of Oxford [800]. Thus, in the following, I will outline the various conflicts of interest that have corrupted medical research, education, and practice, including drug regulators, academic departments, researchers, and practitioners.

Let's start with a short definition of conflicts of interest in medicine. "Conflict of interest arises when an activity is accompanied by a divergence between personal or institutional benefit when compared to the responsibilities to patients and to society; it arises in the context of research, purchasing, leadership, and investments. Conflict of interest is of concern because it compromises the trust of the patient and of society in the individual physician or the medical center" [801]. Dr Howard Brody offers the following criteria for a conflict of interest: "1. The physician has a duty to advocate for the interests of the patient (or public). 2. The physician is also subject to other interests—her or his own, or those of a third party. 3. The physician becomes a party to certain social arrangements. 4. Those arrangements, as viewed by a reasonable onlooker, would tempt a person of normal human psychology to neglect the patient's/public's interests in favor of the physician's (or third party's)" [802]. Although financial conflicts of interest, that is, physicians' financial relationships with the biomedical industry, are presumably the most pervasive and best researched form of conflicts of interest in medicine, others should not be ignored. Non-financial conflicts of interest include, among others, personal or institutional expectations/demands and the desire for prestige and career progression [803].

In biomedical, social and psychological research, it is well established that, to advance in their career, junior scientists are pushed (incentivised) to produce spectacular and novel research findings, as much and as fast as possible, because promotion and tenure in academia are awarded by and large for number of high-impact publications and sum of grants acquired [42, 373, 804]. These incentives impose potent conflicts of interest, as they force researchers to value quantity over quality, may compel them to dredge and misrepresent their data, and to selectively report favourable research findings. In result, most research findings do not replicate and are presumably false or massively exaggerated [46, 48, 50, 493, 496, 510, 805].

In psychotherapy, most researchers strongly identify with a particular school of therapy, for example psychodynamic therapy or cognitive-behavioural therapy. By consequence, researchers devoted to one particular type of therapy have systematically overestimated the efficacy of their own therapy and downplayed the efficacy of the rival therapies, a bias known as the allegiance effect [806, 807]. In medicine, this motivation to advance the interests of a specific professional society or association is better known as the defence (or abidance) of guild interests [808, 809]. Therefore, a critical stance towards treatments and/or disease concepts established within a medical society/association (i.e., the guild) creates a professional conflict of interest, as individuals may risk their reputation and position among colleagues. As aptly stated by Dr. Krumholz,

> "Unfortunately, our profession does not often reward those who question dogma. In fact, there are many episodes throughout the history of medicine and science in which truth was resisted and dogmatic beliefs, however poorly supported by evidence, were imposed by those in a position to do so … We are trained to defer to authority, not to question it … Those who ask difficult questions or challenge conventional wisdom are often isolated. They may find few opportunities to speak and their writings may not be welcome. Compliance with normative behavior may be forced by fear of recrimination. In some cases, junior faculty may fear that support from mentors will be withdrawn or promotions denied". [810]

Iatrogenic harm, that is, prescribed medical treatments that caused harm to patients, is one particular area in medicine that is strongly affected by professional conflicts of interest. As a case in point, let us quickly have a look at a recent study by Bennett and colleagues [811]. Among others, they examined the repercussions (sanctions) clinicians experienced when they published reports of very serious adverse reactions from blockbuster drugs (and one medical device). Of 18 clinicians that alerted professionals and the public about very serious adverse reactions, 11 (61%) experienced personal or professional negative consequences. One professor of medicine lost an academic medical position, one clinician was sued by a pharmaceutical company, five clinicians reported receiving personal threats from executives of pharmaceutical manufacturers, and eight clinicians reported that their integrity and reputation was publicly disparaged.

In the following chapter I will examine in more detail how defensively (and ignorant) the healthcare sector habitually responds when professionals alert to harms from medical interventions. I also detail the denial and minimisation of harm patients typically face when they report damage from medical interventions (i.e. iatrogenic harm), which I understand as a consequence of professional conflicts of interest in medicine.

Denial and Minimisation of Harm

Professional (or guild) interests have resulted not only in marginalisation and discrediting of professionals who warned of serious adverse reactions from established treatments [810–812] but also in a pernicious culture of dismissing patient reports of iatrogenic harms. Very recently, the Cumberlege review exposed pervasive and alarming flaws in the UK healthcare system in response to patients' reports of harm from drugs and medical devices [813]. According to the author, "We have found that the healthcare system—in which I include the NHS [National Health Service], private providers, the regulators and professional bodies, pharmaceutical and device manufacturers, and policymakers—is disjointed, siloed, unresponsive and defensive. It does not adequately recognise that patients are its raison d'etre. It has failed to listen to their concerns and when, belatedly, it has decided to act it has too often moved glacially" [813]. The review provides clear evidence that the medical profession too often shows an alarming disregard for its fundamental ethical principle—first do no harm. According to Helen Haskell, a patient safety advocate commenting on the Cumberlege review,

> "Perhaps most striking was the testimony from hundreds of patients reporting lack of informed consent for their initial treatment, followed by years of dismissal by clinicians and regulators who did not want to associate life altering symptoms or injured children with their medical interventions … The review panel found that healthcare providers' dismissive attitude toward patients was underpinned by a reluctance in all parts of the system to collect evidence on potential harms, by a lack of coordination that would allow clinicians and agencies to interpret and act on that information, and by a culture of denial that failed to acknowledge harm and error, impeding learning and safety". [814]

The Cumberlege review is no exception. A survey conducted by ProPublica in over 1000 US patients who experienced iatrogenic harm yielded similar results [815]. Only 9% of harmed patients who completed the questionnaire said that the hospital (or other treatment facility) voluntarily acknowledged the harm; 10% of hospitals acknowledged under pressure, and nearly all other patients said they were ignored (44%) or responsibility for the harm was denied (31%) by the hospital. The situation was no better at the level of individual healthcare providers: only 13% voluntarily acknowledged the harm, 9% acknowledged under pressure, and almost all other providers ignored the complaint (40%) or denied responsibility (35%). The authors thus concluded, "Many patients described feeling victimized a second time by the way they were treated after experiencing harm. After placing trust in caregivers, they were surprised to encounter stonewalling, denial and blame" [815].

Are these accusations warranted? In my view, and based on my personal experience (persistent problems after urogenital surgery as a child), yes, they are. But don't just take my word for it. Instead let us scrutinise the scientific evidence and see what the literature tells us about denial and minimisation of iatrogenic harm. For instance, in a survey of patients with self-reported adverse drug reactions from statins, the physicians were more likely to deny than to affirm a connection between the reported adverse events and the statin. According to the study authors, "Rejection of a possible connection was reported to occur even for symptoms with strong literature support for a drug connection, and even in patients for whom the symptom met presumptive literature-based criteria for probable or definite drug-adverse effect causality" [816]. This denial of adverse drug effects has far-reaching consequences because it results in significant underreporting and thus belated formal recognition of (and reaction to) drug-related harms. For instance, in a survey of clinicians investigating 65 suspected adverse drug reactions, the authors stressed that not one event was ever reported to an external drug safety (pharmacovigilance) agency [817]. In accordance, a systematic review found that, on average, only 6% of all adverse drug reactions were formally reported, yielding an underreporting rate of 94% [818]. The authors thus concluded "This systematic review provides evidence of significant and widespread underreporting of ADRs [adverse drug reactions] to spontaneous reporting systems including serious or severe ADRs" [818].

Perhaps you may argue that adverse drug reactions are very rare and thus a minor issue for public health. But that's wrong [376, 678]. Adverse drug reactions account for about 5–7% of all hospital admissions, of which most are deemed avoidable [723, 819]. According to a meta-analysis, 7% of all hospitalised patients experienced an adverse drug reaction, and the rate of fatal adverse drug reactions was 0.3%, that is 3 in every 1000 patients, "making these reactions between the fourth and sixth leading cause of death" [820]. That is, although prescription drugs undeniably can be extremely helpful and lifesaving, quite often they can also be very harmful and, sadly, kill many people unnecessarily. The massive underreporting of severe harm from drugs is therefore a serious public health issue, since pharmacovigilance (drug safety evaluation) systems depend on full reporting of suspected adverse drug reactions. Because suspected adverse drug reactions are rarely reported, by consequence, drug regulators all too frequently fail to timely detect and adequately respond to drug safety issues [171, 821].

It has also been shown that pharmaceutical companies deliberately ignored, misrepresented, and underreported suspected adverse drug reactions [376, 458, 822]. Drug regulators heavily rely on the pharmaceutical companies to timely, objectively, and transparently report suspected adverse drug reactions. If they don't, then dangerous (harmful) treatments may remain on the market for too long, causing tremendous damage to hundreds of thousands of patients [678, 811]. But as Dr. Abraham already noted in 2002, "It is demonstrated that a pharmaceutical firm's commitment to search effectively for evidence against the safety of its own product in order to confirm doctors' warnings can have severe limitations" [823]. He was tragically proven right in various high-profile cases such as the Vioxx scandal, where the manufacturer Merck deliberately obscured a clear harm signal for its blockbuster drug rofecoxib (Vioxx) and withheld important safety data from the FDA [797, 824]. Rofecoxib was belatedly withdrawn from the market by Merck in late 2004 for causing major adverse cardiovascular events (e.g., stroke, myocardial infarction) and increasing all-cause mortality, but internal documents released through litigation revealed that the company suspected such a safety issue since the 1990s and definitely knew about the serious cardiovascular harm since mid-2001, that is, long before they officially acknowledged this safety issue [797, 824]. Many thousand lives could have been saved had the pharmaceutical company not systematically engaged in "deflection, silence, denial, suppression, and lying to physicians and the public" [678].

But inadequate post-marketing surveillance is just one among many issues in drug safety regulation. As summarized by Dr. Furberg and colleagues in an article published in the top-tier journal *Archives of Internal Medicine*,

> "The current Food and Drug Administration (FDA) system of regulating drug safety has serious limitations and is in need of changes. The major problems include the following: the design of initial preapproval studies lets uncommon, serious adverse events go undetected; massive underreporting of adverse events to the FDA postmarketing surveillance system reduces the ability to quantify risk accurately; manufacturers do not fulfill the majority of their postmarketing safety study commitments; the FDA lacks authority to pursue sponsors who violate regulations and ignore postmarketing safety study commitments; the public increasingly perceives the FDA as having become too close to the regulated pharmaceutical industry; the FDA's safety oversight structure is suboptimal; and the FDA's expertise and resources in drug safety and public health are limited". [821]

This failure to adequately assess the safety of drugs is well evidenced by the fact that, despite clear harm signals detected during the review of new drug applications, drug regulators approved several drugs with questionable safety profile. By consequence, various of these drugs had to be withdrawn from the market after a while because they had caused too much serious harm [148, 825]. According to a comprehensive analysis by Lasser and colleagues, 8% of all drugs approved by the FDA between 1975 and 1999 acquired one or more serious safety warnings (referred to as black box warnings) and 3% were withdrawn from the market. The probability of acquiring a serious safety warning or being withdrawn from the market after 25 years was a staggering 20% [826]. These alarming figures were consistently replicated in a more recent study focusing on drugs approved by the Canadian drug regulators between 1995 and 2010 [827].

It is also worthy of note that antidepressants are not exempt from belatedly detected serious safety issues requiring their withdrawal from the market. Examples include nomifensine (introduced 1976, withdrawn 1986 due to haematological effects), zimeldine (introduced 1982, withdrawn 1983 due to peripheral neuropathy; never approved in the US), and nefazodone (introduced 1993, withdrawn 2003 due to hepatotoxicity) [148, 825]. In the remainder of this chapter I will focus in detail on professional conflicts of interest in psychiatry in relation to antidepressants and psychiatric drug treatment in general.

Psychiatry Comes to the Defense of Antidepressants

"It is painful to discover how many lives have been harmed and harmed badly when psychiatry is done badly. Psychiatric diagnosis at its worst leads to psychiatric treatment at its worst, and together the combination is a recipe for disaster. The casualties are a living and much-needed rebuke to the field and provide the inspiration and passion for the sizable anti-psychiatry movement. Psychiatry must learn from its bad outcomes and take very seriously the often well-deserved attacks of its critics", wrote Dr. Allen Frances, professor of psychiatry and chair of the DSM-IV workgroup, in his book *Saving Normal* [414]. He wrote these lines because he had a good sense and first-hand experience that psychiatry usually does a poor job when it comes to adequately responding to criticism of careless psychiatric diagnosis and indiscriminate drug treatment. Dr. Peter Gotzsche went even one step further and maintained that the minimisation of drug-related harms in psychiatry amounts to "organised denial" [147]. But why is that?

Drugs are the mainstay of contemporary psychiatry in both research and practice [392, 394, 399, 828]. Psychiatric drugs are the first-line treatment in almost all mental disorders, they spurred the biological revolution, build the foundation of biomedical models, helped to consolidate psychiatry as a medical specialty, and granted the profession generous financial support from the pharmaceutical industry. In short, "Drugs, of course, were the centerpiece of the new [psychiatric] era" [394]. Non-pharmacological interventions typically play a subsidiary role, both in research and practice, and are often considered second-line or adjunct treatments despite proven efficacy and safety as first-line therapies. In view of the fundamental importance of medication in psychiatry, challenging the overreliance on drugs as well as their efficacy and safety, understandably threatens psychiatry's professional (guild) interests [29, 30, 829]. While psychiatrists hardly respond to unfavourable evaluations of psychosocial interventions, they tend to turn out in force when drugs are the target of criticism. That is, whenever researchers or the media question the safety and/or efficacy of popular psychiatric drugs like antidepressants and antipsychotics, not before long various eminent psychiatrists will step in to defend the drugs, quite often harshly, patronising, and with condescending authority [29, 830, 831].

For instance, when in 2017 the UN Special Rapporteur on Human Rights, Dr. Dainius Puras, himself a trained psychiatrist, criticised the excessive frontline use of psychiatric drugs and the overreliance on biomedical models of mental health services, two psychiatrists published a fierce reply titled "Responding to the UN Special Rapporteur's antipsychiatry bias" in the *Australian and New Zealand Journal of Psychiatry*. In the article, they again alleged that "These arguments align with those of the global anti-psychiatry movement" [832]. Unfortunately, this article is no exception, and this pejorative label and similar others were also thrown at me several times. On social media, I was fiercely attacked by various psychiatrists. I was discredited and insulted, I was called "antipsychiatrist", "anti-vaxxer", "pill-shamer", "ideologically biased partisan", "flat-earth-believer", and so on. Perhaps these psychiatrists are not aware that I also wrote critical articles about the evidence base in clinical psychology and psychotherapy [55, 833]. Yet I was never labelled "antipsychology" or "anti-psychotherapy".

The anti-psychiatry argument is very common in debates about the effectiveness of antidepressants and other psychopharmaceuticals (for example, see [22]), and of course it is a strawman and merely serves to stifle a much-needed discussion about overdiagnosis and overprescribing of psychiatric drugs [834]. I am not aware that any academic who wrote critically about psychiatric drug use, including, among others, Drs Moncrieff, Kirsch, Gotzsche, Munkholm, Glenmullen, Jakobsen, Plöderl, Davies, Read, Healy, Bschor, Fava, Cosgrove, Zito, Ioannidis, Warren, Summerfield, Jureidini, Timimi, Kinderman, and, of course myself, identifies as anti-psychiatry. And even if some do, it would by no means invalidate their scientific arguments. Another malicious tactic, very popular during the 1990s but still prevalent today to delegitimise the arguments of critical authors is to associate dissenting views on psychiatric drugs with the sect of Scientology [9, 399]. But this is such a ridiculous accusation that I don't want to further comment on it. Let's instead focus on other (unscientific) accusations.

Another frequent argument purports that authors with a critical stance towards antidepressants and the current drug-centred treatment paradigm of depression are mostly psychologists or doctors without specialised knowledge in psychiatry (for example, see [23]). This is again a strawman and has no bearing on the current debate. And it's also a terribly flawed argument at that. First, and most importantly, even if most critics were psychologists and doctors without specialised knowledge in psychiatry, this would not invalidate their scientific arguments. Second, many (perhaps most) academics who wrote critically about antidepressants (and other psychiatric drugs) are in fact psychiatrists (e.g. Drs Healy, Moncrieff, Steingard, Horowitz, Breggin, Timimi, Munkholm, Frances, Glenmullen, Bschor, Fava, Summerfield, Jureidini). Third, GPs (i.e., doctors without specialised knowledge in psychiatry) treat a much larger portion of people with psychological problems than psychiatrists and, as a group, they also prescribe many more antidepressants (and psychiatric drugs in general) than psychiatrists [575, 639, 725, 835]. Fourth, clinical psychologists are extensively trained in psychopathology and psychiatric nosology, and they often work in inpatient or outpatient psychiatric services, treating patients with mild to very severe mental health problems. Insinuating that they lack specialised knowledge in psychiatry (simply because they have no prescribing rights) is wrong, arrogant, patronising, and possibly just another attempt to retain the power imbalance in the mental health field.

When Dr. Irving Kirsch, professor of psychology at Harvard University, published his three seminal meta-analyses in 1998 [742], 2002 [836] and 2008 [198], demonstrating that antidepressants were just marginally better than placebo, there was a furious outcry from many eminent psychiatrists [11, 605]. An unprecedented media frenzy followed, often sensationalist rather than scientifically balanced and critical. Kirsch became kind of an academic celebrity. In Kirsch's own words, "Somehow, I had been transformed, from a mild-mannered university professor into a media superhero—or super villain, depending on whom you asked" [605]. For the media he was often a superhero, but for most psychiatric professionals he clearly was a super villain. Dr Kirsch was fiercely attacked by various psychiatric organisations, their spokespersons, and many influential academic psychiatrists (including, foremost, key opinion leaders, the product champions working for the pharmaceutical industry). In heated (and sometimes hateful) articles, various critics argued that his findings were biased, that he had applied flawed statistical methods, and that he had intentionally misinterpreted the data (see, for example [21, 837, 838]).

Perhaps the most furious response came in 2012 from the APA in person of the then-president-elect Dr. Jeffrey Lieberman. "Dr. Kirsch is mistaken and confused, and he's ideologically biased in his thinking. He is conducting an analysis and interpreting the data to support his ideologically biased perspective. What he is concluding is inaccurate, and what he is communicating is misleading to people and potentially harmful to those who really suffer from depression and would be expected to benefit from antidepressant medication. To say that antidepressants are no better than placebo is just plain wrong", complained Dr. Lieberman in an interview with Medscape [830].

I received a similar "feedback" on my research from the heads of the Swiss psychiatric association, but more on this below. For now, let's stay with Kirsch, as his work on antidepressants was very influential. Still, I want to clarify a few things: I don't contend that Kirsch's statistical analysis and data interpretation had no inadequacies [839]. Personally, I also don't agree with him that antidepressants are merely active placebos (that is, placebos with physical side effects), for they certainly have psychotropic effects [276, 278]. However, it is debatable whether these psychotropic ("mind-altering") effects clearly help to improve depression in most users [18, 274, 840]. Moreover, it is important to stress that Kirsch's main finding—the marginally small average treatment effect of about 2 points on the Hamilton Depression Rating Scale or an effect size of about 0.3—was independently confirmed by many other research groups, including the FDA, and thus is certainly correct [10, 13, 17, 57, 175, 196, 739].

Criticism of statistical analyses and data interpretation are a crucial part of the scientific process, but I strictly oppose to accusations that Kirsch was driven by malicious motives. It is the offensive (and discrediting) way he was criticised that is absolutely inappropriate in scientific discourse. Unfortunately, ad-hominem attacks and personal insults are no rarity in psychiatry (and medicine in general). Another case in point is the furious attack on Dr. Peter Gotzsche, a high-profile medical researcher and co-founder of the Cochrane collaboration known for his critical stance on psychiatric drugs [147]. The provocative article was written by Dr. David Nutt (professor of neuropsychopharmacology at Imperial College London and former president of the European College of Neuropsychopharmacology; he has extensive financial ties to multiple pharmaceutical companies) together with various other leaders of British psychiatry. These co-authors included Dr. Guy Goodwin (professor of psychiatry at University of Oxford; he also has extensive financial ties to multiple pharmaceutical companies), Dr. Dinesh Bhugra (professor of psychiatry at King's College London), Dr. Seena Fazel (professor of psychiatry at Oxford University), and Dr. Stephen Lawrie (professor of psychiatry at University of Edinburgh). Their article was published in the prestigious journal *Lancet Psychiatry* and in the title of this paper the authors already insinuated that Gotzsche is ideologically biased, posing the rhetorical question "Attacks on antidepressants: signs of deep-seated stigma?" [22]. And in the main text, the authors mockingly asked, "why would Professor Gøtzsche apparently suspend his training in evidence analysis for popular polemic?". The authors concluded their critique by claiming "extreme assertions such as those made by Prof Gøtzsche are insulting to the discipline of psychiatry and at some level express and reinforce stigma against mental illnesses and the people who have them. The medical profession must challenge these poorly thought-out negative claims by one of its own very vigorously" [22]. This is the kind of backlash (repercussion) academics receive when they critically write about psychiatric drugs. And now I'll recount my own story.

My Personal Experience

The president of the Swiss psychiatric association is Dr. Erich Seifritz, professor of psychiatry at the University of Zurich and director of the Psychiatric University Hospital of Zurich (where I did my PhD and habilitation). He was (and presumably still is) dismayed by my research on antidepressants. He complained about me to Dr. Rössler, my former doctorate supervisor and co-author on many of my research papers (including a few papers on antidepressants). Dr. Rössler also happens to be the former director of the Psychiatric University Hospital of Zurich. Anyways, Dr. Seifritz was concerned about two prospective observational studies I conducted with Dr. Rössler showing a prospective association between antidepressant use and worse long-term mental health outcomes, even when carefully controlling for treatment selection (for example depression severity, global functioning, comorbid anxiety disorders, etc.) [220, 841]. Dr. Seifritz also published a commentary to one of these studies, claiming that its methodology was terribly flawed, and "Therefore, the paper is certainly misleading and, furthermore, potentially harmful" [842]. This strong accusation warrants some comments.

The methods we applied were not "terribly flawed". In fact, we used state-of-the-art methodology in observational studies and rigorous statistical adjustments, controlling for much more potential confounders than many previous and subsequent studies did (see, for example [484, 843, 844]). Yet, I do not contend that my studies prove a cause–effect relationship. It is just an observed association, and we were pretty clear about that in the papers [220, 841]. I'm also fine with being criticised. Debate and scrutiny are integral parts of the scientific process. I have written several comments on papers I believe had serious methodological flaws and/or drew conclusions not supported by the data (see, for example [19, 845–847]). One study published in *JAMA Psychiatry* was even retracted by the authors after we had pointed out that their statistical model was inadequate and thus had produced false-positive results [848, 849].

In the case of Dr. Seifritz, however, I have the impression that he was primarily protecting guild interests. At regular intervals, in the media and in the scientific literature, he has been defending the dominant drug-centred treatment paradigm in psychiatry. He is also a passionate promoter of antidepressants and makes a considerable personal income as speaker and adviser for various pharmaceutical companies [850]. Between 2015 and 2019 alone, Dr. Seifritz received general (direct) payments from multiple pharmaceutical companies, including, among others, Janssen, Lundbeck, Servier, Eli Lilly, and Pfizer (all companies are manufacturers of antidepressants), for a total amount of 159,313 Swiss Francs (about 148,620 Euros) [851]. A detailed list of the industry payments to

Dr. Seifritz can be accessed freely online under https://www.pharmagelder.ch/recipient/2590-Erich-Seifritz.html. But still, in his critique of my antidepressant study, Dr. Seifritz asserted that his paper "was conducted in the absence of any commercial or financial relationships that could be construed as a potential conflict of interest" [842]. Really? Since when are extensive financial relationships with antidepressant manufacturers not a "potential conflict of interest", especially in an article concerned with the long-term outcome of antidepressant use? In other words, his conflict of interest declaration was factually wrong and thus a clear violation of publication ethics, for the International Committee of Medical Journal Editors (ICMJE) considers non-disclosure of conflicts of interest as research misconduct [852]. But our disagreements didn't stop here.

In late 2019, a leading Swiss newspaper—Tagesanzeiger—printed a large interview with me [853]. In this interview I talked about the overdefinition and overdetection of depression (which is scientifically well established [117, 450, 481]). I also mentioned the modest efficacy of antidepressants and the high risk of adverse effects like sleep problems and sexual dysfunction (which is scientifically well established [10, 13, 140, 336, 854]). I talked about systematic method biases and selective reporting in antidepressant trials (which is scientifically well established [13, 57, 707]). The journalist also mentioned our meta-analysis on the suicide risk in antidepressant trials [332, 855], so I confirmed that there is mounting evidence that antidepressants may cause suicidal behaviour [328, 329, 715] and that antidepressants can even trigger suicidality in mentally healthy users [9, 325]. I further talked about physical dependence and withdrawal reactions from antidepressants (for which there is strong scientific evidence, even though mainstream psychiatry prefers the euphemistic term "discontinuation syndrome" and mistakenly claims that physical dependence, a prerequisite for withdrawal reactions, does not exist [344, 345, 347, 358]). I also mentioned that financial conflicts of interest are pervasive in psychiatry and general medicine and that they systematically bias the scientific evidence in favour of drugs (which is scientifically well established [592, 772, 794, 856]). And, finally, I talked about the chemical imbalance theory of depression that has never been proven and that is widely considered disconfirmed (as most experts in psychopharmacology agree [26, 595, 624]).

A few days later I attended the annual meeting of the German psychiatric association in Berlin to present a new research paper about flaws and inconsistencies in depression treatment guidelines [259]. This conference is also attended by many psychiatrists and other mental health professionals from Switzerland. There I learned from a colleague from the Psychiatric University Hospital of Zurich that Dr. Seifritz was slightly annoyed with me (to put it politely) because of my interview in the Tagesanzeiger. Back in Zurich, not before long, the Tagesanzeiger send me a yet unpublished reply, or rather, a complaint about my interview signed by the heads of the Swiss psychiatric association, including Dr. Seifritz. The letter was titled "We oppose false claims that unsettle ill people" (my own translation) and basically stated, often in a condescending tone and with several strawman arguments, that everything I said in the interview was utterly wrong, misinformed, and misleading. The newspaper asked me to respond to these serious accusations that questioned my scientific expertise and integrity, and so I wrote a comprehensive rebuttal where I meticulously demonstrated that all I said in the interview was supported by robust scientific evidence as referenced above.

To illustrate how absurd some of the complainants' arguments were, here I present three examples. First, Seifritz and colleagues claimed that there is a complete lack of evidence that GPs would overdiagnose depression, when in fact even GPs admit that depression is overdetected [452]. Moreover, the largest meta-analysis on this issue published in the leading medical journal *Lancet* clearly confirmed that GPs make far more false-positive depression diagnoses (misidentifying non-depressed cases as depressed) than false-negative depression diagnoses (missing depressed cases) [450]. So GPs overdiagnose depression, this is an established scientific finding. Second, Seifritz and colleagues claimed that there is not one industry-sponsored academic chair in Switzerland, when in fact an independent investigation conducted in 2016 revealed over 300 contracts between the industry and several Swiss universities, of which most comprised sponsored academic chairs [857]. For example, Interpharma, a Swiss pharmaceutical industry association, sponsored the academic chair of health economics hold by Professor Stefan Felder at the University of

Basel. But that's not all. Interpharma was also allowed to have a say in the nomination of the chair and rewarded Professor Felder with a signing bonus of 300,000 Swiss Francs (about 280,000 Euros). So once again, Seifritz and colleagues made an evidently false claim. Third, Seifritz and colleagues denied that antidepressants cause physical dependence. Obviously, they were ignorant of the fact that physical dependence arises because the body (including the brain) undergoes adaptations to the presence of a psychotropic drug [343], for example serotonin receptor downregulation following SSRI use as demonstrated in a placebo-controlled neuroimaging study [342]. That is, withdrawal syndromes after drug discontinuation can only occur when the body has physiologically adapted to drug exposure, which is the very definition of physical dependence [344, 858]. Their other arguments were mostly strawmen that have no bearing on my points (e.g. "GPs also prescribe antidepressants for indications like anxiety disorders, sleep problems, eating disorders, pain, and pre-menstrual complaints"), which is why I won't further go into detail.

I send my rebuttal of their reply/complaint to the newspaper and asked the editor that he shall publish it along Seifritz and colleagues' letter in order that the readers may decide for themselves whose claims were misinformed and unevidenced. Unfortunately, for some unknown reason (at least to me), Seifritz and colleagues withdrew their reply so both letters were never published. Instead, a few weeks later the newspaper published an interview with Dr. Seifritz, titled "Antidepressants work", where he once more falsely claimed that antidepressants are effective in *mild* depression and that they *protect* against suicidality [859]. As supporting evidence for the former claim, Seifritz cited a meta-analysis that looked at the efficacy of antidepressants in people with *moderate-to-severe* depression [258]. Besides that inferring efficacy in patients with mild depression from results in patients with moderate or severe depression is poor scientific reasoning, it is also worthwhile to point out that the reported treatment effect in patients with moderate to severe depression in said study was so small that it is of questionable practical relevance to the average patient [20]. As detailed in this book, the best scientific evidence available unequivocally shows that the efficacy of antidepressants has not been established in mild, minor, and subthreshold depression

[152, 256, 261–264]. For this reason, most treatment guidelines, including those of the Swiss psychiatric association co-authored by Seifritz [860], do not recommend antidepressants as first-line treatment in this patient population [181, 232, 233]. And regarding suicidality-protective effects, there is clearly a lack of conclusive evidence that would support such a claim, but mounting evidence to the contrary, in particular in adolescents and young adults [292, 321, 323, 324, 329, 330, 333, 715, 861–864].

Seifritz was also asked about common side effects of antidepressants such as sexual dysfunction and sleep problems. He then claimed that antidepressants have few side effects, and that adverse events are often caused by the underlying depression, and not by the drug. The journalist rightly objected that this explanation is ruled out in a placebo-controlled trial, where side effects are established based on the difference between the placebo group and the antidepressant group, thus the influence of the underlying depression is precluded (since, of course, people in the placebo group also have depression). Seifritz then responded that these between-group differences are small [859]. To put that bold claim into perspective: in antidepressant trials where sexual dysfunction was systematically assessed, the rate of treatment-emergent sexual dysfunction in placebo groups is about 12%, as compared to 70% to 80% in groups of many popular SSRIs and SNRIs. This produces an absolute risk difference of 58–68% and a roughly 6 times increased risk causally related to the pharmacological action of antidepressants [336]. With all due respect, but this is not a small effect, it is a very large effect, and claiming otherwise is disingenuous. In fact, it is the strongest effect the SSRI and SNRI antidepressants have. And this effect is much larger than the therapeutic benefit antidepressants may provide, which, according to response rates, is about 40% in placebo groups as compared to 50% in antidepressant groups, thus producing an absolute risk difference of 10% and a rate ratio of merely 1.25 [140]. Compared to the absolute risk difference (58–68%) and the rate ratio (about 6) for treatment-emergent sexual dysfunction, this is a trivial effect. Finally, with respect to efficacy, Dr. Seifritz reluctantly admitted that the average treatment effect in clinical trials is small, but he confidently asserted that in real-world routine practice the treatment effect would be much larger because clinicians would flexibly adjust the dose when patients don't respond adequately to the drug [859]. This is another false claim, for several meta-analyses of randomised controlled trials have consistently shown that adjusting the dose (mostly dose increase) does not provide any benefit compared to a fixed low or medium dose [268, 269, 272].

By now you certainly get an impression of how researchers who question the benefit–harm ratio of antidepressants are treated by academic leaders and how these eminent professors try to correct the record in the scientific literature and the media. I can assure you that these discrediting attacks certainly keep some researchers from addressing critical research questions and asking inconvenient questions. Several psychiatrists told me in private that they doubt whether the benefits of antidepressants outweigh their harms, especially in people with non-severe depression, but they don't dare to talk about this with their colleagues. Renowned professors like Peter Gotzsche, David Healy, and Irving Kirsch will obviously not surrender to senior psychiatric academics despite serious charges levelled against them (for details, see [9, 11, 147]), but many academics, especially junior researchers, may get intimidated when confronted with such hostile responses and thus prefer to remain silent to not threaten their professional career [810]. Thus, deliberately or not, such furious attacks silence dissenting voices and result in scientific censorship. I will now get into more detail on how the scientific discourse has evolved in two controversial areas of antidepressant safety, that is, physical dependence and withdrawal as well as treatment-emergent suicidality.

Physical Dependence and Withdrawal Reactions from Antidepressants

Shortly after the introduction of the tricyclic antidepressants in clinical practice around 1960, case reports alerted practitioners and researchers that, after discontinuation of the drugs, severe withdrawal symptoms can occur [774, 775]. It was also proposed that withdrawal syndromes were due to neurophysiological adaptations following prolonged drug exposure [346]. Unfortunately, this serious issue remained largely ignored and is poorly understood until this day, but there can be little doubt that antidepressant withdrawal symptoms are caused by neurophysiological adaptations, including downregulation and desensitisation of monoamine receptors [865], a pathomechanism also subsumed under the model of oppositional tolerance [223, 351].

Experts in addiction medicine have long recognised that neurophysiological adaptations to a substance are the defining feature of physical dependence and that withdrawal syndromes (including rebound disorders) resulting from physical dependence can occur with about any central nervous system active substance [344, 858]. According to a consensus statement from the American Academy of Pain Medicine, the American Pain Society, and the American Society of Addiction Medicine, "Physical dependence is a state of adaptation that is manifested by a drug class specific withdrawal syndrome that can be produced by abrupt cessation, rapid dose reduction, decreasing blood level of the drug, and/or administration of an antagonist" [866]. The National Institute on Drug Abuse likewise states "Dependence means that when a person stops using a drug, their body goes through 'withdrawal': a group of physical and mental symptoms that can range from mild (if the drug is caffeine) to life-threatening (such as alcohol or opioids, including heroin and prescription pain relievers). Many people who take a prescription medicine every day over a long period of time can become dependent; when they go off the drug, they need to do it gradually, to avoid withdrawal discomfort. But people who are dependent on a drug or medicine aren't necessarily addicted" [867].

Addiction, by contrast, "is characterized by behaviors that include one or more of the following: impaired control over drug use, compulsive use, continued use despite harm, and craving" [866]. Therefore, "For drugs not associated with abuse potential, an individual may still develop dependence; but again, this would not be classified as an addiction" [344]. And according to the National Institute on Drug Abuse, "a person can be dependent on a drug, or have a high tolerance to it, *without* being addicted to it" (emphasis in original) [867]. So the distinction between physical dependence and addiction is conceptually important, but in everyday language, the two terms are often used interchangeably. Complicating matters further, some patients may indicate that they feel addicted to a drug, but basically refer to physical dependence and withdrawal. According to the Cambridge Dictionary, addiction means "an inability to stop doing or using something, especially something harmful", which is also compatible with the notion of physical dependence. It is thus understandable that some patients may describe dependence and the occurrence of severe withdrawal syndromes as addiction.

But don't blame the patients' use of language. Even physicians, including psychiatrists, often get it wrong. The APA and its appointed experts are presumably among the worst offenders. The confusion about dependence, withdrawal, and addiction is nicely depicted by the various revisions of the APA's diagnostic manual of mental disorders. According to the DSM-III, the occurrence of a withdrawal reaction, that is, a drug-specific syndrome following cessation or dose reduction, was sufficient to diagnose (physical) dependence. That definition of dependence was fundamentally changed with the introduction of DSM-III-R in 1987 [858]. In the new diagnostic manual, a withdrawal reaction was not sufficient to diagnose dependence; behavioural symptoms were newly also required (e.g. much time spend to obtain the drug, uncontrolled use, continued use despite problems) [868]. Most importantly, with the introduction of DSM-III-R, addictive behaviours (i.e. uncontrolled, compulsive drug use) were subsumed under the inappropriate term "dependence" and they remain so to this day. As detailed by Dr. O'Brien, "The word 'dependence' was already in use for many years prior to DSM-III-R to describe the adaptations that occur when medications that act on the central nervous system are ingested with rebound if the medication is discontinued abruptly. If the word also stands for compulsive, uncontrolled, drug-seeking behavior, there is inevitable confusion and patients exhibiting normal tolerance and withdrawal without any evidence of abuse or aberrant behavior are associated with those who meet DSM-III-R 'dependence' criteria" [858]. Thus, indeed a very bad (and consequential) decision by the APA's diagnostic working group.

According to the diagnostic criteria of dependence currently applicable, that is, DSM-5 and ICD-10, even severe and persistent withdrawal syndromes would not classify as dependence. Instead, starting with DSM-IV, a new diagnostic group of drug-specific withdrawal syndromes was introduced. Thus, diagnostic manuals have in fact conflated aspects of addiction and dependence, despite being clearly distinct concepts, but at the same time separated withdrawal from dependence, even though withdrawal is a characteristic feature (or consequence) of physical dependence [858, 866, 868]. Interestingly, the DSM-5 does not include a diagnosis of drug addiction. The only mention of the term addiction is via the label of the nosological category "substance-related and addictive disorders". Thus, instead of providing conceptual clarity and consistency, the current psychiatric diagnostic manuals created an ongoing confusion about dependence, withdrawal, and addiction [132, 868, 869]. The diagnostic manuals are therefore largely responsible for the widespread denial of dependence and withdrawal reactions from antidepressants repeatedly demonstrated by many leading psychiatrists and health organisations (see examples below).

In sum, antidepressants don't cause addiction, but they do cause physical dependence, that is, neurophysiological adaptations to drug exposure, or, in medical jargon, the body's compensatory reaction to a drug's pharmacodynamic effects. It has been shown that even short-term antidepressant use can lead to neurophysiological adaptations [342, 870], so antidepressants evidentially do cause dependence and withdrawal reactions [344, 865, 871]. The failure of the diagnostic manuals to differentiate between dependence (characterised by neurophysiological adaptations and withdrawal) and addiction (characterised by craving and compulsive, uncontrolled drug use), was misused by various mental health professionals and medical organisations to maintain the false belief that antidepressants are not dependence-forming. As you remember, a main objective of the Defeat Depression campaign was to educate the public that antidepressants are not drugs of dependence [425]. In a public statement, RCP and RCGP stated "It is worrying that people may fail to take the medicine in the mistaken belief that it can cause dependence" [132]. Well, the public was right, because that's exactly what the drugs do!

What's really worrying is that the British psychiatric association confused addiction with dependence and that it held the mistaken belief that antidepressants cannot cause dependence, that is, neurophysiological adaptations. Do they at least recognise this misconception now? No, unfortunately not. By relying on the incoherent diagnostic criteria (which confound addiction and dependence), in a recent position statement the RCP still erroneously maintained that antidepressant cannot cause dependence [872]. It is thus past time that psychiatry revises its diagnostic criteria according to the conceptual distinction between dependence and addiction long established in addiction medicine [344, 866, 867]. As urged by Dr. O'Brien, addiction expert at the University of Pennsylvania, "Educators with responsibility for teaching about addiction to medical students and general physicians have to explain that there is a normal physiological response called 'physical dependence', and there is 'addiction', which is drug-seeking behavior called 'dependence' in the DSM" [858]. I would add that they should not only educate general physicians about this confusion, but also psychiatrists (the ones who basically created it).

Various critics, including myself, warned that it took health organisations more than 20 years to acknowledge that benzodiazepines can cause dependence and that now they would show the same pattern of persistent denial with respect to antidepressants [9, 132, 147, 871, 873, 874]. We also expressed concern that psychiatric associations and drug regulators may severely underestimate the true burden of withdrawal syndromes (which result from physical dependence) due to their overreliance on the incoherent diagnostic criteria. For instance, Charles Medawar warned about these failures in a *Nature* article back in 1994 [875]. The response to his letter by Dr. Hugh Freeman, eminent psychiatrist and former editor of the *British Journal of Psychiatry*, confirmed that the profession was completely dismissive of withdrawal syndromes following cessation of antidepressant treatment, confusing physical dependence with addiction and treatment need:

> "During the past 35 years, there has in fact been no evidence that any antidepressants—whatever their structure—cause 'addiction' or 'dependence'. Medawar says there is 'profound confusion' over the meaning of these terms and, if so, he has certainly added to it. Diabetics are dependent on insulin and people with high blood pressure are dependent on hypotensives, in the sense they will become ill again if they stop taking the drugs. Many sufferers from depression are in the same position, but this is totally different from the experience of people who take heroin or cocaine as euphoriants". [876]

Freeman's view was endorsed by various official medical bodies over time. For instance, in 2004 the Committee on Safety of Medicines of the British drug regulator MHRA asserted that "There is no clear evidence that the SSRIs and related antidepressants have a significant dependence liability or show development of a dependence syndrome according to internationally accepted criteria (either DSM-IV or ICD-10)" [874]. Again, these authorities merely relied on the fuzzy (and misleading) diagnostic criteria of dependence that confound physical dependence and addiction. They, too, failed to acknowledge the definition established by experts in addiction medicine, according to which a withdrawal syndrome is a consequence of physical dependence, which in turn is due to drug-specific neurophysiological adaptations.

To prevent that prescribers and consumers link antidepressants with physical dependence, in 1997 Eli Lilly sponsored an expert meeting where it established the term "antidepressant discontinuation syndrome" that would soon replace the more appropriate term "withdrawal syndrome" [358]. In an accompanying summary report of this expert meeting, also sponsored by Eli Lilly, the experts claimed, despite a lack of reliable scientific evidence, that "discontinuation syndromes" were extremely rare, and if they would occur, they were commonly mild, short-lived, and self-limiting [877]. Such claims were confidently reiterated by most leading psychiatrists as if they were established scientific facts and given the seal of authority by reproducing them in official practice guidelines [231, 233]. However, there was never strong scientific evidence in support of these claims and we now know that they are misleading and false [345, 350, 351, 357, 358, 878]. But medical organisations were very slow to react or did not change their position at all. Although NICE and RCP now at least acknowledge that withdrawal syndromes can be severe and long-lasting, the APA still falsely maintains that withdrawal syndromes are rare, typically mild and short-lived [357, 879].

The conviction that antidepressants cannot cause dependence is so deeply entrenched in current medical thinking that various psychiatrists and GPs won't believe their own patients when they mention problems resulting from physical dependence [873, 880, 881]. According to a large patient survey conducted by leading Danish psychiatrists published in 2005, in total 57% of antidepressant users with affective disorders agreed that "When you have taken antidepressants over a long period of time it is difficult to stop taking them" and 56% agreed that "Your body can become addicted to antidepressants". The authors, however, were not willing to accept these experiences, and instead they claimed that antidepressant users are misinformed and have mistaken beliefs. In an all too common patronising tone they concluded "Although all these subjects had been treated in hospital settings they still had major ignorance and negative attitudes, suggesting a need for intensified psychoeducational activities" [882]. No, it is not the patients, it is the psychiatrists who need to be educated about dependence and withdrawal! As Adele Framer, founder of the peer-support website SurvivingAntidepressants.org states, "Prescriber failure to monitor, recognize, and timely address withdrawal symptoms is the motivation for almost all the site membership. In their attempts to go off the drugs, almost all have been told they have relapsed, even the many who suffered brain zaps—a hallmark of withdrawal syndrome—and especially those who have had mysterious symptoms for years, consistent with psychotropic PWS [protracted withdrawal syndrome]" [881].

In 2018, science journalists Carey and Gebeloff [883] wrote in an article for the *New York Times*, that many antidepressant users need to continue drug treatment because the withdrawal symptoms that develop upon dose reduction or cessation are unbearable. "Many, perhaps most, people stop the medications without significant trouble. But the rise in longtime use is also the result of an unanticipated and growing problem: Many who try to quit say they cannot because of withdrawal symptoms they were never warned about", wrote the authors. They further explained "In a recent survey of 250 long-term users of psychiatric drugs—most commonly antidepressants—about half who wound down their prescriptions rated the withdrawal as severe. Nearly half who tried to quit could not do so because of these symptoms. In another study of 180 longtime antidepressant users, withdrawal symptoms were reported by more than 130. Almost half said they felt addicted to antidepressants" [883]. Their evaluation is supported by various other studies, both observational and experimental, which all consistently show that many long-term users are physically dependent on (or feel "addicted to") antidepressants and experience severe withdrawal syndromes when trying to come off the drugs [278, 279, 354, 733–735, 882, 884, 885].

But still, various psychiatrists fiercely objected the *New York Times* article and wrote angry letters to the newspaper. One particularly dismissive commentary was written by Dr. Roy Perlis, editor of the *American Journal of Psychiatry* and published in the very same prestigious journal (the journal is owned by the APA). Disdainfully, Dr. Perlis went on the counterattack. "A recent front-page New York Times article reframed a mental health success story into a conspiracy theory". It followed a long list of unsubstantiated claims and strawman arguments, before he concluded "The increasing number of people receiving standard depression treatments in the United States represents the success of a substantial public health effort. Anything that stands in the way of people seeking treatment requires that we speak up and try to address both the cognitive and affective biases that may prevent effective treatment" [886].

Perhaps, if Dr. Perlis would carefully listen to user complaints about not being able to stop antidepressants due to dependence and withdrawal, instead of lecturing about stigmatisation of drug treatment and cognitive biases, he would understand that there are legitimate concerns about long-term prescriptions in the absence of robust scientific evidence demonstrating that benefits clearly outweigh harms. And what is this obscure "mental health success story" Dr. Perlis is so convinced of? Where is the success of widespread long-term antidepressant use? He certainly knows that in the US the prevalence of depression and anxiety, as well as the suicide rate, are steadily increasing since about 20 years despite evermore people using antidepressants for ever-longer periods [887–890]. I'm terribly sorry, but from a public health perspective, this is anything but a success story [568, 891].

As detailed above, the minimisation and denial of physical dependence and severe withdrawal syndromes upon discontinuation or dose reduction are pervasive and systematic. Nutt and colleagues, in a *Lancet Psychiatry* article, went even one step further and insinuated orchestrated malingering and fabrication of withdrawal syndromes:

> "Indeed, the new antidepressants, especially the selective serotonin reuptake inhibitors, are some of the safest drugs ever made. In our experience, the vast majority of patients who choose to stay on them do so because they improve their mood and wellbeing rather than because they cannot cope

with withdrawal symptoms when they stop. Many of the extreme examples of adverse effects given by the opponents of antidepressants are both rare and sometimes sufficiently bizarre as to warrant the description of an unexplained medical symptom. To attribute extremely unusual or severe experiences to drugs that appear largely innocuous in doubleblind clinical trials is to prefer anecdote to evidence. The incentive of litigation might also distort the presentation of some of the claims". [22]

Obviously, Nutt and colleagues willfully ignored the various double-blind clinical trials demonstrating that withdrawal syndromes are real and frequent, in particular with paroxetine and venlafaxine, and that they can be severe to the point that they cause new affective disorders, serious functioning deficits, and/or emergent suicidality [356, 734, 735, 884, 892, 893], for systematic reviews, see [345, 347, 348].

Thus, in short, there can be no doubt that in clinical practice, antidepressant withdrawal is still frequently dismissed, misdiagnosed (e.g. as relapse, a new mental disorder, functional neurological disorder, or medically unexplained symptoms), and mistreated/mismanaged (e.g. dose escalation, adding other high-dosed psychotropic drugs, fast tapers) [357, 871, 878, 894]. This resonates with the experiences made by many patients documented in online peer-support groups [881]. According to a recent user survey about antidepressant withdrawal, in 12% of cases the doctor denied that the symptoms were related to withdrawal, in 15% the doctors were helpful but inaccurate, 42% were unhelpful and inaccurate and just 1% were helpful (29% did not respond to this question) [880]. It is embarrassing for the medical profession that even psychiatrists who personally experienced severe antidepressant withdrawal had to turn to internet sites like SurvivingAntidepressants.org for guidance when they realised that their education and training was of little help and grossly inadequate [895, 896]. By consequence, arguably the most proficient expert on antidepressant withdrawal is a lay person, the above mentioned Adele Framer, who was personally affected by severe antidepressant withdrawal and who later founded SurvivingAntidepressants.org, as she had to learn the hard way that psychiatrists and general medical practitioners have very little or false knowledge about antidepressant withdrawal [881]. The denial, misdiagnosis, and mistreatment of antidepressant withdrawal by physicians is presumably also the main driver of the constantly increasing memberships of antidepressant withdrawal peer-support groups on the internet [897].

As a case in point, I want to conclude this section with an email from Michelle I received on November 2020. This is one among many similar messages from antidepressant users I frequently receive (many other personal experiences can be found on online peer-support groups such as SurvivingAntidepressants.org). Michelle gave me her consent to reproduce the email verbatim and to quote her first name:

> Dear Dr. Hengartner,
>
> Thank you for your article "Antidepressant Withdrawal: The Tide is Finally Turning". I'm sure you get many emails from people like me but I wanted to express my gratitude for your research and publication. Four months ago, under the supervision of my psychiatrist, I discontinued an SSRI which I had been on for 15 years, prescribed to me as a child for childhood anxiety. I had been feeling pretty good for over a year and wanted to find out what my 'baseline' state was without the drug. In the four months that followed, I experienced depression, anxiety, aggression, and a near-constant and overwhelming feeling of horror I had never felt before. I had not been expecting any symptoms from the drug discontinuation as I assumed these types of 'safe' drugs did not have withdrawal symptoms, and I was definitely not informed by my psychiatrist. After four months that I can honestly describe as the worst of my life, the symptoms remained unbearable and showed no signs of improving and, finally following the urging of both my psychiatrist and therapist, I began taking the SSRI again. I felt relief from my symptoms almost immediately, and within a week back on the SSRI I felt back to 'normal'.
>
> My psychiatrist and therapist have both deemed the last four months a 'relapse' and tried to add a new medication as well as to up the dose on my current medication. I know what I experienced and it was not a relapse—I had never experienced depression or anxiety to that level in my life before. I have also never felt aggression or horror the way I experienced in the last four months. I had also never experienced a depression lasting as long as four months before. Thanks to papers from people like you, I am able to find validation that what I experienced was in fact, withdrawal. I now face the prospect of attempting to more slowly taper off the medication without the support of a psychiatrist. I am also terrified that my brain might be

permanently damaged from 15 years on the medication. There is a serious problem with the way SSRIs are prescribed and with psychiatrists and drug companies refusing to listen to the experiences of the people they are supposed to be helping. Thank you for your work against this.

Best,
Michelle

Treatment-Emergent Suicidality With Antidepressants

In children and adolescents, there is strong evidence from the syntheses of randomised placebo-controlled trials that SSRIs and other new-generation antidepressants increase the risk of suicidal ideation and behaviour [58, 292, 293, 322, 323, 780, 898]. However, as detailed in the chapter "Flaws in antidepressant research", the pharmaceutical industry tried to obscure the harm signal in clinical trials through selective reporting and misrepresentation of suicidal events [322, 323, 715, 770]. Likewise, various influential academics disputed the increased risk of suicidal events in clinical trials based on the results of flawed and methodologically weak ecological studies [899]. Some even claimed that regulatory warnings had led to an increase in youth suicides (for through discussions debunking these erroneous assertions, see [120, 864, 900, 901]).

The risk of treatment-emergent suicidality with antidepressants is less clear in adults. While some meta-analyses of clinical trials found no increased risk of suicidal events, others found increased rates of suicidal behaviour and even suicides [324, 327, 328, 330, 332, 333, 779, 902]. According to the FDA analysis, antidepressants may reduce suicidal ideation and behaviour in older adults [324, 903]. However, and most importantly, not one synthesis of clinical trial data ever found a reduced rate of suicide attempts and suicides with antidepressants relative to placebo in the broader adult patient population. But still various psychiatrists erroneously claim that antidepressants would protect against suicide, commonly based on a few methodologically weak ecological studies and selectively quoted observational studies [899, 904]. However, neither ecological studies nor a recent systematic review of observational studies do provide consistent (and conclusive) evidence that antidepressants protect against suicide in adults [863, 899, 905, 906]. According to our recent meta-analysis of observational studies, exposure to new-generation antidepressants (i.e. SSRIs, SNRIs and atypical antidepressants) was even associated with an increased suicide risk in patients with depression as well as any treatment indication [906].

American and European drug regulators officially acknowledged in the mid-2000s that new-generation antidepressants increase the risk of suicidality in children, adolescents, and young adults [903]. However, according to Dr. Healy [9, 715] drug regulators failed to adequately investigate (and recognise) this pernicious safety issue, especially in adults, even though a harm signal was reported by various researchers during the early 1990s [326, 776, 907]. Healy is not the only one to criticise the drug regulators for their hesitance to recognise a putative causal association between antidepressant use and increased risk of suicidality. When the FDA drug safety evaluator Dr. Andrew Mosholder reported to the FDA leadership that, according to his analysis of placebo-controlled clinical trials submitted to the agency, antidepressants increase the risk of suicidality in youth, his superiors criticised his findings as "premature and based on unreliable data" and they "barred him from reporting his conclusion to an FDA advisory committee" [908]. Among those FDA leaders questioning Mosholder's evaluation was Dr. Thomas Laughren, then director of the Division of Psychiatry Products. He presented Mosholder's analysis, but "stressed the unreliability of the data instead of the possible risk from the drugs" [908].

Most importantly, "For more than a decade Dr. Laughren endorsed industry's denials of an increased suicide risk for consumers of SSRI antidepressants. He dismissed safety concerns raised by FDA medical reviewers, including a reviewer who reported a seven-fold greater incidence of suicidality in children prescribed sertraline (Zoloft®). Dr. Laughren stated in a memo dated October 25, 1996: 'I don't consider these data to represent a signal of risk for suicidality for either adults or children'" [909]. Another eight years had to pass until the FDA formally acknowledged an increased risk of suicidality with antidepressants in children and adolescents, and in total ten years to expand their safety warning to young adults.

Researchers, safety advocates, and journalists who dared to suggest that new-generation antidepressants may increase the risk of suicide not only in children, but also in adults, were frequently reprimanded or sanctioned by academic departments, psychiatric organisations, and influential psychiatrists [9, 147, 812, 910]. For instance, in late 2002, Dr. Healy lost his future appointment as director of the University of Toronto's Mood and Anxiety Disorder Clinic and a professorship at the university's department of psychiatry after he had delivered a lecture where he also raised the question whether SSRIs may increase the risk of suicide among certain patients. In response this this lecture, within a week he received an email from the University of Toronto unilaterally rescinding their employment offer [812].

Two more examples. When in February 2013 a German television programme reported on the suicide risk with new-generation antidepressants, the German psychiatric association immediately responded with a public statement and a press release asserting that "antidepressants help to prevent suicides" [861]. In support of this claim they cited only one analysis of clinical trials that did not even examine suicide attempts or suicides, while deliberately ignoring the various studies specifically assessing suicide attempts and suicides that found no protective effect or even increased risk with antidepressants relative to placebo. Finally, Nutt and colleagues, in their fierce attack against Dr. Gotzsche, also dismissed the possibility that antidepressants might increase the suicide risk and in accordance with the chairs of the German psychiatric association, suggested that antidepressants protect against suicide:

> "Suicide kills about 6000 people every year in the UK. Most of these people are depressed and more than 70% are not taking an antidepressant at the time of death. Blanket condemnation of antidepressants by lobby groups and colleagues risks increasing that proportion. In countries where antidepressants are used properly, suicide rates have fallen substantially". [22]

I was repeatedly confronted with similar arguments on social media and during peer review of my studies on the risk of treatment-emergent suicidal events in antidepressant trials [332, 333, 855]. In fact, this is the preferred line of reasoning of many psychiatrists and thus can be found in various other prominent articles (see for instance [899, 904]). This typical argumentation by Nutt and colleagues is thus worthy of closer inspection.

First, suicide indeed kills many people, of which many (though by far not all) were depressed and not on antidepressants. However, this does not answer the question whether antidepressants protect against suicide. Alternatively, one could also argue that about 30% were taking antidepressants and it did not prevent them from suicide. So how can Nutt and colleagues imply that the 70% not on antidepressants had benefitted from the drugs? Of course, they cannot (or should not) draw such a conclusion from these data, which is why this is a very poor and misleading argument. This is akin to claiming that smoking does not cause lung cancer for only about 10–15% of current smokers will develop lung cancer, while 85–90% will not [911].

Second, suggesting that regulatory warnings about the risk of treatment-emergent suicidality with antidepressants would paradoxically increase the suicide rate is lacking robust scientific evidence and thus is largely unsubstantiated [912–915]. Authors arguing that the regulatory warnings about treatment-emergent suicidality in youth had resulted in increased suicide rates in this population selectively cited and/or misrepresented studies that were terribly flawed and ignored more thorough analyses that clearly disconfirmed these findings [120, 864, 901].

Third, and related to the point above, Nutt and colleagues cite one international ecological study that found that increased antidepressant prescribing was correlated with lower suicide rates. Such studies examine associations on the group level (here per countries), but not on the individual person level, and thus are prone to serious biases and cannot demonstrate cause–effect relationships [864, 916]. Moreover, the evidence from ecological studies is highly inconsistent and inconclusive [905, 917, 918]. Two systematic reviews concluded that the evidence from ecological studies provides little or no support for the view that increased antidepressant prescribing had led to a reduction in suicide rates [863, 919]. It is also worthy of note that one of the largest international ecological studies published prior to Nutt and colleagues' article found that increased antidepressant prescribing was associated with higher suicide rates [920], which is completely the opposite finding to the study Nutt and colleagues selectively preferred to cite. Thus, not only did Nutt and colleagues overemphasise the finding from a single ecological study, they also failed to acknowledge that the evidence from ecological studies is fully inconsistent and of very limited validity.

Fourth, and perhaps most importantly, Nutt and colleagues completely ignore the findings from studies with the highest certainty in evidence, that is, meta-analyses of clinical trials. None of these studies found that antidepressants protect against suicide, and in various analyses the suicide rate was numerically (and in some also statistically significantly) higher in the antidepressant group relative to the placebo group [324, 329–333, 779, 902]. Their complete disregard for clinical trial data is striking all the more, as a few lines below they alleged, quite incorrectly, that withdrawal reactions and other serious adverse events have not been demonstrated in doubleblind clinical trials, thus relating such harms to the drugs would mean to prefer "anecdote to evidence" [22]. According to their own argumentation, it follows that Nutt and colleagues prefer anecdote to evidence when it comes to the alleged suicide-protective effects of antidepressants.

But authors were not only reprimanded for contending that antidepressants may increase the suicide risk, some were also fiercely criticised for correctly pointing out that antidepressants barely protect against suicide. For instance, in 2019, US psychiatrist Dr. Amy Barnhorst published an article titled "The empty promise of suicide prevention—Many of the problems that lead people to kill themselves cannot be fixed with a little extra serotonin" in the *New York Times*. In this opinion paper, Barnhorst maintained that in most cases antidepressants won't protect against suicide, for suicide is often the tragic consequence of an impulsive reaction to desperation caused by socio-environmental adversity. She thus concluded "We need to address the root causes of our nation's suicide problem—poverty, homelessness and the accompanying exposure to trauma, crime and drugs" [921]. Although this article was not inherently critical of antidepressants, it provoked an angry response by Dr. Jeffrey Lieberman, a dinosaur of US psychiatry, chair of the psychiatry department at Columbia University and former president of the APA.

The next day the article was published, Dr. Lieberman wrote on Twitter "Amy Barnhorst doesn't read scientific literature or skipped training. This article is wrong. Suicide is largely preventable, if proper measures taken and prescription drug provided. New York Times please vet authors better". At the end of his tweet he then tagged the APA (@APAPsychiatric). Dr. Barnhorst responded ironically with "I skipped training". Several commentators were appalled by Dr. Lieberman's condescending and hostile tweet. For instance, an anonymous psychiatrist (@FightOn49er) wrote "This is not how we speak to colleagues we disagree with. You are a department chair at Columbia! Do better, Dr. Lieberman!" and Dr. Leah DeSole, a clinical psychologist, stated "Thank you for this comment. I'm glad Jeff cares deeply about this topic! However, let's remember to prize civility, professionally and personally, in our tweets". Dr. Lieberman then immediately responded to her with "All for civility except in the case of misinformation that puts lives at risk, especially when purveyed by a professional who wears the patina of credibility" (see the whole Twitter conversation here: https://twitter.com/FightOn49er/status/1122183796806148098).

It is incomprehensible that Dr. Lieberman makes such bold and defamatory claims, given that the US has just experienced the highest suicide rate since World War II (14.2 suicides per 100,000 people in 2018 [888]) and despite the fact that evermore people, currently about 70% of people with serious psychological distress, receive mental health treatment (mostly drug treatment) [477]. Likewise, among US veterans diagnosed with a mental disorder and receiving mental health treatment (again, by and large drug treatment), the suicide rate is alarmingly high (about 68 per 100,000 people) and has remained largely constant over time [922]. Thus, if suicide was preventable the way Dr. Lieberman pretends (or wishes) it to be, then why do mental health services in the US fail so terribly at it? Certainly not because they would insufficiently prescribe antidepressants and other psychiatric drugs.

Considering the disturbing surge of suicides that runs parallel to the increasing societal problems in the US (e.g. poverty, inequality, drug abuse), should Dr. Lieberman not at least be open to suggestions that the current biomedical approach to suicide-prevention is inadequate or at least insufficient? Would we not expect that someone like Dr. Lieberman would critically reflect on the terrible impression his defensive and defamatory tweets make on the public and other mental health professionals? It's not that Dr. Lieberman would just be some brash medical student; he is a leading professor of psychiatry and former president of the most powerful psychiatric association in the world, the APA. With all due respect, but if this really is the best answer academic psychiatry has to offer, then the profession's guiding biomedical paradigm truly is in crisis [390, 392].

Now, this was certainly not the first time Dr. Lieberman revealed a complete disregard for constructive debate and respectful conversation. I have already detailed above how he denigrated Dr. Kirsch as "mistaken and confused" and "ideologically biased in his thinking" [830]. In his habitual manner to insult people who do not share his drug-centred views, he is by no means an outlier. In my view such desperate ad hominem attacks are the norm rather than the exception, and as detailed above, they come disproportionally often from leading academics. Unfortunately, instead of engaging in a constructive debate based on empirical evidence and scientific arguments, when it comes to defending the alleged benefits and the mass prescription of antidepressants (and other psychiatric drugs), many psychiatrists resort to derision, delegitimisation, defamation, misrepresentation, strawman arguments, and unevidenced claims. No wonder that these "debates" yield nothing but anger and anguish, but never new insights, critical reflection, or scientific progress. In short, this behaviour is utterly unscientific. Such responses are thus best conceived of as defences of guild interests and claims to leadership and power [30, 810, 923]. Readers familiar with the philosopher of science Dr. Thomas Kuhn and his famous book *The Structure of Scientific Revolutions* probably will also consider such hostile responses as desperate defences of an incommensurable scientific paradigm [924].

Corporate Bias

Medicine has made incredible progress over the course of the twentieth century, especially in the first half. Medical breakthroughs, for example, antibiotics, insulin, vaccines, chemotherapy, surgical innovations, immunosuppressants, and antiretrovirals had a huge impact on the prevention and treatment of various life-threatening diseases. In step with these major advancements, the healthcare sector grew massively. In the late twentieth century, healthcare services and biomedical research became a highly competitive and lucrative multi-billion-dollar market. Innovative surgical techniques were introduced, sophisticated imaging procedures were developed, many new drugs were marketed, managed care plans were developed, and patients became healthcare consumers. Although the prevention, detection, diagnosis and treatment of various diseases had advanced considerably, many experts expressed concern over problematic developments in modern biomedicine that increasingly put commercial and professional interests over public health, patient safety, academic freedom, and research integrity [29, 59, 171, 375–377, 379, 381, 382, 650, 659, 767, 812].

The pharmaceutical industry is arguably the main perpetrator and its list of transgressions (i.e. healthcare fraud and scientific misconduct) is long and shocking [376, 428, 925]. As reported by Public Citizen, in the US alone, pharmaceutical companies paid a total of $38.6 billion in penalties for 412 settlements reached with the federal and state governments in the 27 years from 1991 through 2017 [926]. Unlawful promotion of drugs accounted for the most financial penalties (US$11.3 billion, 29% of all financial penalties). GlaxoSmithKline and Pfizer were the worst offenders; these two companies paid more financial penalties than any other companies ($7.9 billion and $4.7 billion, respectively). Although these tremendous sums are impressive, "Financial penalties continued to pale in comparison to company profits, with the $38.6 billion in penalties from 1991 through 2017 amounting to only 5% of the $711 billion in net profits made by the 11 largest global drug companies during just 10 of those 27 years (2003–2012)" [926].

According to the most recent analysis adjusted for inflation, among 26 major pharmaceutical companies, 22 (85%) had financial penalties in the US for illegal activities for the period 2003 to 2016. The combined value of financial penalties during this 14-year period totaled a staggering $33 billion. Eleven of the 26 companies accounted for 88% of the total penalties, of which the worst offenders were GlaxoSmithKline ($9.8 billion), Pfizer ($2.9 billion), Johnson & Johnson ($2.7 billion), Abbott Laboratories ($2.6 billion), Merck ($2.1 billion) and Eli Lilly ($1.8 billion). But even for GlaxoSmithKline, the shocking $9.8 billion in total penalties amounted to a mere 1.6% of its total revenues. For the other companies listed above, this proportion was less than 0.8% [925]. Thus, although some companies paid tremendous penalties for illegal activities (mostly pricing violations, off-label marketing, and kickbacks), these penalties are trivial in comparison to the companies' huge revenues and may be accepted as common (out-of-pocket) business expenses. As stated by Jureidini and McHenry, "Expensive litigation, for the industry, is just part of the price of doing business" [29]. It has thus been suggested that courts should not only punish the companies, but also the corporate executive officers [927]. When the directors of pharmaceutical companies would face jail for illegal corporate activities, perhaps then, and only then, the companies would change their way of doing business.

There is no doubt that pharmaceuticals are an incredibly lucrative business [388], and the pharmaceutical industry found many ways—both legal and illegal—to increase its profits. The very meaning of corporate bias is that through their extensive financial power, the pharmaceutical industry can exert substantial control over the healthcare sector by influencing health policy, drug regulation, medical associations, consumer organisations, academic departments, and individual prescribers. Pharmaceutical products can be very helpful and lifesaving, but in many indications they are largely ineffective and various drugs caused more harm than good [171, 376, 383]. In any case, there is compelling scientific evidence that the benefits of drugs have been systematically exaggerated while harms were downplayed or ignored. Many drugs are massively overused and inadequately prescribed, largely due to aggressive pharmaceutical marketing and promotion (to both doctors and the public) as well as the industry's influence over continuing medical education, academic medical departments and the research landscape [376, 381, 428, 459, 928]. However, don't think that the medical profession was solely fooled and betrayed by the pharmaceutical industry as insinuated by various authors, for example by Dr. Ben Goldacre in his book "Bad pharma: how drug companies mislead doctors and harm patients" [428]. It is not just a one-way direction, where industry is the bad guy and doctors the naïve but well-meaning dupes. Medicine was quite often complicit in this widespread deception/exploitation of patients and the public because it regularly and eagerly partnered with the industry [459]. As succinctly articulated by Dr. Matheson, "Is medicine the manipulated victim of the pharmaceutical corporations, or their colleague in corruption? The answer, of course, is both. Sometimes medicine is pharma's unwitting dupe, sometimes its eager bedfellow" [659].

The pervasive and detrimental effect of corporate bias is perhaps best illustrated by the opioid epidemic in the United States that, as of 2019, has accounted for about 770,000 deaths over the past 20 years [929]. According to the Centers for Disease Control and Prevention (CDC), the opioid crisis is the "worst drug overdose epidemic in history" [930]. Notably, this epidemic was not caused by a pathogen, it is a man-made plague for which the pharmaceutical industry and its allies are largely responsible [929]. The main causes of the opioid epidemic are aggressive pharmaceutical marketing, misleading/deceptive industry-sponsored medical education programs, bribes and kickbacks offered to doctors for prescribing opioids, the downplaying/denial of the drugs' potential for addiction, the promotion of pain as a fifth vital sign, and the creation of pain advocacy groups to advance the industry's corporate agenda [929–931]. According to Dr. Jonathan Marks, a professor of bioethics, humanities, and law,

> "There is overwhelming evidence that the opioid crisis—which has cost hundreds of thousands of lives and trillions of dollars (and counting)—has been created or exacerbated by webs of influence woven by several pharmaceutical companies. These webs involve health professionals, patient advocacy groups, medical professional societies, research universities, teaching hospitals, public health agencies, policymakers, and legislators. Opioid companies built these webs as part of corporate strategies of influence that were designed to expand the opioid market from cancer patients to larger groups of patients with acute or chronic pain, to increase dosage as well as opioid use, to downplay the risks of addiction and abuse, and to characterize physicians' concerns about the addiction and abuse risks as 'opiophobia'". [928]

A recent legal settlement proves that the marketing strategies of the pharmaceutical industry were utterly unethical and illegal. In October 2020, the US Justice Department announced that Purdue Pharma, maker of the highly addictive opioid oxycodone (OxyContin), has agreed to plead guilty to criminal charges related to its marketing of oxycodone. The company faces penalties of roughly $8.3 billion [932].

The opioid crisis tragically illustrates how pharmaceutical corporate bias can damage patient safety and public health. Is the situation different in psychiatry? I contend it's not, and many experts in evidence-based medicine, public health, and bioethics agree [28–30, 147, 414, 767, 768, 771, 933]. For instance, Dr. Barry Blackwell, a psychopharmacologist and member of the International Network for the History of Neuropsychopharmacology, gloomily wrote in 2017:

> "Industry has taken over and corrupted clinical trials, bribed academics to be complicit, infiltrated medical education and its curricula, seduced professional and consumer organizations, lobbied politicians to relax regulations and partially funded the FDA, influencing its decisions, meanwhile vastly inflating the populations at alleged risk for mental disorders and the willingness of physicians to medicate them, a process aided and abetted by the DSM diagnostic system coupled with misleading advertising direct to the public and dubious marketing strategies for gullible doctors". [934]

Dr. Scull, a historian of medicine, also wrote a damning summary on the issue of corporate bias in psychiatry:

> "And so to scandal. He who pays the piper calls the tune, and to a quite extraordinary extent, drug money has come to dominate psychiatry. It underwrites psychiatric journals and psychiatric conferences (where the omnipresence of pharmaceutical loot startles the naive outsider). It makes psychiatric careers, and many of those whose careers it fosters become shills for their paymasters, zealously promoting lucrative off-label uses for drugs whose initial approval for prescription was awarded on quite other grounds. It ensures that when scandals surface universities will mainly turn a blind eye to the transgressions of those members of their staff who engage in these unethical practices. And it controls psychiatric knowledge in multiple ways. Its ghostwriters produce peer-reviewed 'science' that surfaces in even the most prestigious journals, with the most eminent names in the field collaborating in the deception. Researchers sign confidentiality agreements, and inconvenient data never see the light of day. The very categories within which we think about cognitive and emotional troubles are

> manipulated and transformed to match the requirements of the psychiatric marketplace. Side effects, even profound, permanent, perhaps fatal side effects, are ignored or minimised. Fines may be levied when somnolent regulators are finally prompted into action, or damages paid where aggressive class action lawyers force hitherto suppressed findings into the public arena, but the profits already booked far exceed these costs of doing business". [394]

Although provocatively articulated, Dr. Scull's assessment is accurate and empirically well supported. Numerous articles and books confirm that psychiatric research and practice are strongly biased towards the commercial interests of the pharmaceutical industry [27–29, 67, 399, 414, 768, 856, 935–937]. More specifically, the marketing departments of the pharmaceutical companies are the powerhouse in psychiatry. As outlined by Dr. Healy,

> "the [pharmaceutical] marketing department starts once a compound has been discovered. Marketing decides whether a new drug will be an antidepressant rather than an anxiolytic or a treatment for premature ejaculation. Marketing determines which journals with which lead authors clinical trials will appear in. Marketing recruits academics, including geneticists, neuroimaging specialists and social psychiatrists, to consultancy and speaker panels, and makes friends for the company. The marketing department supports educational events by putting on symposia, sponsoring speakers and bringing psychiatrists to international meetings. The work of the marketing departments is to create ‚evidence' and establish consensus". [938]

Now, a few things warrant clarification before I move to the next sections. First and foremost, it is important to stress that a financial conflict of interest does not imply that a physician (be it an academic or practitioner) is necessarily biased in his judgement. And, of course, it does by no means indicate that someone is corrupt or bought by industry. Biases resulting from conflicts of interest don't need to be conscious and explicit. Often, perhaps predominantly, they are unconscious and implicit. However, there can be no doubt that, overall, financial conflicts of interest lead to more industry-favourable assessments, biased benefit–harm evaluations and medical overuse, that is, overdiagnosis and overprescribing [14, 28, 29, 379, 380, 458, 459, 800, 939–941].

Just like a manager of a football team more often interprets an ambiguous situation in favour of his/her own team compared to an independent observer (e.g., whether an intervention was a foul or not, whether the ball was out or not), so do pharmaceutical company employees and physicians working for the industry (e.g. as speakers and/or consultants) interpret ambiguous data more often in favour of the industry compared to independent experts without industry ties. And just like in sports (e.g. a footballer diving to obtain a penalty kick for his team), when success (or profit) depends on a decisive action, not so uncommonly there are also clear instances of dishonesty, deception, and fraud in the pharmaceutical marketplace [29, 771, 822, 824, 933]. But let us hear from an insider. Dr. Matheson worked in pharmaceutical marketing between 1994 and 2010. He rightly admits that pharmaceutical companies have contributed to many major breakthroughs in medicine (the recent development of vaccines for the new coronavirus disease being just one example). "On the one hand, it remains my belief that pharmaceutical research and development efforts are capable of great good", wrote Matheson [659]. But there is also another, dark and troubling side of drug company influence. "On the other hand, pharmaceutical *marketing* is anathema to science, corrupting to medicine, wasteful to economies, and harmful to patients, and I must acknowledge the moral difficulty that for many years I sold my intellect in its service. Pharma itself, of course, has never truly acknowledged its underbelly of secrets, half-truths, corruption, power, and death, and it flaunts the language of ethics like a silk cummerbund over a paunch. If it is a lie to dissemble, distort, or omit, then pharma must be considered a liar whose subtle falsehoods stock the annals of medicine" [659].

Most stakeholders thus agree that financial conflicts of interest can and do have a detrimental impact on healthcare, but some physicians are reluctant to accept it or try to minimise the problem. In fact, a few opponents even suggested that conflict of interest policies and regulation may harm medicine (for a critique of these notions, see [942]). In view of the compelling scientific evidence demonstrating a most likely causal association between financial conflicts of interest and positions, assessments and prescribing patterns that are systematically biased in favour of the industry, such concerns are empirically unfounded and misleading [592, 593, 772, 794–796, 799, 943–948].

As aptly summarised by Drs Steinbrook, Kassirer, and Angell, all three being former editors of the leading *New England Journal of Medicine*,

> "Judges are expected to recuse themselves from hearing a case in which there are concerns that they could benefit financially from the outcome. Journalists are expected not to write stories on topics in which they have a financial conflict of interest. The problem, obviously, is that their objectivity might be compromised, either consciously or unconsciously, and there would be no easy way to know whether it had been. Yet Rosenbaum and Drazen [opponents of conflict of interest policy and regulation] seem to think it is insulting to physicians and medical researchers to suggest that their judgment can be affected in the same way. Doctors might wish it were otherwise, but none of us is immune to human nature". [942]

I will now detail how the pharmaceutical industry exerts influence over psychiatry (and medicine in general) at all levels, starting with drug regulators, then turning to academic departments, researchers, medical journals, and concluding with medical organisations and prescribers/practitioners.

Drug Regulators

"The regulatory state and the pharmaceutical industry work largely in partnership and behind a cloak of secrecy", wrote Dr. Abraham in 2008 [949]. His view is strongly endorsed by many others. For instance, based on an investigation of some 1600 FDA inspection and enforcement documents conducted by *Science*, it was concluded that the agency's oversight of clinical research was "lax, slow, and secretive" [950]. In an investigation published earlier the same year in *JAMA*, Dal-Re and colleagues reported on FDA inspections that revealed clear research misconduct in two influential industry-sponsored pre-marketing (phase III) clinical trials (ARISTOTLE and RECORD4), comprising alterations of patient records, data falsification, failure to fully report adverse events and noncompliance with protocol procedures [951]. Consequently, the FDA excluded results from one trial (RECORD4) in their benefit–harm evaluation but granted license approval for the investigational drug and the flawed trial results were published by the sponsor. Despite being clearly fraudulent, the trial publication was cited over 1100 times and was included in meta-analyses and clinical practice guidelines. The results from the second fraudulent trial (ARISTOTLE) were not excluded from the FDA assessment and the agency granted a license approval for the investigational drug. The trial publication was cited more than 6900 times and was included in many meta-analyses and clinical practice guidelines. The FDA never communicated its detection of research misconduct in these two influential trials to doctors or the public. The authors thus concluded, "FDA trial inspection reports have been largely hidden from public view, but access to information on the integrity and quality of clinical trials that underpin a product's assessment is critical, particularly when irregularities or misconduct are identified. Public availability of these reports is required to meet current standards for clinical trial transparency and uphold the integrity of the scientific evidence base" [951].

By now you have certainly realised that we cannot uncritically rely on the scientific literature, that approved drugs are both effective and safe. Most concerning, however, is that drug regulators appear to increasingly protect the commercial interests of the industry rather than public health and patient safety, which is unequivocally a manifestation of corporate bias [825]. This process was also coined regulatory capture, "a variable and dynamic effect of corporate bias that describes a shift in policy by government agencies away from regulation in the interests of patients and public health to prioritization of the private interests of the regulatees instead" [952]. That is, drug regulators frequently act in ways that benefit the industry rather than patients and the public. As stated by Dr. Vinay Prasad in an interview with *Science*, the "FDA is a regulatory agency charged with protecting the public's best interests. But at times it behaves like an attorney working on behalf of the [pharmaceutical] companies" [950]. Such accusations are by no means new and there is quite compelling evidence that they are well founded.

For instance, in 2004, Dr. David Graham, then associate director of the FDA's Office of Drug Safety, testified to US Congress that he was urged by his superiors "to not warn the public about dangers of drugs like Vioxx" [716]. Recognising his responsibility as a drug safety analyst, he warned the public nonetheless, but then was "marginalized by FDA management and not asked to participate in the evaluation of any drug safety issues". The following year he stated that "FDA is inherently biased in favor of the pharmaceutical industry. It views industry as its client, whose interest it must represent and advance. It views its primary mission as approving as many drugs as it can, regardless of whether the drugs are safe or needed" [716]. He is not an isolated case. Dr Curt Furberg, a member of the FDA's drug safety advisory committee and a prominent authority on drug safety, was forbidden to participate in FDA hearings on the safety of COX-2 inhibitors after he made remarks towards the media that valdecoxib (Bextra) may cause heart attacks and strokes just like rofecoxib (Vioxx), a drug from the same class recently withdrawn from the market by its manufacturer Merck for this specific safety reason [953].

Finally, Dr Ronald Kavanagh is a former FDA reviewer of psychiatric drugs who was fired from his position in 2008 for whistleblowing [716]. In an interview he said about his former employer: "While I was at FDA, drug reviewers were clearly told not to question drug companies and that our job was to approve drugs … If we asked questions that could delay or prevent a drug's approval—which of course was our job as drug reviewer—management would reprimand us, reassign us, hold secret meetings about us, and worse … Sometimes we were literally instructed to read a 100–150 page summary and to accept drug company claims without examining the actual data, which on multiple occasions I found directly contradicted the summary document" [29]. These three examples indeed suggest that there is systematic and pervasive corporate bias (regulatory capture) at the FDA. But let us look a bit deeper at these issues.

A survey among FDA scientists found "pervasive and dangerous political influence" at the FDA [954]. In particular, 40% of the 997 respondents said they fear retaliation for voicing safety concerns in public, and 18% indicated that they had been asked to inappropriately exclude or alter technical information or conclusions from the data for non-scientific reasons in an FDA scientific document. Only 47% believed that the FDA routinely provides complete and accurate information to the public, and 81% agreed that the public would be better served if the independence and authority of the FDA post-market safety systems were strengthened. Commercial interests resulting in inappropriate acts (or attempts) to reverse, withdraw, or modify FDA determinations or actions was endorsed by 60% of the respondents. Finally, 20% said they "have been asked explicitly by FDA decision-makers to provide incomplete, inaccurate, or misleading information to the public, industry, media, and elected officials" [954].

How strong are the ties between drug regulators and the pharmaceutical industry? This is the question I will now address. Let us first have a look at how the major drug regulatory agencies are funded. Both FDA (US) and EMA (Europe) obtain more than half of their budget through industry fees. EMA is funded by industry fees rising from 20% in 1995 to 75% in 2010, whereas the FDA is funded by industry fees reaching 50% by 2002 and over 60% by 2010 [825]. In 2017, altogether 79% of the FDA budget was paid for by the biomedical industry through required user fees [955]. The British Medicines and Healthcare products Regulatory Agency (MHRA) is entirely (100%) funded by industry. The industry pays these fees to drug regulators in return for accelerated drug regulatory review times [956]. For instance, the FDA faces a 6-month deadline for priority drug reviews and a 10-month deadline for most other drugs. If the agency doesn't adhere to these deadlines, the pharmaceutical companies won't pay the fees. So, does this financial pressure affect the quality of the reviews and regulatory decisions? Yes, it likely does. According to a comprehensive analysis, drugs approved just before deadline had a higher rate of post-approval safety problems, including market withdrawals, serious safety warnings, and safety alerts. According to the authors, the study "suggests that the deadlines may impede quality by impairing late-stage deliberation and agency risk communication" [957].

But what about the directors of drug regulatory agencies? Are they personally tied to the industry? Yes, many are [956]. For instance, Dr. Scott Gottlieb was chief executive (commissioner) of the FDA from 2017 to 2019. He was known for having extensive financial relationships with the industry over his professional career [958]. Before he became the highest FDA official, he had served on the boards of various pharmaceutical companies. He was also a fervent advocate of accelerated and permissive drug approvals. "What we can't have is an FDA that's ruled by statistics over medicine," he once said. "Americans deserve a less cautious FDA, and an FDA that actively embraces advances in science" [958]. This is quite a strange statement for a drug regulator, for how can drug development and evaluation advance without sound statistical methods? In other words, Gottlieb preferred fast (permissive) drug approvals over stringent (cautious) benefit–harm evaluations. Understandably, the industry loved him for such a pro-business position, and he was swiftly rewarded: soon after he left the FDA in 2019, he joined Pfizer's board of directors [959].

You think Dr. Gottlieb is an outlier? He clearly is not. That leading officials and senior scientists leave the FDA to work for the pharmaceutical industry is very common and has also been described as the "FDA's revolving door" [960]. According to Drs Hayes and Prasad, "This employment pattern may raise concern that, although regulators intend to act always in the best interest of the public, the frequent opportunity for subsequent employment with the industry may serve to dissuade them from being too oppositional or critical" [961]. Dr. Gottlieb certainly had strong ties to the industry, but there are even more extreme examples [956]. For instance, before Dr. Ian Hudson became director of the British Medicines Control Agency in 2001 and later chief executive of the MHRA, he was worldwide safety director of SmithKline Beecham (now GlaxoSmithKline), one of the largest pharmaceutical companies worldwide. Among his many tasks as safety director for SmithKline Beecham, he was also responsible to defend the safety of paroxetine in court, claiming that the use of paroxetine could not be related causally to any suicidal or homicidal event [9]. However, note that in the mid-2000s, drug regulators concluded that paroxetine can cause suicidality in children and adolescents [786]. Likewise, an independent evaluation of paroxetine trials demonstrated a probability of 98–99% (i.e. close to certainty) that paroxetine use in adults is associated with an increased risk of suicide attempts relative to placebo [328]. Would you trust a former drug company director like Dr. Hudson to defend public health and patient safety against the industry's commercial interests? Let me ask differently. Would a former director of an oil company be the right person to lead an environmental protection agency? But back to the FDA…

Dr. Thomas Laughren was team leader of FDA's Psychiatric Drug Product Division from 1983 to 2005 and from then on director of this division until his retirement in late 2012. Throughout his career at the FDA, he had maintained close collaborations with the pharmaceutical industry, and some of his industry-collaborations were highly controversial [716, 909]. For instance, Dr. Laughren participated in various industry-sponsored consensus panels and conferences promoting polypharmacy and expanded use of psychiatric drugs for unapproved indications (i.e. off-label use). He also advocated for broadening diagnostic criteria in approved indications and authored several articles on these controversial topics with some of industry's highest paid key opinion leaders and even with pharmaceutical company directors such as Eli Lilly's chief medical officer Dr. Leigh Thompson [909]. Having such a loyal ally among the FDA leadership certainly is a great asset for the pharmaceutical industry, but is this in the public's best interest? Unfortunately, corporate bias (or regulatory capture) isn't limited to directors.

Although the FDA makes the final decision whether to approve or reject a new drug application or whether an approved drug should be withdrawn from the market or receive a safety warning, the agency strongly relies on the benefit-harm assessments provided by its Drug Advisory Committees. These committees comprise external experts, mostly leading academic physicians, and they quite often have financial relationships with the manufacturers of the drugs under consideration. Do these conflicts of interest influence the experts' judgements? Yes, they probably do [961, 962]. For instance, in a Drug Advisory Committee meeting from 2004 discussing the safety of COX-2 inhibitors (including rofecoxib), it was shown that 10 of the 32 voting panel members had financial ties to manufacturers of COX-2 inhibitors, including receipt of speaking or consulting fees or research support. If the 10 members with financial conflicts of interest had not been allowed to vote, a majority of the panel would have voted to withdraw two of the COX-2 inhibitors from the market. However, with their votes included, a majority of the panel was in favour to keep these drugs on the market [963]. Since then the FDA has slightly tightened its conflict of interest policy, so pharmaceutical companies now increasingly adopt "after-the-fact compensation"—rewarding influential physicians who voted in favour of the company's drug with speaking and consulting honoraria or research support after regulatory agencies came to a decision [964]. I will now leave the drug regulators and turn to academic research and publishing.

Academic Medical Departments, Researchers, and Medical Journals

Fabbri and colleagues conducted a review on the influence of industry sponsorship on the research agenda. Based on the scientific evidence, they concluded "Corporate interests can drive research agendas away from questions that are the most relevant for public health. Strategies to counteract corporate influence on the research agenda are needed, including heightened disclosure of funding sources and conflicts of interest in published articles to allow an assessment of commercial biases. We also recommend policy actions beyond disclosure such as increasing funding for independent research and strict guidelines to regulate the interaction of research institutes with commercial entities" [651]. Testoni and colleagues also conducted an analysis of the health and biomedical sciences and found that bioindustry, in collaboration with a few elite universities, largely sets the research agenda. They concluded, "Overall, the main focus of the prevailing HBMS [health and biomedical sciences] agenda appears to be set on therapeutic and specifically pharmacological intervention involving the use of novel drugs or innovative molecular biology techniques. At the same time, prevention and assessment of socio-environmental factors influencing disease onset are almost absent … A more balanced research agenda, together with epistemological approaches that consider socio-environmental factors associated with disease spreading, could contribute to being better prepared to prevent and treat more diverse pathologies and to improve overall health outcomes" [965]. Likewise, in psychiatry it is well established that the pharmaceutical industry exerts control over the research landscape by supporting research projects centred on its commercially favoured topics (e.g. treatment efficacy instead of drug safety, see [78, 772]). Moreover, industry support has also created a marked power imbalance between different research fields, resulting in a strong bias towards research on psychopharmacology and the neurosciences at the expense of environmental, social, and psychological research [390, 392].

Through funding entire fields of research, the biomedical industry has the power to influence health policy, healthcare provision, and clinical decision making. Many academic medical departments and biomedical research institutes are sponsored, entirely or in part, by the pharmaceutical industry [29, 30, 812]. For instance, the Lundbeck Foundation, owner of Lundbeck Pharmaceuticals, sponsors the professorships for six leading Danish neuroscientists, three at Aarhus University and three at the University of Copenhagen [966]. The Swiss pharmaceutical association Interpharma sponsors a professorship in health economics at the University of Basel [857]. Eli Lilly financially supports the Centre for Addiction and Mental Health, a prestigious psychiatric university hospital in Toronto [812]. The Sackler family, owner of Purdue Pharma, established the Sackler Graduate School of Biomedical Sciences at Tufts University and funded the Raymond and Beverly Sackler Institute for Biological, Physical and Engineering Sciences at Yale University [29, 928]. And so the list goes on… Now, let's have a closer look at the academic medical departments, the alleged purveyor of research integrity and academic freedom.

Anderson and colleagues examined the academic affiliations of directors board members of the largest pharmaceutical companies [967]. They found that 94% of the US pharmaceutical companies had at least one directors board member who concurrently held a leadership position at an US academic medical center. The leadership positions included university presidents, deans, hospital or health system executive officers, and clinical department chairs or center directors. In a subsequent analysis, the authors found that pharmaceutical company directors were affiliated with 19 of the top 20 National Institute of Health funded medical schools and all the 17 top ranked US hospitals [968]. Among the 279 academically affiliated pharma directors, 121 were professors, 85 were trustees, and 73 were leaders (e.g. university chief executive officers, university presidents and vice presidents, and deans or presidents of medical schools). Finally, Campbell and colleagues showed that among the department chairs of US medical schools, 60% of the respondents had some form of personal relationship with industry, including serving as a consultant (27%), being a member of a scientific advisory board (27%), a paid speaker (14%), an officer (7%), a founder (9%), or a member of the board of directors (11%) [969].

Based on these findings it is difficult to conceive of how leading academic medical departments can fully adhere to the principles of both research integrity and academic freedom. In my view these principles are necessarily compromised when academic leaders are bound by contract to increase the profits of a pharmaceutical company and to act in the company shareholders' best interest. Let me ask a few pertinent questions. Do you think that a pharmaceutical company would tolerate that one of its directors, in his/her role as chair of an academic medical department, decides to focus on the long-term harms associated with the prescription drugs the company markets? Do you think the company would appreciate if he/she is devoted to research on psychosocial interventions as cost-efficient alternatives to the costly drugs his/her company produces? Or do you think the company would be pleased if he/she wants to specialise in the topics of illegal marketing, unethical drug promotion, and research misconduct—transgressions his/her company has been charged with? Assuming that this academic leader adheres to scientific integrity, that is, objectivity, honesty, and transparency, do you think that his/her research output is in accord with the vested interests of the pharmaceutical company he/she is a member of the directors board? If you can't answer all these questions in good faith with "Yes", then you understand why contemporary academic medicine is compromised by pervasive corporate bias [29, 59, 380, 812].

The majority of biomedical research, especially clinical trials, is sponsored by the private for-profit industry [656, 970, 971]. In addition, most principal investigators in drug trials have financial ties to the pharmaceutical industry [592]. Ebrahim and colleagues showed that 79% of meta-analyses of antidepressants have financial conflicts of interest, either because they were sponsored by the industry or the authors were industry employees or had financial ties to the industry [772]. According to a systematic review of randomised placebo-controlled antidepressant trials for depression published between 1980 and 2011, 97% of trials were sponsored by the pharmaceutical industry [194]. The comprehensive meta-analysis of active-controlled (head-to-head) and placebo-controlled antidepressant trials for depression conducted by Cipriani and colleagues found that 78% were funded by the pharmaceutical industry [141]. However, the latter figure is likely an underestimate, for the study sponsor was not declared in all trials [13]. Moreover, even if a drug trial is demonstrably not industry-sponsored, at least one study author commonly has financial relationships with the pharmaceutical industry. Unfortunately, these conflicts of interest are quite often not fully disclosed in journal articles [29, 972, 973]. Thus, there are just very few, if any, reports of antidepressant trials that have no financial conflict of interest, even when the trials were governmentally funded. To illustrate how pervasive industry relationships often are in governmentally funded trials, I will present two of the arguably most important non-industry sponsored antidepressant trials below.

STAR*D was the largest and with a cost of $35 million the most expensive antidepressant trial ever conducted. It was sponsored by the NIMH, lending it credibility as a governmentally funded, independent trial unaffected by industry's commercial interests. However, this is far from the truth. Even though STAR*D was not sponsored by the pharmaceutical industry, financial conflicts of interest were pervasive, for 9 of the 12 authors listed on the main publication had extensive ties to the pharmaceutical industry, including speakers, advisory, and consultancy board memberships, receipt of research grants, and even equity holdings [974]. Shown below is the conflict of interest statement. You will easily notice that, in close competition with the conflict of interest statement in the APA depression practice guideline pasted farther below, this is the longest paragraph of the entire book:

> "Dr. Rush has served as an advisor, consultant, or speaker for or received research support from Advanced Neuromodulation Systems, Inc.; Best Practice Project Management, Inc.; Bristol-Myers Squibb Company; Cyberonics, Inc.; Eli Lilly & Company; Forest Pharmaceuticals, Inc.; Gerson Lehman Group; GlaxoSmithKline; Healthcare Technology Systems, Inc.; Jazz Pharmaceuticals; Merck & Co., Inc.; the National Institute of Mental Health; Neuronetics; Ono Pharmaceutical; Organon

USA Inc.; Personality Disorder Research Corp.; Pfizer Inc.; the Robert Wood Johnson Foundation; the Stanley Medical Research Institute; the Urban Institute; and Wyeth-Ayerst Laboratories Inc. He has equity holdings in Pfizer Inc and receives royalty/patent income from Guilford Publications and Healthcare Technology Systems, Inc. Dr. Trivedi has served as an advisor, consultant, or speaker for or received research support from Abbott Laboratories, Inc.; Akzo (Organon Pharmaceuticals Inc.); Bayer; Bristol-Myers Squibb Company; Cephalon, Inc.; Corcept Therapeutics, Inc.; Cyberonics, Inc.; Eli Lilly & Company; Forest Pharmaceuticals; GlaxoSmithKline; Janssen Pharmaceutica; Johnson & Johnson PRD; Meade Johnson; the National Institute of Mental Health; the National Alliance for Research in Schizophrenia and Depression; Novartis; Parke-Davis Pharmaceuticals, Inc.; Pfizer Inc; Pharmacia & Upjohn; Predix Pharmaceuticals; Sepracor; Solvay Pharmaceuticals, Inc.; and Wyeth-Ayerst Laboratories. Dr. Wisniewski has received research support from the National Institute of Mental Health and served as an advisor/consultant for Cyberonics, Inc. Dr. Nierenberg has served as an advisor, consultant, or speaker for or received research support from Bristol-Myers Squibb Company; Cederroth; Cyberonics, Inc.; Eli Lilly & Company; Forest Pharmaceuticals Inc.; Genaissance; GlaxoSmithKline; Innapharma; Janssen Pharmaceutica; Lichtwer Pharma; the National Institute of Mental Health; the National Alliance for Research in Schizophrenia and Depression; Neuronetics; Organon, Inc.; Pfizer Inc; Sepracor; Shire; Stanley Foundation; and Wyeth-Ayerst Laboratories. Dr. Stewart has served as an advisor, consultant, or speaker for or received research support from Eli Lilly & Company; GlaxoSmithKline; Organon USA Inc.; Shire; and Somerset. Dr. Warden has received research support from the National Institute of Mental Health and has equity holdings in Bristol-Myers Squibb Company and Pfizer, Inc. Dr. Thase has served as an advisor, consultant, or speaker for AstraZeneca; Bristol-Myers Squibb Company; Cephalon, Inc.; Cyberonics, Inc.; Eli Lilly & Company; Forest Laboratories, Inc.; GlaxoSmithKline; Janssen Pharmaceutica; Eli Lilly & Company; Novartis; Organon, Inc.; Pfizer Pharmaceutical; Sanofi Aventis; Sepracor, Inc.; Shire US Inc.; and Wyeth Pharmaceuticals. Dr. Lavori has served as an advisor, consultant, or speaker for or received research support from Bristol-Myers Squibb Company; Celera Diagnostics Inc; Cyberonics, Inc.; the Department of Veterans Affairs; Forest Pharmaceuticals, Inc.; GlaxoSmithKline; Leaf Cabrezer Hyman and Bernstein; the National

Institutes of Health; and Neuronetics, Inc. Dr. McGrath has served as an advisor, consultant, or speaker for or received research support from Eli Lilly & Company; GlaxoSmithKline; Lipha Pharmaceuticals; the National Institute of Mental Health; the National Institute on Alcohol Abuse and Alcoholism; New York State Department of Mental Hygiene; Organon, Inc.; Research Foundation for Mental Hygiene (New York State); and Somerset Pharmaceuticals. Dr. Rosenbaum has served as an advisor, consultant, or speaker for or received research support from Astra-Zeneca; Boehringer-Ingelheim; Bristol-Myers Squibb Company; Cephalon; Compellis; Cyberonics; EPIX; Forest; GlaxoSmithKline; Janssen; Lilly; MedAvante; Neuronetics; Novartis; Orexigen; Organon; Pfizer, Inc; Roche Diagnostics; Sanofi; Schwartz; Somaxon; Somerset; Sepracor; Shire; Supernus; and Wyeth. He has equity holdings in Compellis, Medavante, and Somaxon. Dr. Sackeim has served as an advisor, consultant, or speaker for or received research support from Cyberonics, Inc.; Eli Lilly & Company; Magstim Ltd.; MECTA Corporation; Neurocrine Biosciences Inc.; Neuronetics Inc.; NeuroPace Inc.; and Pfizer Inc. Dr. Kupfer has served as an advisor, consultant, or speaker for or received research support from Amersham; the Commonwealth of Pennsylvania; Corcept Corporated; Eli Lilly & Company; F. Hoffmann-La Roche Ltd.; Forest Pharmaceuticals; Lundbeck; the National Institute of Mental Health; Novartis; Pfizer, Inc; Servier Amerique; and Solvay/Wyeth. He has equity holdings in Body Media and Med Avante and receives royalty income from Oxford University Press. Dr. Fava has served as an advisor, consultant, or speaker for or received research support from Abbott Laboratories; Alkermes; Aspect Medical Systems; Astra-Zeneca; Bayer AG; Biovail Pharmaceuticals, Inc.; BrainCells, Inc.; Bristol-Myers Squibb Company; Cephalon; Compellis; Cypress Pharmaceuticals; Dov Pharmaceuticals; Eli Lilly & Company; EPIX Pharmaceuticals; Fabre-Kramer Pharmaceuticals, Inc.; Forest Pharmaceuticals Inc.; GlaxoSmithKline; Grunenthal GmBH; J & J Pharmaceuticals; Janssen Pharmaceutica; Jazz Pharmaceuticals; Knoll Pharmaceutical Company; Lichtwer Pharma GmbH; Lorex Pharmaceuticals; Lundbeck; MedAvante, Inc.; Novartis; Nutrition 21; Organon Inc.; PamLab, LLC; Pfizer, Inc; PharmaStar; Pharmavite; Roche; Sanofi/Synthelabo; Sepracor; Solvay Pharmaceuticals, Inc.; Somerset Pharmaceuticals; and Wyeth-Ayerst Laboratories. He has equity holdings in Compellis and MedAvante. Dr. Niederehe, Dr. Lebowitz, and Mr. Luther report no competing interests". [974]

The second example is the TADS trial, already discussed in the chapter "Flaws in antidepressant research", which was also sponsored by the NIMH. This placebo-controlled trial assessed the efficacy of fluoxetine and cognitive-behavioural therapy alone and in combination in adolescents with depression [782]. The financial disclosures in the main article are shown below, and you will notice that many authors had financial relationships with Eli Lilly, the manufacturer of fluoxetine, including speaker, consultancy, and research payments:

> "Dr March has served on the speaker's bureau for Pfizer and Lilly and has received research support from Lilly, Pfizer, and Wyeth. Dr Findling has received research support from Bristol-Myers Squibb, Forest, GlaxoSmithKline, Lilly, Nature's Herbs, Organon, Pfizer, Solvay, Somerset, and Wyeth; been a consultant for Bristol-Myers Squibb, Forest, GlaxoSmithKline, Lilly, Pfizer, Somerset, and Wyeth; and served on the speaker's bureau for Bristol-Myers Squibb, GlaxoSmithKline, Lilly, and Wyeth. Dr Waslick has received research support from Lilly. Dr Walkup has received research support and honoraria from Lilly. Dr Kastelic has received honoraria from Pfizer. Dr Kratochvil has received reseach support from Lilly, Forest, and GlaxoSmithKline; been a consultant for Lilly; and served on the speaker's bureau for Lilly. Dr Harrington has received research support from Lilly, Pfizer, and Astra-Zeneca. Dr Leventhal has been a consultant, received research support, and served on the speaker's bureau for Lilly. Dr Emslie has received research support from Lilly, Organon, and RepliGen; been a consultant for Lilly, GlaxoSmithKline, Forest Laboratories, Pfizer, and Wyeth-Ayerst; and served on the speaker's bureau for McNeil". [782]

Now of course you may argue that I cherry picked a few extreme examples that confirm my argument. But that's not the case. Extensive financial ties to industry are the rule rather than the exception among leading psychiatric academics. We just didn't know (or recognised) for too long. But when reporting of financial conflicts of interest became mandatory in most medical journals in the early 2000s, it was revealed how pervasive financial conflicts of interest are among academic physicians. In 2000, Dr. Angell, then editor-in-chief of the *New England Journal of Medicine*, had a very hard time to find a psychiatric academic without financial relationships to the pharmaceutical industry for an editorial on an antidepressant trial published in the journal. "But as we spoke with research psychiatrists about writing an editorial on the treatment of depression, we found very few who did not have financial ties to drug companies that make antidepressants" she noted in consternation in an article titled "Is academic medicine for sale?" [59].

An analysis of conflict of interest disclosure forms filed by 273 speakers at the APA's annual meeting in 2008 collectively told of 888 consulting contracts and 483 contracts to serve on speakers' bureaus between academic psychiatrists and pharmaceutical companies [30]. Although disclosures of conflicts of interest at scientific conferences and on scientific publications give a first impression of how pervasive the financial relationships between academic medicine and industry are, they don't show the whole picture. The monetary amount of industry payments is not stated in such declarations, and as detailed above, many academics do not (fully) disclose their ties to industry [972, 973]. The true extent (and amount) of physicians' financial ties to industry became only fully known when the US Physician Payments Sunshine Act introduced by Senator Charles Grassley in 2007 was enacted in 2010. The Sunshine Act led to public databases that list all industry payments to US physicians (see Open Payments Database and Dollars for Docs). Although certainly a major breakthrough in a long quest for more transparency in medicine, the new legislation was strongly opposed by various stakeholders [975]. Probably for good self-serving reasons, because the Sunshine Act revealed not only how extensive the financial relationships of many leading academics are, but also how pervasive concealment and non-disclosure of industry payments is among academics, both in general medicine and in psychiatry. Let's look at some disturbing findings.

Norris and colleagues assessed all US physicians who received more than US$ 100,000 from industry in the period 2009 to 2010 according to the public industry-payments database Dollars for Docs. There were in total 373 US physicians who had received more than $100,000 from the industry in that calendar year, of which 117 (31%) were psychiatrists (a disproportionally large rate). 147 of these 373 physicians who received large industry payments had published at least one scientific article between January 2009 and March 2011. On average, there were 8 publications per physician. Only 77% of all physicians provided a conflict of interest disclosure in the article, 23% did not. Even worse, among publications with disclosure, 41% falsely reported that the physician had no financial conflicts of interest to disclose, and in 28% of publications, a conflict other than the payments listed in the Dollars for Docs database was disclosed. Thus, in merely 31% of all publications with a conflict of interest statement the industry relationships were correctly disclosed [976].

Things have not changed since 2009/2010. In a more recent study, Tau and colleagues [973] compared financial relationships listed in the Open Payments Database with those disclosed by US-based academic physicians who were lead-authors of clinical drug trials published between 2016 and 2018 in three leading medical journals. Altogether 85% of lead-authors had received general (i.e. personal) payments from the industry (excludes research support) and the median annual sum received was $62,472. Only 5% of authors disclosed all financial relationships reported in the Open Payments Database, 60% disclosed only parts of the reported payments, and 20% disclosed none of the received payments. Moreover, in 8% of industry-sponsored trials, the lead authors had not disclosed personal payments from the study sponsor, which is a grave violation of publication ethics and a form of scientific misconduct [852]. The study authors thus concluded "These findings could raise concerns about the authors' equipoise toward the trial results and influence the public perception of the credibility of reported data" [973].

The Sunshine Act also unveiled various instances of concealment and serious underreporting of industry payments among leading US psychiatry professors. For instance, in the early 2000s, Dr. Melissa DelBello was professor of psychiatry at the University of Cincinnati and lead author of an influential trial of quetiapine (an atypical antipsychotic) in adolescents with bipolar disorder sponsored by AstraZeneca (the manufacturer of quetiapine). When she was asked by a journalist how much industry funding she received, she responded, "Trust me, I don't make much" [933]. However, towards her employer (the University of Cincinnati) she had disclosed $100,000 from AstraZeneca. Perhaps she indeed considered this substantial sum small in comparison to what her colleagues typically receive, which would not be reassuring. But it gets even worse, for AstraZeneca reported paying her $238,000, that is, more than double the amount Dr. DelBello had declared towards her employer.

Or take Dr. Joseph Biederman, who in the early 2000s, was an exceptionally prominent professor of psychiatry at Harvard University. He played a leading role in establishing both the diagnosis of paediatric bipolar disorder and aggressive antipsychotic treatment in kids with this diagnosis. He had received research support from 15 different pharmaceutical companies and served as speaker and adviser to 7 of them, including Eli Lilly and Janssen Pharmaceuticals (subsidiary of Johnson & Johnson), which produce the blockbuster antipsychotics olanzapine (Zyprexa) and risperidone (Risperdal). He was also director of the Johnson & Johnson Center for Pediatric Psychopathology Research at Massachusetts General Hospital and lead-author of various industry-sponsored drug trials in children and adolescents [977]. When asked by a journalist how much he receives from industry he refused to tell. But a Congressional investigation then revealed that he had failed to disclose towards his employer (Harvard University) large payments he had received from various pharmaceutical companies [933]. From 2000 to 2007, Dr. Biederman earned at least $1.6 million in consulting fees from various drug makers but failed to report all but $200,000 to Harvard University. Surely such large-scale deception is shocking and casts a dark shadow on his character. But how about this: in a deposition between Dr. Biederman and lawyers for the states, he was asked what rank he held at Harvard. "Full professor", he answered. "What's after that?" asked a lawyer. "God", Dr. Biederman responded [977]. I leave this uncommented.

And then there is also the infamous case of Dr. Charles Nemeroff, who in the early 2000s was professor and chair of psychiatry department at Emory University. He had extensive financial ties to multiple pharmaceutical companies and was one of the world's most influential psychiatrists (see also chapter "The transformation of depression"). The magazine *The Economics of Neuroscience* had Dr. Nemeroff on the cover of its September 2000 issue, designating him the "Boss of Bosses" and asking in the headline "Is the Brash and Controversial Charles Nemeroff the Most Powerful Man in Psychiatry?" [9]. Anyway, from 2000 to 2007, Dr. Nemeroff earned more than $2.8 million in consulting fees from various drug makers and failed to report at least $1.2 million of that income to his university. According to a Congressional investigation, he also violated federal research rules. For instance, Dr. Nemeroff signed a letter dated July 15, 2004, promising Emory University administrators that he would earn less than $10,000 a year from GlaxoSmithKline to comply with federal rules to act as principal investigator on NIH research projects investigating GlaxoSmithKline's antidepressants. But in that year alone, he actually had earned $170,000 in income from GlaxoSmithKline [978]. From 2004 to 2008, while receiving NIH grants to study GlaxoSmithKline's antidepressants, Dr. Nemeroff accepted and failed to report at least $500,000 in fees and expenses from GlaxoSmithKline [933].

If you think that this systematic concealment and nondisclosure of industry payments had negative consequences for these key players, then you might be surprised to hear that they still are prominent professors and chairs of psychiatry departments. Drs DelBello and Biederman remained in their positions at University of Cincinnati and Harvard University, respectively, as if nothing happened. Dr. Nemeroff was prohibited by Emory University from submitting NIH grants for two years and in 2009 he resigned from Emory University. However, just one month later, aided by the then-director of the NIMH, Dr. Insel (a good friend of Dr. Nemeroff), and with his guarantee that he could freely apply for NIH grants, Dr. Nemeroff became chair of psychiatry at the University of Miami [933]. So, all's well that ends well for Dr. Nemeroff.

But leaving the deception of universities and federal research funders aside, do industry payments to academics influence their work? That is, do industry payments to medical academics bias the scientific evidence in favour of the industry? Yes, they most certainly do. As detailed by Antonuccio and colleagues, "Company-sponsored experts, whether they are researchers or educators, are by definition company employees. They will be retained only if they offer consistently favorable treatment to the company's products" [24]. This view has been endorsed by various other experts (see, for instance, [29, 405, 406]). Most importantly, this is not just some kind of a controversial assumption, it is a conclusion strongly supported by the scientific literature. There is compelling evidence demonstrating that authors with financial conflicts of interest report more industry-favourable findings and conclusions than authors without ties to industry [592, 794, 799, 944, 946–948, 963]. Put differently, authors with financial conflicts of interest systematically overstate treatment benefits and minimise harms. This should come as no surprise, as you certainly don't bite the hand that feeds you. And what holds true for individual academics probably also holds true for publishers of medical journals and journal editors [28, 29, 979]. So let's have a look.

Medical journals, and the organisations that publish (or own) them, make a substantial proportion of their revenues from drug advertisements [979, 980]. For instance, in 1997, the Massachusetts Medical Society, owner of the leading *New England Journal of Medicine*, made 21.3% of its annual total revenue from drug advertisements in its main journal. The American Medical Association made 10.4% of total revenue from drug advertisements in its top-tier *Journal of the American Medical Association* (*JAMA*), and the American College of Physicians earned 12.9% of its annual total revenue from drug advertisements in its top-tier journal *Annals of Internal Medicine* [981]. The pharmaceutical companies thus can (and already did) exert pressure on medical journals, especially when they publish articles critical towards the effectiveness of blockbuster drugs, knowing that to some extent the owners of these journals financially depend on their advertisements and other profitable avenues such as industry-sponsored journal supplements [29, 979, 980].

But there is another important factor that makes some medical journals financially dependent on the pharmaceutical industry. Drug companies commonly order large amounts of expensive reprints of their articles when a trial yields favourable results that the company can efficiently promote to physicians to increase prescribing of their drug. According to Dr. Smith, former editor of the *British Medical Journal* (*BMJ*), Merck bought 900,000 reprints of an article about the effectiveness of rofecoxib (Vioxx) published in the *New England Journal of Medicine* at a cost estimated to be between $700,000 and $836,000 to promote the drug [982]. A comprehensive analysis of six top-tier medical journals by Lundh and colleagues showed that industry-sponsored trials were more frequently cited and thus significantly contributed to the journals' high impact factors. In addition, income from the sales of article reprints contributed to 3% and 41% of the total income for the *BMJ* and the *Lancet* in 2005–2006 [983]. These findings confirm that some leading medical journals, and by consequence their publishers, strongly depend on the pharmaceutical industry. Influential industry-sponsored trials not only increase the journals' impact factors, they also guarantee the owners of the journals substantial revenues. But the ties between medical journals and the pharmaceutical industry don't end here.

A last important source of conflicts of interest in medical journals are financial relationships of journal editors with the industry. Liu and colleagues [984] reported that 51% of editors of influential US medical journals had received general payments in 2014 (including fees for consulting, speaking, travel, lodging, and consumption) from US pharmaceutical and medical device manufacturers. The mean general payment per editor in that year was $27,564. The five largest general payments to individual editors in the calendar year 2014 were $11.0 million, $1.3 million, $554,162, $355,923, and $325,860. The authors also found large differences between general medicine and various specialties. In high impact general medicine journals, the mean general payments to journal editors was $3899. In cardiology, the mean general payment per editor was $225,556, in orthopaedics it was $92,828, and in endocrinology $63,612. By contrast, in family medicine it was $690, in paediatrics $397, in surgery $246, in general internal medicine it was $54, and in pathology only $11. With a mean of $4371 in general industry-payments, editors of psychiatry journals ranked somewhere in the middle range. There were, in addition, a mean of $37,330 per editor for research support, but since research payments don't count as direct personal income, they were not studied in detail.

An analysis for the year 2015 consistently confirmed these findings [985]. The study found that 46% of editors of influential US medical journals had personal financial ties to the US pharmaceutical and device industry. The median number of general payments per editor was 9 and the median amount of total payments received was $4364. Consulting fees contributed most to the total amount of general payments received. Among US journal editors with industry relationships, 48% received payments more than $5000 in that year, and altogether 38% made more than $10,000 from consulting fees alone. In sum, about half of US journal editors make a personal income from industry payments, and in about half of these, payments are substantial, that is, larger than $5000 a year. A few editors make even a tremendous income from general industry payments, tens thousands of dollars, mostly due to consulting fees. Therefore, various experts requested that journals should disclose the (financial) conflicts of interest of their editors, as is mandatory for authors, so that readers can appraise how strongly journal editors are tied to the industry [980, 986].

Medical Organisations, Medical Education, and Clinical Practice

Just as many academic departments and academic physicians have financial ties to industry, sometimes multiple and very strong ones, so do medical organisations. In 2015, UK professional healthcare organisations received 2189 payments worth in total $12.5 million from the pharmaceutical and device industry. These payments were mostly contributions to costs of events (67.6%) and donations and grants (29.7%) [987]. The leaders of medical organisations likewise have strong financial relationships with the industry. Moynihan and colleagues [988] analysed the financial relationships of leaders of US medical associations from 2017 to 2019 and found that, overall, 72% of these leaders had financial ties to the pharmaceutical and device industry (among leaders with a medical degree, the rate was even 80%). The median amount of industry payments among leaders was $31,805 for the period 2017–2019. The authors further found large differences between specialties. While the rate of leaders with financial ties to industry was 93% for both the Infectious Diseases Society of America and the Orthopaedic Trauma Association, it was 61% for the American College of Physicians and "only" 37% for the American Psychiatric Association (APA). But let's look a bit closer at the latter organisation.

As detailed throughout this book, the APA has, quite understandably, frequently and intensively collaborated with the pharmaceutical industry (given that drugs are the centrepiece in psychiatric research and practice). The pharmaceutical companies are also omnipresent at the APA's annual meetings where they promote their products in various sponsored symposia and huge exhibition halls [394, 399]. Alarmingly, quite often these drug promotions are in violation with APA or FDA rules, for example due to promotion of off-label prescribing [989]. But for the APA, the partnership with the industry in its annual meetings is highly profitable. With the pharmaceutical companies paying for symposia, the exhibition booths, and funding social activities, meeting revenues rose from $1 million in 1980 to $3.1 million in 1990, $11.3 million in 2000, and reaching $16.9 million in 2004, producing a net profit of $9.8 million for the APA in that latter year [30]. In 2000 and 2006, altogether 29% of the APA's annual revenues came from industry, while in 2008 that percentage slightly dropped to 21%. The APA also has two affiliates, the American Psychiatric Foundation and the American Psychiatric Institute for Research and Education, which both are financially heavily supported by the pharmaceutical industry [30].

The arguably most influential achievement of the APA is its diagnostic manual, the DSM, which defines which behaviours and feelings are considered pathological and thus in need of treatment. Given that the pharmaceutical industry can legally promote psychiatric drugs only for approved indications as set out by DSM diagnoses, the manual had and still has a strong impact on the prescribing of drugs. Lowering the diagnostic threshold of a given disorder and/or introducing new disorders and diagnostic labels can massively broaden the market for psychiatric drugs and provide opportunities to expand lucrative drug patents [63, 67, 414, 429, 937, 990]. Understandably, the pharmaceutical industry has a huge interest in how and what the DSM defines as a mental disorder.

Although the pharmaceutical industry does not directly fund the DSM, drug company influence is pervasive in the DSM [991]. Altogether 57% of the DSM-IV task force members had financial ties to pharmaceutical companies. In the DSM-5, that rate even rose to 69%. Financial ties to industry are also the norm in the diagnostic work group members, that is, the experts responsible for the revision of disorder categories and inclusion of new disorders within a diagnostic category. For instance, 100% of the DSM-IV mood disorder work group members had financial relationships with industry. In the DSM-IV anxiety disorders work group, the rate was 81%, and in the DSM-IV schizophrenia and other psychotic disorders work group the rate was 100%. The rates for the corresponding DSM-5 work groups were 67%, 57%, and 83%. Thus, the proportion of work group members with financial ties to industry slightly dropped from DSM-IV to DSM-5, but the rates remained substantial. Overall, three-fourths of the DSM-5 work groups had a majority of members with financial ties to the pharmaceutical industry [991].

Another very influential publication of the APA are its treatment guidelines. Cosgrove and colleagues analysed three major APA clinical practice guidelines applicable in 2008—the schizophrenia, bipolar disorder, and major depressive disorder guidelines. Altogether 90% of guideline authors had a financial relationship with at least one pharmaceutical company. In both the bipolar disorder and schizophrenia guidelines, the rates were 100% each, whereas in the major depressive disorder guideline the rate was 60%. Strikingly, none of the authors' financial conflicts of interest were disclosed in the clinical practice guidelines. Among the authors with industry relationships, most received research funding (78%) and consultancy fees (72%). Altogether 17% of guideline authors with industry relationships also held equity in a drug company that manufactured the drugs identified in the practice guidelines [992].

In a subsequent study, Cosgrove and colleagues analysed the financial conflicts of interest in 14 major depressive disorder clinical practice guidelines, including the APA's most recent edition. In 6 guidelines (43%) no author had financial ties to the industry. In 5 guidelines (36%) a minority of authors had industry relationships and in 3 guidelines (21%) a majority of authors had industry relationships. The latter category also included the APA practice guideline, of which all 6 authors had multiple ties to the pharmaceutical industry. In accordance with the scientific evidence, 9 of 14 guidelines did not recommend antidepressants as first-line treatment in mild depression, but 5 did (among those the APA guideline). Most importantly, while 4 of 5 guidelines (80%) recommending antidepressants as first-line treatment in mild depression had significant financial conflicts of interest (defined as majority of members or the chair of the work group according to the Institute of Medicine), only 3 of 9 guidelines (33%) not making such a recommendation had significant financial conflicts of interest [993]. Thus, as consistently demonstrated in the literature detailed above, authors with financial ties to industry more often draw conclusions and make recommendations that favour the pharmaceutical companies' commercial interests [592, 799, 944, 946–948].

But how extensive are the financial conflicts of interest in the APA depression practice guideline? Below you see the conflicts of interest disclosure of the six authors of the current APA depression practice guideline, Drs. Alan Gelenberg (chair), Marlene Freeman, John Markowitz, Jerrold Rosenbaum, Michael Thase, and Madhukar Trivedi:

> "The Work Group on Major Depressive Disorder reports the following potentially competing interests for the period from May 2005 to May 2010: Dr. Gelenberg reports consulting for Eli Lilly and Company, Pfizer, Best Practice, AstraZeneca, Wyeth, Cyberonics, Novartis, Forest Pharmaceuticals, Inc., GlaxoSmithKline, ZARS Pharma, Jazz Pharmaceuticals, Lundbeck, Takeda Pharmaceuticals North America, Inc., eResearch Technology, Dey Pharma, PGxHealth, and Myriad Genetics. He reports serving on speakers bureaus for Pfizer, GlaxoSmithKline, and Wyeth. He reports receiving research grant funding from Eli Lilly and Company, Pfizer, and GlaxoSmithKline. He reports stock ownership in Healthcare Technology Systems. Dr. Freeman reports that she received research support from the Meadows Foundation, the National Institute for Mental Health, the U.S. Food and Drug Administration, the Institute for Mental Health Research, Forest, GlaxoSmithKline and Eli Lilly and Company (investigator initiated trials), and Pronova Biocare (research materials). She received an honorarium for case-based peer-reviewed material for AstraZeneca's website. She reports consulting for Ther-Rx, Reliant, and Pamlab. She reports receiving an honorarium for speaking at an APA continuing medical education program that was sponsored by Forest and an honorarium for speaking at a continuing medication education program sponsored by KV Pharmaceuticals. She reports receiving an honorarium from Leerink Swann for participating in a focus group. Dr. Markowitz reports consulting for Ono Pharmaceutical Co., Ltd. (2005). He reports receiving research support from Forest Pharmaceuticals, Inc. (2005). He reports receiving grant support from the National Institute of Mental Health (2005–2013), the National Alliance for Research in Schizophrenia and Depression (2005), and MINT: Mental Health Initiative (2005). He reports receiving royalties from American Psychiatric Publishing, Inc. (2005–2010), Basic Books (2005–2010), Elsevier (2005–2010), and Oxford University Press (2007–2010). Dr. Rosenbaum reports attending advisory boards for Bristol-Myers Squibb, Cephalon, Cyberonics, Forest Pharmaceuticals, Inc., Eli Lilly and Company,

MedAvante, Neuronetics, Inc., Novartis, Orexigen Therapeutics, Inc., Organon BioSciences, Pfizer, Roche Diagnostics, Sanofiaventis, Shire, and Wyeth. He reports consulting for Auspex Pharmaceuticals, Compellis Pharmaceuticals, EPIX Pharmaceuticals, Neuronetics, Inc., Organon BioSciences, Somaxon, and Supernus Pharmaceuticals, Inc. He reports receiving honoraria from lectureships for Boehringer Ingleheim, Bristol-Myers Squibb, Cyberonics, Forest Pharmaceuticals, Inc., Eli Lilly and Company, and Schwartz Pharma. He was involved in the creation of the Massachusetts General Hospital Psychiatry Academy (MGH-PA) and has served as a panelist in four satellite broadcast programs. MGH-PA programs that have industry support are always multi-sponsored, and curriculum development by the Academy is independent of sponsorship; the curricula from January 2005 to March 2009 included sponsorship support from AstraZeneca, Bristol-Myers Squibb, Cephalon, Eli Lilly and Company, Forest Pharmaceuticals, Inc., GlaxoSmithKline, Janssen Medical Affairs LLC, Ortho-McNeil Pharmaceutical, sanofiaventis, Shire, and Wyeth. He reports equity holdings in Compellis Pharmaceuticals, MedAvante, and Somaxon. Dr. Thase reports that he provided scientific consultation to AstraZeneca, Bristol-Myers Squibb, Eli Lilly & Company, Forest Pharmaceuticals, Inc., Gerson Lehman Group, GlaxoSmithKline, Guidepoint Global, H. Lundbeck A/S, MedAvante, Inc., Neuronetics, Inc., Novartis, Otsuka, Ortho-McNeil Pharmaceuticals, PamLab, L.L.C., Pfizer (formerly Wyeth-Ayerst Laboratories), Schering-Plough (formerly Organon), Shire U.S., Inc., Supernus Pharmaceuticals, Takeda (Lundbeck), and Transcept Pharmaceuticals. He was a member of the speakers bureaus for AstraZeneca, Bristol-Myers Squibb, Eli Lilly and Company, GlaxoSmithKline, Pfizer (formerly Wyeth-Ayerst Laboratories), and Schering-Plough (formerly Organon). He received grant funding from Eli Lilly and Company, GlaxoSmithKline, the National Institute of Mental Health, the Agency for Healthcare Research and Quality, and Sepracor, Inc. He had equity holdings in MedAvante, Inc., and received royalty income from American Psychiatric Publishing, Inc., Guilford Publications, Herald House, Oxford University Press, and W.W. Norton and Company. His wife was employed as the group scientific director for Embryon (formerly Advogent), which does business with Bristol-Myers Squibb and Pfizer/Wyeth. Dr. Trivedi reports that he was a consultant to or on speaker bureaus for Abbott Laboratories, Inc., Abdi Ibrahim, Akzo (Organon Pharmaceuticals, Inc.), AstraZeneca, Bristol-Myers Squibb Company,

> Cephalon, Inc., Cyberonics, Inc., Eli Lilly and Company, Evotec, Fabre Kramer Pharmaceuticals, Inc., Forest Pharmaceuticals, GlaxoSmithKline, Janssen Pharmaceutica Products, L.P., Johnson & Johnson P.R.D., Meade-Johnson, Medtronic, Neuronetics, Otsuka Pharmaceuticals, Parke-Davis Pharmaceuticals, Inc., Pfizer, Inc., Sepracor, Shire Development, Solvay Pharmaceuticals, VantagePoint, and Wyeth-Ayerst Laboratories. He received research support from the Agency for Healthcare Research and Quality, Corcept Therapeutics, Inc., Cyberonics, Inc., Merck, National Alliance for Research in Schizophrenia and Depression, National Institute of Mental Health, National Institute on Drug Abuse, Novartis, Pharmacia & Upjohn, Predix Pharmaceuticals (Epix), Solvay Pharmaceuticals, Inc., and Targacept". [231]

The massive amount of industry relationships among authors of the APA major depressive disorder clinical practice guideline is by no means an exception. A systematic review found that the majority of clinical practice guidelines had authors with industry affiliations, including consultancies (authors with relationship, range 6–80%), research support (4–78%), equity/stock ownership (2–17%), or any financial conflict of interest (56–87%) [994]. In a seminal study by Choudhry and colleagues from 2002, 192 authors of 44 North American and European clinical practice guidelines on various conditions were surveyed. Altogether 87% of authors had financial relationships with the pharmaceutical industry. On average, the guideline authors had ties to 11 different companies. But these financial conflicts of interest were in the vast majority not disclosed in the guidelines. Moreover, while only 7% of the guideline authors thought that their own relationship with the pharmaceutical industry influenced their own recommendations made, 19% of authors (i.e. more than double) thought that their co-authors' recommendations were influenced by their industry relationships [995].

A more recent analysis of 114 clinical practice guidelines from various countries by Kung and colleagues showed that the scientific quality of most clinical practice guidelines is poor [996]. Fewer than half of the guidelines surveyed met more than 50% of the Institute of Medicine quality standards. For instance, scientific evidence supporting recommendations was lacking in 35% of guidelines, 76% failed to include an information scientist and a formal quality of evidence rating was missing in 24%. Moreover, financial conflicts of interest were pervasive (71% of chairs and 91% of co-chairpersons had industry relationships) and often not disclosed. Thus, even when guidelines contain author conflict of interest disclosures, these are all too often incomplete. A recent analysis of 18 clinical practice guidelines providing recommendations for 10 high-revenue medications found that 26% of guidelines authors who received payments from industry did not fully disclose these payments. Altogether 7.5% of authors declared no financial conflicts of interest but were found to have industry relationships [997]. In another analysis of North American practice guidelines for hyperlipidaemia or diabetes, it was shown that among guideline authors who formally declared no conflicts of interest, 11% had one or more industry relationships [998]. Financial relationships between the medical organisations that produce the guidelines and the industry are also very common but rarely declared in the guidelines [999, 1000].

Bindslev and colleagues examined 45 guidelines from 14 Danish specialty societies published between July 2010 and March 2012 and found that 96% of guidelines had one or more authors with a conflict of interest. Of 254 guideline authors, 53% had a conflict of interest. The most common conflicts of interest were being a consultant, an advisory board member, or a company employee. Disturbingly, only one guideline (2%) disclosed author conflicts of interest and the quality of the guidelines was generally poor [1001]. The situation is no better in the depression domain. Based on their evaluation of 11 clinical practice guidelines for major depressive disorder, Zafra-Tanaka and colleagues concluded "Most of evaluated CPGs [clinical practice guidelines] did not take into account the patient's viewpoints, achieved a low score in the rigor of development domain, and did not clearly state the process used to reach the recommendations" [1002]. In accordance, Bennet and colleagues found that only 4 of 17 (24%) practice guidelines for depression in children and adolescents met minimal quality standards and only 2 (12%) were rated high quality [1003].

Among the few notable exceptions of high-quality documents is the NICE depression guideline, for both adults and youth. It has comparably few conflicts of interest and adheres to high quality standards, including a grading of recommendations, assessment, development and evaluations, a risk of bias assessment, and discussion of the clinical significance of treatment effects [1002, 1003]. But unfortunately, the norms are highly conflicted guidelines of inadequate scientific rigour. A prototypical example of these poor-quality documents is the APA major depressive disorder clinical practice guideline [231]. It is among the many guidelines that have massive financial conflicts of interest (see above). It is also of poor scientific quality, as the methodology used to reach recommendations as well as to grade the strength of recommendations is based on expert consensus (which is problematic in general and especially in view of the authors' extensive ties to the pharmaceutical industry), a literature search strategy is not mentioned, a list of included studies is not available, and a risk of bias assessment is not provided. Moreover, the APA depression guideline does not evaluate or discuss the clinical significance of treatment effects, and 20% of the references are incongruent with the recommendations [1002, 1004]. But there are even more limitations.

All six authors of the APA depression guideline are professors of psychiatry with a main research interest in psychopharmacology and biological psychiatry. General practitioners who treat the majority patients with depression were not included in the panel. Also missing on the panel were methodologists, public health experts, nurses, patients, as well as non-medical practitioners, including psychologists and social workers. Altogether 9% of all cited research and 13% of references supporting the recommendations were co-authored by the six guideline authors. Finally, the independent panel that reviewed the guideline for bias had undisclosed financial ties to pharmaceutical companies that manufacture antidepressants [1004]. Unsurprisingly, the APA depression guideline much more often recommends antidepressants as first-line treatment than other depression guidelines [1002], even for mild depression, where the effectiveness of antidepressants has not been demonstrated. In fact, the APA depression guideline is the only one among 14 guidelines studied that makes an explicit recommendation for antidepressants in mild depression, paradoxically giving this recommendation the highest rating of certainty level [1004]. Finally, the paediatric depression guideline of the American Academy of Child and Adolescent Psychiatry [1005] is equally hampered by massive conflicts of interest and poor quality standards [1003].

In sum, although clinical practice guidelines have become very influential in modern evidence-based medicine, they typically are of poor scientific quality and are subject to pervasive (and often undisclosed) conflicts of interest [996, 1000–1003]. Understandably, various experts expressed concern about the proliferation of and adherence to such unreliable practice guidelines [990, 1006, 1007]. As aptly summarised by Shaneyfelt and Centor in a *JAMA* editorial in 2009,

> "The most widely recognized bias is financial. Guidelines often have become marketing tools for device and pharmaceutical manufacturers … Other biases are also important. The specialty composition of a guideline panel likely influences guideline development. Specialty societies can use guidelines to enlarge that specialty's area of expertise in a competitive medical marketplace. Federal guideline committees may focus on limiting costs; committees influenced by industry are more likely to shape recommendations to accord with industry needs. Guidelines have other limitations. Guidelines are often too narrowly focused on single diseases and are not patient focused. Patients seldom have single diseases, and few if any guidelines help clinicians in managing complexity … Guidelines are not patient-specific enough to be useful and rarely allow for individualization of care. Most guidelines have a one-size-fits-all mentality and do not build flexibility or contextualization into the recommendations … Only when likely biases of industry and specialty societies have been either removed or overcome by countervailing interests can impartial recommendations be achieved … If all that can be produced are biased, minimally applicable consensus statements, perhaps guidelines should be avoided completely. Unless there is evidence of appropriate changes in the guideline process, clinicians and policy makers must reject calls for adherence to guidelines. Physicians would be better off making clinical decisions based on valid primary data". [1008]

More recently, Dr. Ioannidis, a leading expert in evidence-based medicine, echoed these obvious limitations and biases of clinical practice guidelines:

> "Thus, these guidelines writing activities are particularly helpful in promoting the careers of specialists, in building recognizable and sustainable hierarchies of clan power, in boosting the impact factors of specialty journals and in elevating the visibility of the sponsoring organizations and their conferences that massively promote society products to attendees. However, do they improve medicine or do they homogenize biased, collective, and organized ignorance? Well-conducted unbiased guidelines can be useful. However, most published guidelines have one or more red flags that either make them overtly unreliable or should at least raise suspicion among potential users. The list of red flags includes sponsoring by a professional society with substantial industry funding, conflicts of interest for chairs and panel members, stacking, insufficient methodologist involvement, inadequate external review, and noninclusion of nonphysicians, patients, and community members". [1009]

Above I have detailed how the pharmaceutical industry can influence physicians' prescribing behaviour by supporting academic departments, senior researchers, medical organisations, and both the clinical practice guidelines and diagnostic manuals they produce. Another powerful avenue for drug companies to influence prescribing is through sponsoring continuing medical education and the speakers at these events and by promoting their products directly to physicians through marketing lectures (typically sponsored lunches/dinners with slide presentations) and office visits from pharmaceutical sales representatives [428, 588, 1010–1012]. These are the topics I will now turn to.

To remain current with the rapidly changing healthcare practices and medical treatments, physicians regularly attend continuing medical education. The aim of these educational events is to ensure that physicians are up to date with the best practices in modern healthcare. The best practices (or standards of care) should of course be in the interest of patients and the public. Alas, continuing medical education is not exempt from unduly influences that serve the commercial interests of the pharmaceutical and device industry rather than the best interests of patients and the public. Corporate bias in continuing medical education is introduced through the industry's financial support of educational events, the invited speakers at these events, and the academic departments, medical societies or specialised companies organising these events [428,

1013–1015]. Unfortunately, most physicians are not aware of these influences. As recently stressed by Dr. Fugh-Berman, "Although awareness of individual conflicts of interest and ethical problems with physician-industry relationships has increased, few people realise just how much continuing education is used for product promotion" [1012].

Internal industry documents released through litigation or whistle-blowing clearly show that pharmaceutical companies misuse educational events to promote their drugs, including illegal off-label prescribing [29, 1016]. For instance, both Forest Laboratories and GlaxoSmithKline sponsored educational events to promote off-label prescribing of their antidepressant drugs escitalopram and paroxetine, respectively, for unapproved adolescent depression [29]. According to the scientific evidence there can be little doubt that industry-funding of educational events introduces bias, resulting in unbalanced assessments of drug treatments that overstate benefits and minimise harms [428, 1011, 1012, 1017]. Key opinion leaders, the top-ranked academic experts on industry payroll, are the preferred speakers at such educational events. However, their role is highly controversial, for they make a substantial personal income from promoting the pharmaceutical companies' products to physicians and the public [29, 406, 428]. Various authors thus contend that key opinion leaders significantly contribute to the corruption of medicine [1018] and that all too often, they risk becoming "drug representatives in disguise" [405]. But what about the many practitioners? Do they also have financial relationships with the biomedical industry? And how are they influenced by the industry?

In 2014, 52% of all US physicians received at least one general payment from the industry for a total value of $1.94 billion (excludes research support). General payments slightly declined recently but remained considerable. In 2018, 45% of all US physicians received at least one general payment for a total value of $1.82 billion. The median annual payment per physician was $216 and the mean payment was $4606 [1019]. In addition, US pharmaceutical companies spend almost twice as much money on drug promotion compared to research and development [1020]. Marketing to physicians accounts for most promotional spending of the pharmaceutical industry. From 1997 through 2016, spending for direct-to-physician marketing increased from $15.6 billion to

$20.3 billion, of which $5.6 billion were due to pharmaceutical detailing [433]. The latter is a euphemistic term for drug promotion, which often takes place at sponsored lunches or dinners. Physicians also frequently receive visits from pharmaceutical sales representatives who promote their company's drugs and distribute free drug samples and gifts. Is this problematic? Yes, it is! Research has consistently shown that these promotions are often unbalanced and that risks/harms are rarely mentioned, even for drugs that carry serious safety warnings [588, 1021, 1022]. Perhaps you remember the promotional material GlaxoSmithKline provided to its sales representatives related to its fraudulent study 329, which stated that paroxetine "demonstrates remarkable efficacy and safety in the treatment of adolescent depression", despite a lack of meaningful benefits and significantly increased risk of suicidal behaviour [29]. So you certainly get an impression of how unbalanced and biased such drug promotions by sales representatives often are.

Nevertheless, you may rightly argue that everybody (including physicians) knows that promotional messages are typically exaggerated, regardless of whether they come from a car manufacturer, watchmaker, or pharmaceutical company. You may thus rightly object that most physicians are well aware that pharmaceutical sales representatives exaggerate (or misrepresent) the benefit–harm ratio of the drugs they sell. However, the scientific evidence does not consistently support this view. According to the literature, most physicians perceive pharmaceutical sales representatives and industry-sponsored continuing medical education events as important and accurate sources of drug information and scientific knowledge, but views are divided and some physicians also have sceptical attitudes towards industry influence [1010, 1011, 1017, 1023, 1024]. The main issue is that physicians think they can discern biased promotional messages from accurate scientific evidence, but they often fail to do so [1012, 1025, 1026]. As emphasised by Sah and Fugh-Berman, "although physicians believe they can extract objective information from sales pitches, they routinely fail to distinguish between correct and incorrect information provided by sales representatives" [1027].

As I already detailed elsewhere, it comes without saying that most physicians aren't intentionally corrupted by gifts and sponsored meals, even though there are certainly a few who willingly accepted bribes and kickbacks [1028–1030]. Nevertheless, the rare cases of deliberate over-prescribing and/or mistreatment in exchange for money and/or gifts are not the main public health issue. The crucial question is whether all these shiny gifts, the sponsored dinners at fancy locations, sponsored conference travel and location, the constant interactions with handsome sales representatives delivering catchy marketing messages, and the regular attendance of industry-sponsored continuing medical education events, unconsciously influence physicians' prescribing behaviours. That is, do physicians unintentionally prescribe more drugs, sometimes inappropriately, due to these pervasive pharmaceutical marketing strategies?

Let us first examine if physicians believe that their prescribing behaviour is influenced by the pharmaceutical industry. This question is easy to answer, for the scientific evidence is very clear and consistent about that. Only a minority of physicians think that their interactions with the pharmaceutical industry, including receipt of gifts and payments, have an impact on their own prescribing behaviour, but they consider their physician colleagues more susceptible to pharmaceutical marketing strategies than themselves [588, 1010, 1011, 1024]. For instance, in one study, 39% of physicians agreed that industry promotions and contacts did influence their own prescribing behaviour, but 84%, that is more than double, believed that other physicians are affected [1031]. As you might remember, we saw the same pattern in relation to perceived bias in clinical practice guidelines, where only 7% of authors thought that their own relationships with the pharmaceutical industry influenced their recommendations, but 19%, again more than double, conceded their co-authors were influenced by industry ties [995]. Of course, it cannot both be true that most physicians are unbiased and many other physicians are biased. So what's happening here?

This inconsistency (i.e., "I'm not influenced by industry but my colleagues are") is most likely the result of cognitive-motivational biases and suggests that individual physicians considerably underestimate the influence industry has over their own prescribing behaviour [1027, 1032]. If true, then there should be strong and consistent evidence of an association between industry relationships (e.g. gift receipt, contact with pharmaceutical sales representatives) and prescribing behaviour that subserves the industry's commercial interest (i.e. more prescriptions, preference for costly, patented drugs). But before I detail the scientific evidence, let's just quickly recapitulate that the pharmaceutical companies spend billions of dollars every year for direct-to-physician marketing [433, 1020]. They would certainly not spend such vast sums if there would be no return on investment. That is, their tremendous marketing efforts must result in increased drug sales (and profits), otherwise they would cut down spending on marketing. So you probably sense what's coming …

A compelling body of scientific evidence indeed consistently shows that the more gifts physicians receive, the more they interact with pharmaceutical sales representatives, and the more they attend industry-sponsored continuing medical education and promotional events, the more drugs they prescribe (often off-label, i.e. for non-approved indications), the costlier the drugs they prescribe (patented drugs instead of much cheaper but equivalent generic drugs), and the more inappropriate the prescriptions are (i.e. nonadherent to best practice) [1033–1037]; for systematic reviews, see [796, 798, 943, 1010].

In conclusion, there can be little doubt that direct-to-physician pharmaceutical marketing alters physicians' drug prescribing, increasing the rate of low-value, inappropriate and unnecessary prescriptions. Pharmaceutical marketing leads to harmful overprescribing and therefore can have a detrimental impact on public health and patient safety, as tragically evidenced by the US opioid epidemic [928, 929, 931]. Although few physicians think that their interactions with the industry influence their treatment decisions, the scientific evidence strongly indicates the opposite. Most physicians are not aware that pharmaceutical companies can change their prescribing behaviour through subtle marketing strategies, indicating that this is an unintentional, subconscious act [1012, 1027]. For the same reason, mere disclosure of industry relationships won't prevent (or remove) the biases resulting from financial conflicts of interest [1038]. As succinctly summarised by Mitchell and colleagues in a systematic review recently published in the top-tier journal *Annals of Internal Medicine*:

> "We present evidence that receipt of financial payments from industry is consistently associated with increased prescribing. This association has been identified across a broad range of physician specialties, drug classes,

and prescribing decisions. In addition, evidence of a temporal association and dose-responsiveness strongly suggests a causal relationship. We also found evidence, consistent with prior studies, that industry payments are associated with increased use of lower-value drugs. Taken together, our results support the conclusion that personal payments from industry reduce physicians' ability to make independent therapeutic decisions and that they may be harmful to patients. The medical community must change its historical opposition to reform and call for an end to such payments". [796]

This leads us directly to the last chapter, "Solutions for reform".

6

Solutions for Reform

Before I offer some thoughts (and suggestions) as to how we could try to make better, I want to briefly summarise my main points, by clearly pointing out what my arguments are and what not. I constantly had the experience, in the scientific literature and personally (e.g. during peer review and via newspapers and social media), that people are frequently attacked with strawmen, false accusations, and misrepresentations of their arguments. For instance, when I contend that most negative emotional states physicians (especially GPs) diagnose with major depression are mild or subthreshold, I frequently get an angry response from psychiatrists that I deny the suffering of people with severe depression and that I minimise the burden of a serious psychiatric disorder. But that's absolutely not my argument. I acknowledge that some forms of depression are very serious and debilitating and I recognise the burden of severe clinical depression. But it's a strawman argument, because saying that most forms of depression are mild or subthreshold does not call into question that severe depression exists. Of course, severe depression is real, and in my view it's a medical condition in need of treatment. But fortunately, these serious conditions lie at the extreme end of a spectrum and they are relatively rare compared to the many more people diagnosed

M. P. Hengartner, *Evidence-biased Antidepressant Prescription*,
https://doi.org/10.1007/978-3-030-82587-4_6

with major depression who have non-serious, transient symptoms and self-limiting, minor impairments.

Starting in the 1970s and reaching a peak in the 1990s, academic psychiatry made strong efforts that GPs better detect the broad (and heterogeneous) concept of depression. The predominant view back then was that depression is severely under-recognised and underdiagnosed in primary care. Many educational events and awareness campaigns were run in order to remedy what was felt to be one of the biggest issues in mental healthcare. The pharmaceutical industry strongly supported these efforts, for the broadening of the diagnostic criteria of depression and increased detection of depressive states also massively extended the market for antidepressants. Depression became an overinclusive condition largely treated in primary care, in particular by GPs, and a new generation of antidepressants, the SSRIs, were heralded as miracle drugs, as quick and safe chemical cures for a broad array of emotional problems, ranging from stress, sorrow, insecurity, anxiousness, sadness up to the rare manifestations of severe (melancholic) depression. The GPs followed psychiatry's (and the pharmaceutical industry's) instructions and eagerly diagnosed depression in their patients, mostly accompanied with a prescription for an SSRI. And so depression became one of the most frequent medical conditions, both in the community and in primary care, and antidepressants the best-selling drug class [63, 93, 393].

Yet many forms of what GPs diagnose as depression are normal emotional reactions to common problems of living, the sadness and despair that sometimes come with human life when we lose a friend, partner, or family member, when lifelong dreams shatter or an important project fails, something we worked hard for, with devotion and passion. After such events, it quite often happens that we are sad and heartbroken, we may lose pleasure and interest in some activities, ruminate, have negative thoughts about ourselves, we sleep badly and lack appetite. Sometimes this state can go on for a few weeks, but usually we adapt after some time, readjust, and fully recover. And many (perhaps most) people stay well afterwards (unless they are hit by a new critical life event). I know this from personal experience. And there is strong scientific evidence that such emotional reactions, even if acutely intense and burdensome, typically have a good long-term outcome [480–482].

Feeling intense sadness, discontent, fatigue, and lack of pleasure or interest is not necessarily pathological, under many circumstances it is perfectly normal. Ultimately, it is what makes us human: caring, compassionate people with feelings, hopes, and dreams. Labelling such emotional reactions categorically as mental disorders, handing over a diagnosis of major depression and an antidepressant prescription, medicalises unhappiness (or distress) and leads to a pharmaceuticalisation of life [3, 5, 453, 1039, 1040]. By consequence, there is clear and unequivocal scientific evidence that depression is overdiagnosed [450] and that antidepressants are massively overused [105, 117, 127].

This does not mean, however, that all people with clinical depression are correctly diagnosed and receive adequate treatment. Even severe forms of depression can go undetected and remain untreated, thus underdiagnosis and undertreatment undeniably also is a reality [105]. Nevertheless, severe/serious depression is much less frequent than mild/minor depression [115, 116, 463]. Likewise, only a small proportion of people have chronic or highly recurrent depression, some have a few recurrences and about half of all people fully recover after a first episode and remain well long-term [190, 471]. Thus, without denying that depression can be a serious and persistent disorder in a minority of people, the claim that depression is typically severe and chronic is factually wrong. Except from benefitting the pharmaceutical industry, which has long realised that marketing the disease is more profitable than marketing the treatment, I see absolutely no reason why we should scare people with a false (or inaccurate) depiction of how depression typically manifests in the general population and in primary care patients.

Another misleading (unevidenced) claim about depression is the notion that it is a brain disorder. Thus far, any convincing scientific evidence that depression is caused by a clearly defined pathology/dysfunction in the brain is lacking [395, 1041, 1042]. This is not to say that neurobiological factors are not involved in the expression (and experience) of depression symptoms. Of course they are, because without a brain we would not be able to have emotions. But this by no means implies that an abnormality in the brain must be the cause of negative emotions [395, 396]. An extreme variant of the brain disorder notion is the chemical imbalance or monoamine (serotonin) deficiency theory.

Although long very popular in mainstream psychiatry and still endorsed by various academics and practitioners, there has never been strong scientific support for it and many experts argue that it has been disconfirmed [26, 595, 624]. However, as a marketing strategy, the chemical imbalance notion was (and still is) priceless to the pharmaceutical industry, as it helped to erroneously promote antidepressants as essential chemical cures that fix an underlying neurobiological pathology [596, 1043].

However, the effectiveness of antidepressants does not live up to those high expectations. It took some time, though, to find this out, because pharmaceutical companies persistently engaged in selective reporting of favourable efficacy outcomes: trials with positive results were published, often multiple times, whereas trials with negative results were hidden or published as positive after dredging the data [57, 174, 1044]. The so-called key opinion leaders, influential academic psychiatrists on industry payroll, significantly contributed to this distortion of the evidence base and engaged in uncritical promotion of antidepressant mass prescribing [9, 29], even in patient populations where the benefit–harm ratio is largely unfavourable, for example, in children and adolescents [120, 784] and in adults with mild depression [181, 455].

We also know that antidepressant trials are plagued with many serious methodological limitations, including preselected and unrepresentative samples, very short duration of merely 6–8 weeks, removal of early placebo responders, inadequate handling of study dropouts (missing values), and unblinding of clinical investigators [13, 144, 163, 707]. All of these limitations most likely bias the results in favour of antidepressants, thus leading to exaggerated efficacy estimates and underestimation of harms [18, 54, 695]. Antidepressants certainly can have some therapeutic effects (e.g. sedation or activation), but if benefits clearly outweigh harms in most patients with moderate-to-severe depression remains uncertain [13, 18, 102, 140]. Moreover, antidepressants have no meaningful benefits in patients with mild, minor, and subthreshold depression, which is why most treatment guidelines do not recommend antidepressants as first-line treatment in this patient population [181, 232, 233].

That said, I do not contend that antidepressants have no psychotropic effects. They certainly have, and users typically sense these mental changes [274]. So when I say that antidepressants are often not much better than placebo, I do not imply that antidepressants are inert. Depending on their pharmacological action, antidepressants can have more sedating or activating effects [273, 274], and all can (and often do) cause some form of emotional numbing [276–278]. The reason why antidepressants fail to separate from placebo in about every second trial, and overall demonstrate only a small benefit, is that these psychotropic effects do not necessarily improve depression. Whereas one patient may benefit from sedation, another may perceive this mental state as unpleasant/harmful. Activation may help some people to overcome anhedonia and psychomotor retardation, but in others it may cause adverse reactions such as agitation, insomnia, and even suicidal behaviour. Likewise, emotional numbing may be helpful or even lifesaving to some patients in the short-term to overcome acute distress, but in the long-term it is often perceived as harmful and a main reason for quitting treatment [1045, 1046]. As a result, patient views on the helpfulness of antidepressants vary greatly. Just slightly above half of users (50–60%) are satisfied with their antidepressant and consider the medication helpful, whereas the rest (40–50%) feel no benefit or even perceive the drug as harmful [276, 365, 366].

My last main argument is that evidence-based medicine is subject to pervasive conflicts of interest and corporate bias. Many physicians are closely tight to the companies that market the drugs they research and prescribe. But the industry is not only a manufacturer of medical products, it is also the main sponsor of a large segment of the healthcare sector. Through their immense financial and political power, the pharmaceutical industry has considerable influence over drug regulators, academic medical departments, medical organisations, patient and consumer organisations, and individual prescribers. These pervasive industry relationships introduce systematic bias in medical research, education, and practice, and eventually result in overtesting, overdiagnosis, and overtreatment, thus harming patients and the public [171, 377, 379, 380, 458]. Psychiatry, and in particular the domain of depression, are of course not exempt from these undue industry influences.

This does not mean that all medical interventions (including psychiatric treatments) are per se harmful. I am convinced they are not. Insinuating that I hold such a view would be a terrible (and malicious) misrepresentation of my arguments. Medicine has made great achievements, often in partnership with the pharmaceutical industry. Medical interventions can cure (or prevent) serious illnesses and save lives. This is beyond dispute. But the history of medicine, including the most recent, is also replete with examples where established medical interventions have, on balance, done more harm than good [383, 645, 647]. Moreover, a treatment that may be life-saving in some patients can also badly harm many more patients when uncritically promoted and inadequately prescribed outside a specific, narrowly defined patient population or when used in unapproved indications [414, 428, 458, 928, 1047]. This is also beyond dispute. Antidepressants likely fall into this category, for they are mostly prescribed to patients who are unlikely to benefit, that is, the majority of adult patients with mild, minor and subthreshold depression, patients with bipolar depression, youth and old adults with depression and/or anxiety symptoms, and unapproved (off-label) indications in all age groups [105, 117, 119, 129, 301, 1048–1050].

Moreover, the scientific evidence clearly shows that corporate bias has resulted in the approval and marketing of ineffective or harmful drugs, the provision of unnecessary medical interventions, and the denial or minimisation of iatrogenic harm [171, 379, 380, 428, 949]. Case in points are the Vioxx scandal (involving Merck) [824], the OxyContin scandal (involving Purdue Pharma) [931], the Tamiflu scandal (involving Roche) [1051], and, most pertinent to the topic of this book, the Paxil/Seroxat scandal (involving GlaxoSmithKline) [770, 785, 786]. The Thalidomide disaster (involving Chemie Grünenthal) is deliberately not included here, as it occurred before stringent premarketing drug evaluation was in place [1052].

Another detrimental consequence of the pervasive financial relationships between medicine and the biomedical industry is the growing public mistrust in medical organisations and the healthcare system. Mistrust can prevent people from accepting (and using) medical interventions with clearly evidenced effectiveness. Instead, people who lost confidence in biomedicine may prefer unevidenced (inferior) treatments or reject medical interventions altogether. Such a mistrust in the medical profession has most likely also contributed to peoples' rejection of essential vaccines, which may jeopardise (or damage) public health [1053, 1054]. The public mistrust in psychiatry is, at least in part, also attributable to media reports about the pervasive industry relationships among eminent academic psychiatrists and their concealment/nondisclosure of massive financial conflicts of interest [978, 1055–1058]. It is quite understandable that people get suspicious about an alleged new wonder treatment when they learn that the professor praising the new drug at medical conferences, in journal articles, and in the media earns tens of thousands dollars per year in consultancy and speaker fees from the company selling this drug.

Restoring Confidence in the Depression Domain

The creation of "major" depression with the introduction of the DSM-III turned out as a big failure, resulting in an overinclusive, heterogeneous, and fuzzy concept of clinical depression [4, 6, 7, 410]. The diagnostic threshold was put so low and the criteria defined so broadly that a substantial portion of the population experiencing normal (adaptive) emotional reactions to problems of daily life, including occupational failures, financial strain, conflicts in relationships or the loss of a beloved person, now fulfils the diagnostic criteria of major depression [3, 5]. That is, many conditions diagnosed as major depression are neither major nor a mental disorder in its fundamental meaning, that is, "a dysfunction in the psychological, biological, or developmental processes underlying mental functioning" as set out by the DSM-5 [1059]. Put differently, the validity of major depression is severely compromised by overdefinition.

But not only is the validity of major depression poor, the diagnosis is also unreliable. The DSM-5 field trials [421] clearly demonstrated that the diagnostic reliability of major depressive disorder is disconcertingly low, with a Kappa coefficient of 0.28. This coefficient indicates that two psychiatrists agreed that a patient has depression between 4% and 15% of the time and that in most cases they disagreed and came to divergent conclusions. That is, even highly trained and specialised psychiatrists "have a hard time agreeing on who does and does not have major depressive disorder" [422]. If even specialists are that undecided what major depression is and which patient has it, then just think of how uncertain diagnoses are when issued by GPs [450] and when diagnoses are based on structured interviews administered by lay people (such as the Composite International Diagnostic Interview; CIDI), as is standard practice in epidemiological studies to estimate the prevalence of depression (e.g. [476]). Therefore, in lieu of an "epidemic of depression" one could rightly also be worried about an epidemic of dubious (unreliable) diagnoses and questionable prevalence rates (see also [410, 489, 491]).

Another important factor related to the point above is overdetection, meaning that many people receiving a diagnosis of depression do not event meet the overinclusive (low-threshold) criteria of major depression [450]. The fuzzy boundary between normal sadness/distress and major depression has led to a high rate of false-positive depression diagnoses, largely driven by specialty groups and depression awareness campaigns that constantly pressured GPs and the public to be on the look-out for depression and to interpret common stress symptoms and low mood as undetected (masked) depression in need of (long-term) drug treatment [25, 132, 404, 452]. This process was further fuelled by the proliferation of screening questionnaires that massively overestimate the presence and severity of depression [436–438].

By consequence, the majority of people now using antidepressants for depression, also referred to as the worried well, do not have clinical depression [3, 105, 117, 447]. That is, millions of people are treated with antidepressants (mostly SSRIs) from which they unlikely benefit but are put at a high risk of bothersome adverse effects, especially treatment-emergent sexual dysfunction and sleep disturbances [336, 339, 854, 1060]. In addition, many people remain on antidepressants long-term, which can cause excessive weight gain [340, 1061] and severe withdrawal reactions that mimic depression relapses or new emerging mental disorders when people try to come off the drugs [217, 218, 732]. Unnecessary antidepressant use can thus harm patients and public health. It also leads to a misallocation of limited healthcare resources and may thus inadvertently contribute to the underserving of people with serious clinical depression who are most in need of medical services but often don't receive minimally adequate psychiatric treatment, let alone legal, financial, and psychosical support [105, 106]. So what to do about it? What's the remedy?

Several authors suggested that the diagnosis of melancholic depression as a distinct mood disorder should be reinstated [4, 255]. I agree that melancholic depression is a useful concept, but unless psychiatry abandons the diagnosis of major depression, I see no benefit in establishing melancholic depression as a separate diagnosis, for it would largely overlap with the severe spectrum of major depression. Instead, following seminal research by Wakefield and Horwitz, I propose that the diagnostic criteria of major depression should be revised according on their study results [481, 1062, 1063]. In the absence of suicidal ideation or behaviour, psychotic symptoms, and marked psychomotor retardation, I suggest that episodes of sadness/despair related to bereavement and other losses (e.g. job loss, separation) that last no longer than two months should not be classified as a depressive disorder. These conditions are best understood as uncomplicated, normal emotional reactions to critical life events, and not as mental disorders, that is, medical conditions. Just as it is a normal, adaptive process to grieve the loss of a beloved person, be it due to death or separation, it is also normal that people grieve the loss of an occupation, position, project, or cherished activity. Most importantly, even when grieving (i.e. the process of adapting and readjusting after a loss) takes longer than two months, eventually mood will spontaneously improve and almost all people affected fully recover [5, 482, 1064].

These diagnostic revisions would depathologise (normalise) benign and temporary episodes of distress/despondency that should not be defined as mental disorders necessarily in need of psychiatric treatment. Watchful waiting (i.e. explanation, reassurance, and monitoring) is probably the best way GPs (and mental health specialists) manage these unproblematic (benign) episodes if people seek healthcare. This is also the current evidence-based recommendation to treat mild forms of depression [181, 233, 410]. Aerobic exercise is also a safe and effective intervention in mild, non-serious depression [1065, 1066]. However, drug treatment and/or psychotherapy is indicated when mood worsens, impairment/distress exacerbates, or serious dysfunctional (pathognomonic) symptoms develop (i.e. suicidal ideation or behaviour, psychotic symptoms, or marked psychomotor retardation).

The proposed redefinition of unproblematic (benign) depression episodes as normal emotional reactions to critical life events would also substantially lower the prevalence of depression and relieve pressure from healthcare providers and the public who are constantly cautioned about the risks of untreated depression. Attention and resources can then be concentrated more efficiently on the people with serious clinical depression that are truly in need of medical treatment and psychosocial support, including medication, psychotherapy, social work, and legal assistance. Safe housing and income support, if needed, are a basic requirement which every society should be willing to offer if economically possible. Of course, intensive treatment and support are costly, which is why we need to set the priorities right and guarantee that we do not waste limited healthcare resources for the treatment of depression episodes that are neither pathological nor in need of treatment. Therefore, I also second Thombs and Ziegelstein, who urged that "Primary care doctors should not screen their patients for depression" [444], for routine application of depression screening questionnaires in primary care does not provide any meaningful benefit but may increase the rate of false-positive diagnoses and unnecessary drug treatment [441, 442, 1067].

GPs prescribe the majority of antidepressants [725, 835] and often are the only treatment providers in depression [105, 639]. However, GPs have very limited time for their patients, on average only 10 to 15 minutes per visit in Europe and North America [1068]. By consequence, the patients' involvement in decision making is typically very poor in depression care [1069, 1070]. All too often, the short consultation time is used for a hasty (premature) depression diagnosis and an antidepressant prescription, even in cases where clinical depression is unlikely or when diagnostic criteria are not met [105, 117, 414, 452]. Fortunately, patient involvement in decision making can be improved by shared decision-making interventions and, crucially, longer consultation time [1071]. If physicians had more time to listen to their patients, to educate and reassure them that mild and subthreshold depression is typically benign and improves spontaneously within a few weeks, and if patients were more involved in treatment decisions, then probably we would see less antidepressant prescriptions for mild/subthreshold depression episodes where the drugs' benefit–harm ratio is, on average, unfavourable.

Another promising approach to curb the inadequate (unnecessary/harmful) prescribing of antidepressants in people with non-serious, mild and transient depression is to abandon once and for all the chemical imbalance or serotonin deficiency notion of depression. There is no convincing empirical support for a dysfunction in the monoamine neurotransmitter system as a cause of depression, and a lot of evidence that clearly disconfirms this hypothesis [26, 595, 596, 637]. Yet to this day the chemical imbalance theory is circulated widely, in educational materials and advertisements, and endorsed by many GPs, antidepressant users, and the general public [369, 617, 618, 1072]. This is very problematic, for patients who believe their depression is caused by a chemical imbalance have more pessimistic expectations about recovery [617, 1073]. Users who hold chemical imbalance beliefs are also reluctant to stop antidepressant treatment and prefer to remain on the drugs indefinitely, even when long-term treatment is not indicated [611–613]. Considering the well-established common adverse effects of long-term antidepressant treatment, including sexual dysfunction, weight gain, and sleep disturbances [273, 339], nonindicated long-term use is likely harmful. That is, the unsubstantiated chemical imbalance notion may propel unnecessary, harmful long-term antidepressant treatment and must thus be abandoned.

On a related note, in accordance with several other experts, I contend that there is no convincing scientific evidence that depressive disorders (and common mental disorders in general) are brain disorders [393, 395, 396, 506]. Unless researchers discover a demonstrable abnormality/pathology in brain function or structure causally related to the emergence of depression (i.e. a neurobiological prognostic marker), this notion remains an unconfirmed hypothesis. As extensively discussed in this book, thus far such evidence is completely lacking (for a recent systematic review, see [1042]). But still many eminent authors boldly assert that mental disorders are the result of a brain abnormality/pathology [524, 530], and the public has largely accepted this unproven hypothesis [541, 542]. The brain disorder notion is a broader conceptualisation of the chemical imbalance theory of depression and likewise comes at a substantial price. According to the best evidence available, the belief in a neurobiological cause of mental disorders likely increases stigma and negative attitudes towards mental disorders, both among the general public and mental health professionals [620, 622, 1074]. Neurobiological reductionism also led to a one-sided, narrow and unbalanced research agenda with potentially negative consequences for clinical practice and public mental health [392, 396, 503, 540, 1075].

Except from neurological conditions, for example dementia and stroke, which can cause serious psychopathological symptoms, common mental disorders such as depression and anxiety are not associated with a demonstrable brain disorder [392, 561, 1041]. Along with others, I thus suggest that the media, researchers, and practitioners no longer purport that mental disorders are brain disorders [396, 506]. Unless future research provides reliable and convincing scientific evidence for a neurobiological cause, it is best to avoid the brain disorder notion. Instead, people should be told that for sure brain functions are involved in the expression and experience of negative (or burdensome) mental states such as depression and anxiety. Without a brain we were not able to have emotions, but there is no evidence thus far that depression and anxiety are due to a specific neurophysiological abnormality or pathology (e.g. a dysfunction in brain circuits or neurochemistry). Just because negative emotions are contingent on brain activity does not imply that negative emotional states, even when severe and debilitating, are indicative of a brain disorder. Brain functions are also altered when we experience positive, highly pleasant emotions such as being in love with someone [1076]. By the reasoning of the mental-disorders-are-brain-disorders advocates, as far as brain functions are altered when we are in love with someone, this mental state would also qualify as a brain disorder.

The experience of negative emotions, even intense and prolonged ones, is an evolved psychological mechanism. That is, negative emotions are deeply embedded in human nature and typically (not always) originate from a healthy, normal, and well-functioning brain in response to specific environmental triggers (including interpersonal experiences). Just think of grief or embarrassment, for example. Likewise, it is not inherently abnormal to temporarily respond with intense sadness and anhedonia (i.e. loss of pleasure and interest) after a critical life event [5]. It is not because intense sadness, anhedonia, and accessory symptoms (e.g. sleep problems, lack of appetite, concentration difficulties) lasting longer than two weeks were defined as a major depression episode (i.e., a mental disorder) that this condition by consequence becomes a brain disorder. This is especially true when depression develops following one or more critical life events, as it often does [1077, 1078]. And it is not because intense sadness and anhedonia correlate with alterations in brain function, that this mental state is due to a brain disorder. As discussed by Dr. Miller [396], alterations in people's social network affect physical health, yet no one would seriously contend that physical illness is a social network disorder.

How well antidepressants work in moderate to severe depression, and if that effect is clinically (or practically) relevant, is still not conclusively answered [13, 20]. Due to publication bias and selective reporting, it is difficult to estimate the true treatment effects based on the scientific literature [102]. It is thus essential that all trials are pre-registered in a public trial registry and that the results for all pre-specified outcomes are fully reported according to the study protocol [428, 1079]. But that's likely not enough, for without access to clinical study reports it is impossible to verify whether adverse events or study dropouts were correctly recorded, classified, and transparently reported in journal articles [87, 665]. Independent researchers should thus have unrestricted access to the raw data for cross-evaluations and verification of study results [29, 653]. The re-analysis of study 329, a paroxetine trial in adolescents sponsored by GlaxoSmithKline, the manufacturer of paroxetine, has clearly shown that re-analyses of the raw data can lead to fundamentally altered conclusions [322, 770]. The data from influential clinical trials that have a significant impact on medical practice should thus be available to independent researchers who want to examine (and validate) the accuracy of the trial results.

But this is just a first step to obtain reliable, accurate, and fully reported data. The issues with antidepressant trials run much deeper, for the validity of the trial results is questionable. As comprehensively detailed in this book, there are many and often systematic biases in antidepressant trials, including preselected, unrepresentative samples, very short observation periods, unblinding of outcome assessors (and study participants), and comedication with sedative-hypnotic drugs. What are thus needed are pragmatic real-world effectiveness trials with representative samples and long-term follow-up (i.e. at least six months). Using an active placebo (i.e. a pill that has no psychotropic effect but may cause nausea and other typical side effects) would avoid or substantially minimise unblinding bias. But since active placebos are ethically problematic in long-term trials, low-intensity active control groups such as guided self-help may also be adequate comparators (in addition to clinical management with inert pill placebo).

Also, doctors prefer to evaluate the efficacy of antidepressants in relation to core depression symptoms, but to patients, quality of life appears to be more important [1080, 1081]. To evaluate whether antidepressants can truly make a difference in the life of people with depression, patient-centred outcomes such as quality of life, including among others general wellbeing, ability to work, and relationship satisfaction, are indeed more relevant than core depression symptoms. The advantage of quality of life measures over depression symptom rating scales is that they balance benefits and harms of antidepressants. Given that the therapeutic effects of antidepressants (i.e. suppression of negative emotions, sedation and/or activation) may be offset by their adverse effects (e.g. sleep problems, agitation, emotional numbing, drowsiness, sexual dysfunction, weight gain), an outcome measure that captures both therapeutic and adverse drug effects provides the better indicator of overall effectiveness. Quality of life measures fulfil these criteria and may thus help to elucidate whether the small therapeutic benefits of antidepressants outweigh their harms in moderate to severe depression.

Regardless of whether depression symptoms or quality of life are used as the primary outcome, it is essential that researchers do not exclusively rely on statistical significance testing to evaluate the benefits of antidepressants [18]. Whether antidepressants really make a difference depends on whether their treatment effects are clinically (or practically) important in magnitude, and not merely on a statistically significant result [15]. Unfortunately, this crucial issue has long been neglected and there is still no consensus on how large a treatment effect has to be to make a minimally important difference [133, 139]. However, based on our recent analysis of estimates of a minimally important difference, we showed that antidepressants fail to clearly exceed even liberal lower-bound estimates and thus concluded that the clinical (or practical) relevance of antidepressants in moderate to severe depression remains uncertain [20].

I further suggest that clinical trials should contain a taper period of at least four weeks to empirically examine the incidence and severity of withdrawal syndromes following discontinuation of antidepressant treatment. There is an increasing body of scientific evidence demonstrating that severe withdrawal syndromes may affect a substantial portion of antidepressant users [345, 347, 357]. Physicians must thus inform patients about potential withdrawal reactions from antidepressants when different treatment options for depression are discussed. In this respect it is also important to stress that in the acute treatment of non-severe depression, there are various scientifically established alternatives to antidepressants that are equally effective but have fewer side effects. These include psychotherapy, physical exercise, and St John's Wort [202, 203, 1082–1084]. With respect to long-term benefits, that is, sustained remission and relapse prevention, the scientific evidence consistently shows that psychotherapy is more effective and better tolerated than antidepressants [205, 206, 209–211]. Given that most treatment recommendations are based on short-term trials, this is an important aspect that is often ignored in clinical practice. It also indicates that psychotherapy should be preferred to antidepressant treatment in moderate depression [212]. Finally, in accordance with common treatment recommendations [231–233], the combination of psychotherapy and antidepressants is likely the most effective treatment strategy in the acute treatment of severe depression because adding psychotherapy to antidepressants not only improves efficacy but also treatment acceptability, meaning that patients improve more and are less likely to terminate treatment prematurely [204]. In the long-term, combination therapy is also more effective than antidepressants alone, but the evidence is inconclusive as to whether combination therapy is meaningfully better than psychotherapy alone [212, 213].

What to do about corporate bias and conflicts of interest? First of all, medicine should acknowledge and proactively engage with treatment-related (iatrogenic) harms, instead of systematically denying or minimising this serious and quite prevalent public health issue [459, 678]. The healthcare system should not ignore or silence patients who report suspected treatment-related harms [815, 816]. As detailed by Haskell, "healthcare providers' dismissive attitude toward patients was underpinned by a reluctance in all parts of the system to collect evidence on potential harms, by a lack of coordination that would allow clinicians and agencies to interpret and act on that information, and by a culture of denial that failed to acknowledge harm and error, impeding learning and safety" [814]. Likewise, clinicians/researchers who inform the public about serious adverse drug reactions should not have to fear personal and/or professional consequences (repercussions), for example the loss of an academic position or litigation [811, 812]. As stressed by Dr. Krumholz, a professor of medicine at Yale University,

> "When I entered medicine, I did not realize that there was such intense pressure to conform. But we learn early on that there is a decorum to medicine, a politeness. A hidden curriculum teaches us not to disturb the status quo. We are trained to defer to authority, not to question it. We depend on powerful individuals and organizations and are taught that success does not often come to those who ask uncomfortable questions or suggest new ways of providing care. The sense of danger that we feel when we question authority is not unfounded. Those who ask difficult questions or challenge conventional wisdom are often isolated. They may find few opportunities to speak and their writings may not be welcome. Compliance with normative behavior may be forced by fear of recrimination. In some cases, junior faculty may fear that support from mentors will be withdrawn or promotions denied … I have grown to appreciate those who will stand up despite the risks or in the face of efforts to silence them. Promoting the best science and the best advocacy for patients and the public sometimes entails risk. Change does not come easily to a system and there is resistance to those who may seek to make the system safer, more effective, and more patient-centered through new ideas or the articulation of uncomfortable truths." [810]

Asking questions about the effectiveness of antidepressants is one of those "uncomfortable questions", and critically writing about adverse effects of antidepressants such as treatment-emergent suicidality or withdrawal syndromes is indeed by and large "not welcome" in psychiatry and may prompt fierce (sometimes hateful) reactions. I also found myself on the receiving end of such attacks and I am definitely no exception [9, 11, 147]. Questioning the benefit–harm ratio of antidepressants has made many critics powerful enemies. For examples of such fierce reactions from leading psychiatrists, see for example [22, 23, 830]. Unfortunately, leaders in medicine often attempt to defend the status quo in their specialty, that is, the standards of care, and thus may try to censor or marginalise authors who question the benefit–harm ratio of first-line treatments [810]. A willingness to dispassionately engage with authors who raise "uncomfortable questions" clearly must be encouraged more in medicine. Defensiveness, denial, and dismissal are not the way forward to improve public health and patient care. The history of medicine, even the most recent one, constantly reminds us that some novel medical interventions that were considered safe and effective and thus established as new standard of care (i.e. best medical practice) eventually turned out to be ineffective or harmful [383, 645, 647].

Given that the prior probability of a novel medical treatment to be truly safe and effective is low, and due to systematic biases in the conduct and reporting of research, it necessarily follows that a novel treatment likely does not work in real-world routine practice for many (perhaps most) patients even when the scientific evidence suggests that it allegedly does [171, 172, 383, 458]. Antidepressants may also fall into this broad category of medical treatments with very limited effectiveness and questionable benefit–harm ratio in a majority of patients treated with them in routine practice, especially those with non-severe depression [8, 9, 11–13, 18, 102, 135, 140].

At the core of uncertain or questionable standards of care lies what Ioannidis and colleagues coined the "medical misinformation mess", which they ascribe to four key problems: "First, much published medical research is not reliable or is of uncertain reliability, offers no benefit to patients, or is not useful to decision makers. Second, most healthcare professionals are not aware of this problem. Third, they also lack the skills necessary to evaluate the reliability and usefulness of medical evidence. Finally, patients and families frequently lack relevant, accurate medical evidence and skilled guidance at the time of medical decision-making" [660]. The authors also offer a solution to these problems: "Increasing the reliability of available, published evidence may not be an imminently reachable goal. Therefore, efforts should focus on making healthcare professionals more sensitive to the limitations of the evidence, training them to do critical appraisal, and enhancing their communication skills so that they can effectively summarize and discuss medical evidence with patients to improve decision-making. Similar efforts may need to target also patients, journalists, policy makers, the lay public and other healthcare stakeholders" [660]. Similar recommendations were made by Cosgrove and colleagues specifically with respect to antidepressants for depression [142].

The professional or guild interests detailed above (i.e., defending the standards of care in ones' specialty) often come along with financial conflicts of interest, for most medical organisations and academic medical departments have strong ties to the pharmaceutical industry. Not only do many medical organisations and departments depend on financial support from the industry [987], several leaders of these organisations and departments are also members of the directors' boards of pharmaceutical companies or serve the industry as consultants and speakers [967, 969]. Moreover, about half of all physicians receive general (non-research) payments from the industry [1019]. Physicians who interact with pharmaceutical companies typically believe they are not influenced by industry [1010, 1027]. However, the scientific evidence clearly says otherwise: physician–industry interactions, which largely involve financial relationships, systematically bias medical education, research, and practice in favour of the industry's commercial interests [379, 428, 592, 593, 796, 946–948, 1011]. Thus, let's see how we could possibly reduce biases resulting from physicians' (financial) relationships with the pharmaceutical industry.

When confronted with conflicts of interest disclosure and regulation, some physicians react defensively and resentful [942, 975]. To them the mere notion that industry relationships (be it contact with pharmaceutical sales representatives, attending industry-sponsored medical education events, payments for meals and lodging, or consulting and speaking fees) could influence their decisions is an insult to the profession. The mistaken belief that physicians are immune to industry influence stems from the misconception that bias is the result of an intentional, conscious act of corruption. Although this rarely happens, most bias results from unintentional, subconscious effects of industry relationships. As summarised by Sah and Fugh-Berman:

> "Most physicians view the favoring of self-interest over profession obligations with repugnance. Physicians express indignation at the suggestion that accepting gifts or compensation affects therapeutic choices because they understand that such an exchange would mean they have made a deliberate decision to act unethically. Physicians, who would never, for example, engage in a *quid pro quo* exchange of money for prescriptions,

may believe that such a conscious and genuine commitment to ethical behavior renders them immune to commercial influence. This righteous but wrong assumption derives from not knowing that many psychological processes occur below conscious awareness". [1027]

The most important psychological process that explains why physicians who receive payments/gifts from the pharmaceutical industry tend to behave in ways that benefit the industry's commercial interests–sometimes at the expense of patient safety and/or public health—is reciprocity, the urge to return favours [939, 1027, 1038]. Although this largely subconscious process has been repeatedly stressed in the literature, and despite the fact that industry-payments to physicians are consistently associated with changes in prescribing behaviour and treatment recommendations in favour of the industry, most physicians refuse to accept that their relationships with industry could influence them. That is, the vast majority of physicians perceive their interactions with industry as largely unproblematic and inconsequential. In fact, most physicians consider industry relationships indispensable and advantageous, a clear benefit for patients and public health [942, 1010, 1011]. This firm belief is surprising. Let me ask a few questions. Would physicians accept that a judge has a financial (or personal) relationship with the defendant he/she needs to rule for or against? Would physicians accept that a referee in a world cup final is a member of the directors' board of one the teams? Would physicians accept that a member of a public committee that awards a mandate to an organisation owns stocks in that particular organisation? I don't think so … But then, why do physicians believe that, contrary to other conflicted decision makers, they are immune to bias?

Now of course physicians are not stupid, and they certainly understand the concept of conflict of interest. For instance, a large majority of physicians agrees that industry-supported medical education can introduce bias [1017]. But still, most physicians regularly attend such events. This inconsistency between attitudes and behaviour of course generates dissonance. To resolve dissonance, physicians use a variety of denials and rationalisations. These include to avoid thinking about the conflict of interest, to disagree that industry relationships affect physician behaviour, to deny responsibility for the problem, to enumerate techniques for remaining impartial, and to reason that industry relationships are educational and benefit patients [1023]. As detailed above, nothing could be farther from the truth. Therefore, let me stress it again: industry relationships lead to increased, costly, and inappropriate (low-quality) drug prescribing [796, 798, 1010]. Put differently, direct-to-physician marketing does not improve prescribing. It does not benefit patients or the public. The only ones that truly benefit from direct-to-physician marketing are the pharmaceutical companies that increase their profits. And this is also the reason why the pharmaceutical industry is willing to invest billions of $ every year in direct-to-physician marketing, accounting for most promotional spending overall [433].

As Dr. Howick states, "a main cause of the current problems with evidence seems to be … an asymmetry of the relationship between rationality (evidence) and power (financial bias), with financial bias being by far the stronger, and strong enough to beat evidence" [649]. So how do we curb biases in medical education, research, and practice resulting from industry payments to physicians and medical organisations? The standard approach is conflict of interest disclosure. However, while transparency is necessary, it is evidently insufficient [380]. In fact, various experts argue that conflict of interest disclosure may even exacerbate bias, since authors who disclose their financial relationships with the industry may thus feel that they have a blanket check to make extreme (biased) assertions [1038, 1085, 1086]. Therefore, let's be clear: mere transparency won't solve this problem.

The main issue is that pharmaceutical companies are required to test the efficacy and safety of their own products before receiving marketing approval. And of course, they are conflicted. The have much to gain from favourable trial results, but much to lose from unfavourable trial result. As stressed by Dr. Ioannidis, "corporations should not be asked to practically perform the assessments of their own products. If they are forced to do this, I cannot blame them, if they buy the best advertisement (i.e., 'evidence') for whatever they sell" [377]. The conduct and evaluation of pivotal pre-marketing trials should thus be performed by independent, governmental research institutes funded through industry fees. Next, it is also important that the leading academic physicians who participate in regulatory advisory meetings and/or who later make treatment recommendations as authors of practice guidelines are unconflicted. That is, they should not be allowed to have financial relationships with the companies whose products they are supposed to assess critically and objectively in their role as independent experts. Unfortunately, many of these leading experts are not truly independent, for often they have long-standing and close relationships with pharmaceutical companies, working for them as consultants and speakers, and sometimes they are also stockholders or members of the directors board [961, 963, 994, 1001]. Corporate bias affects not only research, but also education and practice [171, 579, 825, 1012]. In all these domains, the end goal should be financial independence from commercial interests. A detailed list of recommendations to curb bias resulting from financial conflicts of interest was recently published by Moynihan and colleagues [380]. As I fully endorse them, these are quoted verbatim in Table 6.1 below.

I want to close this book with a previously expressed plea for "scientific debate instead of beef" [16]. The furious and polarised disputes about the validity of the concept of depression and the utility (and role) of antidepressants in its treatment are neither fruitful nor do they help patients or the public. We need balanced and evidence-based scientific evaluations. We need to acknowledge that not all depression episodes are the same and thus not one intervention fits all. The overinclusive, fuzzy, and heterogeneous diagnosis of major depression is neither clinically useful nor conceptually valid. We need to depathologise normal emotional reactions to critical life events and problems of daily life, but at the same time recognise that severe (melancholic) depression is a serious psychiatric disorder in need of treatment. A blanket condemnation of antidepressants is inappropriate and not in the patients' best interest, for some adults with severe (serious) clinical depression may benefit from antidepressants. On the other hand, in people with mild and subthreshold depression the drugs' benefit–harm ratio is likely unfavourable. Particular caution is also warranted in minors and old adults, where antidepressants should be prescribed sparingly and only to the most seriously ill. Moreover, denying or minimising antidepressants' adverse effects is unethical and a threat to patient safety and public health. Informed decision-making is therefore key. It is important to inform patients that, even in moderate to severe adult depression, the therapeutic effects are, on average, modest and that

Table 6.1 Possible solutions to end corporate bias in medical research, education, and practice adopted from Moynihan and colleagues [380]

Domain	Recommendation
Research	Governments require independent production of evidence used for healthcare decision making, including the evaluation of new treatments, tests, and technologies
	Governments require that public healthcare organisations, including regulatory and health technology assessment agencies, receive no industry funding and that their advisers have no financial relationships with industry
	Groups conducting research synthesis, including systematic reviews, ensure reviewers have access to all information on study methods and all relevant study results, including clinical study reports, and are conducted without industry funding and by authors with no financial relationships with companies that could benefit from the outcomes
Education	Professional, advocacy, or academic groups engaged in educational activities for health professionals or the public or advocacy affecting regulatory or policy decisions, move to end reliance on industry funding and end financial relationships between their leadership and industry
	National governments work with professional associations and licensing bodies to develop policies that ensure educational activity supported by industry cannot contribute to accreditation of health professionals
	Medical journals and their editors move to end reliance on healthcare industry income
Practice	Professional groups, hospitals, health services, and governments prohibit marketing interactions between industry and decision makers, including practising professionals, and actively support development of healthcare information independent of commercial interests
	Professionals, policy makers, and the public move to reliance on practice guidelines produced and written by groups that have no financial relationships with industry and that have access to evidence, including research synthesis, free of industry influence
	Research funding bodies and academic institutions modify academic metrics and incentives explicitly to reward academic collaboration with public agencies and civil society groups as well as industry

antidepressants can cause serious harm, including both rare (e.g. cardiac arrhythmias, hyponatremia) and common adverse drug reactions (e.g. sleep problems, sexual dysfunction).

The fierce personal attacks that various leading psychiatrists led on researchers that raised important safety and efficacy issues also cast the specialty of psychiatry in an unfavourable light. Dismissing (and denigrating) researchers who ask uncomfortable questions may propel public and professional reservations about psychiatry. Such reservations are certainly also fostered by the strong and pervasive ties between psychiatry and the pharmaceutical industry, which often were (and quite often still are) systematically concealed and obfuscated. My last plea is therefore for more independent, patient-oriented research on antidepressants, especially into relevant long-term treatment outcomes, such as quality of life and social functioning. To quote a famous phrase from Dr. Douglas Altman: "We need less research, better research, and research done for the right reasons" [1087]. We also need to free medical education from unduly industry influences, and we definitely need to curb industry relationships among psychiatric organisations, academic leaders, scientific publishers, guideline authors, diagnostic work group members, and individual prescribers. With this book I hope to have made a small contribution to an evidence-based, judicious, and cautious prescribing of antidepressants in depression without fuelling blanket condemnation of this popular drug class.

References

1. Shorter E. Before Prozac: the troubled history of mood disorders in psychiatry. Oxford: Oxford University Press; 2008.
2. Lieberman JA. Why do we continue to doubt antidepressants' efficacy? Medscape. June 27, 2018.
3. Dowrick C, Frances A. Medicalising unhappiness: new classification of depression risks more patients being put on drug treatment from which they will not benefit. BMJ. 2013;347:f7140.
4. Ghaemi SN, Vohringer PA, Vergne DE. The varieties of depressive experience: diagnosing mood disorders. Psychiatr Clin North Am. 2012;35(1):73–86.
5. Horwitz AV, Wakefield JC. The loss of sadness: how psychiatry transformed normal sorrow into depressive disorder. Oxford: Oxford University Press; 2007.
6. Lorenzo-Luaces L. Heterogeneity in the prognosis of major depression: from the common cold to a highly debilitating and recurrent illness. Epidemiol Psychiatr Sci. 2015;24(6):466–72.
7. Parker G. Beyond major depression. Psychol Med. 2005;35(4):467–74.
8. Gotzsche PC. Why I think antidepressants cause more harm than good. Lancet Psychiatry. 2014;1(2):104–6.

M. P. Hengartner, *Evidence-biased Antidepressant Prescription*,
https://doi.org/10.1007/978-3-030-82587-4

9. Healy D. Let them eat Prozac: the unhealthy relationship between the pharmaceutical industry and depression. New York: New York University Press; 2004.
10. Jakobsen JC, Katakam KK, Schou A, Hellmuth SG, Stallknecht SE, Leth-Moller K, et al. Selective serotonin reuptake inhibitors versus placebo in patients with major depressive disorder. A systematic review with meta-analysis and Trial Sequential Analysis. BMC Psychiatry. 2017;17(1):58.
11. Kirsch I. The emperor's new drugs: exploding the antidepressant myth. London, UK: Bodley Head; 2009.
12. Moncrieff J. Are antidepressants as effective as claimed? No, they are not effective at all. Can J Psychiatry. 2007;52(2):96–7.
13. Munkholm K, Paludan-Muller AS, Boesen K. Considering the methodological limitations in the evidence base of antidepressants for depression: a reanalysis of a network meta-analysis. BMJ Open. 2019;9(6):e024886.
14. Hengartner MP. Methodological flaws, conflicts of interest, and scientific fallacies: implications for the evaluation of antidepressants' efficacy and harm. Front Psychiatry. 2017;8:275.
15. Hengartner MP. What is the threshold for a clinical minimally important drug effect? BMJ Evid Based Med. 2018;23:225–7.
16. Hengartner MP. Scientific debate instead of beef; challenging misleading arguments about the efficacy of antidepressants. Acta Neuropsychiatr. 2019;31(4):235–6.
17. Hengartner MP, Jakobsen JC, Sorensen A, Ploderl M. Efficacy of new-generation antidepressants assessed with the Montgomery-Asberg Depression Rating Scale, the gold standard clinician rating scale: a meta-analysis of randomised placebo-controlled trials. PLoS One. 2020;15(2):e0229381.
18. Hengartner MP, Plöderl M. Statistically significant antidepressant-placebo differences on subjective symptom-rating scales do not prove that the drugs work: effect size and method bias matter! Front Psychiatry. 2018;9:517.
19. Hengartner MP, Plöderl M, Braillon A, Jakobsen JC, Gluud C. Sertraline in primary care: comments on the PANDA trial. Lancet Psychiatry. 2020;7(1):17.
20. Hengartner MP, Plöderl M. Estimates of the minimal important difference to evaluate the clinical significance of antidepressants in the acute

treatment of moderate-to-severe depression. BMJ Evid Based Med. 2021. https://doi.org/10.1136/bmjebm-2020-111600.
21. Moller HJ, Bitter I, Bobes J, Fountoulakis K, Hoschl C, Kasper S, et al. Position statement of the European Psychiatric Association (EPA) on the value of antidepressants in the treatment of unipolar depression. Eur Psychiatry. 2012;27(2):114–28.
22. Nutt DJ, Goodwin GM, Bhugra D, Fazel S, Lawrie S. Attacks on antidepressants: signs of deep-seated stigma? Lancet Psychiatry. 2014;1(2):102–4.
23. Vinberg M. Misinformed, misconducted, misguided and misrepresented meta-analyses. The use of antidepressants (AD) in major depressive disorders (MDD). Bipolar Disord. 2020;22(8):862–3.
24. Antonuccio DO, Burns DD, Danton WG. Antidepressants: a triumph of marketing over science? Prev Treat. 2002;5(1):25.
25. Gardner P. Distorted packaging: marketing depression as illness, drugs as cure. J Med Humanit. 2003;24(1–2):105–30.
26. Lacasse JR, Leo J. Serotonin and depression: a disconnect between the advertisements and the scientific literature. PLoS Med. 2005;2(12):e392.
27. Applbaum K. Getting to yes: corporate power and the creation of a psychopharmaceutical blockbuster. Cult Med Psychiatry. 2009;33(2):185–215.
28. Fava GA. Financial conflicts of interest in psychiatry. World Psychiatry. 2007;6(1):19–24.
29. Jureidini J, McHenry LB. The illusion of evidence-based medicine: exposing the crisis of credibility in clinical research. Adelaide: Wakefield Press; 2020.
30. Whitaker R, Cosgrove L. Psychiatry under the influence. London: Palgrave Macmillan; 2015.
31. Angst J, Dobler-Mikola A, Binder J. The Zurich study—a prospective epidemiological study of depressive, neurotic and psychosomatic syndromes. I. Problem, methodology. Eur Arch Psychiatry Neurol Sci. 1984;234(1):13–20.
32. Angst J, Paksarian D, Cui L, Merikangas KR, Hengartner MP, Ajdacic-Gross V, et al. The epidemiology of common mental disorders from age 20 to 50: results from the prospective Zurich cohort study. Epidemiol Psychiatr Sci. 2016;25(1):24–32.
33. Rössler W, Riecher-Rössler A, Angst J, Murray R, Gamma A, Eich D, et al. Psychotic experiences in the general population: a twenty-year prospective community study. Schizophr Res. 2007;92(1–3):1–14.

34. Moore TH, Zammit S, Lingford-Hughes A, Barnes TR, Jones PB, Burke M, et al. Cannabis use and risk of psychotic or affective mental health outcomes: a systematic review. Lancet. 2007;370(9584):319–28.
35. Rössler W, Hengartner MP, Angst J, Ajdacic-Gross V. Linking substance use with symptoms of sub-clinical psychosis in a community cohort over 30 years. Addiction. 2012;107(6):1174–84.
36. Forstmeier W, Wagenmakers EJ, Parker TH. Detecting and avoiding likely false-positive findings—a practical guide. Biol Rev Camb Philos Soc. 2017;92(4):1941–68.
37. Gelman A, Loken E. The statistical crisis in science. Am Sci. 2014;102(6):460–5.
38. Sainani KL. The problem of multiple testing. PM R. 2009;1(12):1098–103.
39. Simmons JP, Nelson LD, Simonsohn U. False-positive psychology: undisclosed flexibility in data collection and analysis allows presenting anything as significant. Psychol Sci. 2011;22(11):1359–66.
40. Wicherts JM, Veldkamp CLS, Augusteijn HEM, Bakker M, van Aert RCM, van Assen MALM, et al. Degrees of freedom in planning, running, analyzing, and reporting psychological studies: a checklist to avoid p-hacking. Front Psychol. 2016;7:12.
41. Ioannidis JP. Why science is not necessarily self-correcting. Perspect Psychol Sci. 2012;7(6):645–54.
42. Nosek BA, Spies JR, Motyl M. Scientific utopia: II. Restructuring incentives and practices to promote truth over publishability. Perspect Psychol Sci. 2012;7(6):615–31.
43. Pashler H, Harris CR. Is the replicability crisis overblown? Three arguments examined. Perspect Psychol Sci. 2012;7(6):531–6.
44. Yong E. Replication studies: bad copy. Nature. 2012;485(7398):298–300.
45. Bakker M, van Dijk A, Wicherts JM. The rules of the game called psychological science. Perspect Psychol Sci. 2012;7(6):543–54.
46. Begley CG, Ellis LM. Drug development: raise standards for preclinical cancer research. Nature. 2012;483(7391):531–3.
47. Francis G. Publication bias and the failure of replication in experimental psychology. Psychon B Rev. 2012;19(6):975–91.
48. Ioannidis JP. Why most published research findings are false. PLoS Med. 2005;2(8):e124.
49. Ioannidis JP, Panagiotou OA. Comparison of effect sizes associated with biomarkers reported in highly cited individual articles and in subsequent meta-analyses. JAMA. 2011;305(21):2200–10.

50. Prinz F, Schlange T, Asadullah K. Believe it or not: how much can we rely on published data on potential drug targets? Nat Rev Drug Discov. 2011;10(9):712.
51. Cohen J. The earth is round (p < .05). Am Psychol. 1994;49(12):997–1003.
52. Dwan K, Altman DG, Arnaiz JA, Bloom J, Chan AW, Cronin E, et al. Systematic review of the empirical evidence of study publication bias and outcome reporting bias. PLoS One. 2008;3(8):e3081.
53. Hengartner MP. Estrogen-based therapies and depression in women who naturally enter menopause before population average. JAMA Psychiatry. 2016;73(8):874.
54. Hengartner MP. Subtle scientific fallacies undermine the validity of neuroendocrinological research: do not draw premature conclusions on the role of female sex hormones. Front Behav Neurosci. 2017;11:3.
55. Hengartner MP. Raising awareness for the replication crisis in clinical psychology by focusing on inconsistencies in psychotherapy research: how much can we rely on published findings from efficacy trials? Front Psychol. 2018;9:256.
56. Melander H, Ahlqvist-Rastad J, Meijer G, Beermann B. Evidence b(i) ased medicine—selective reporting from studies sponsored by pharmaceutical industry: review of studies in new drug applications. BMJ. 2003;326(7400):1171–3.
57. Turner EH, Matthews AM, Linardatos E, Tell RA, Rosenthal R. Selective publication of antidepressant trials and its influence on apparent efficacy. N Engl J Med. 2008;358(3):252–60.
58. Whittington CJ, Kendall T, Fonagy P, Cottrell D, Cotgrove A, Boddington E. Selective serotonin reuptake inhibitors in childhood depression: systematic review of published versus unpublished data. Lancet. 2004;363(9418):1341–5.
59. Angell M. Is academic medicine for sale? N Engl J Med. 2000;342(20):1516–8.
60. Lexchin J. Those who have the gold make the evidence: how the pharmaceutical industry biases the outcomes of clinical trials of medications. Sci Eng Ethics. 2012;18(2):247–61.
61. McGauran N, Wieseler B, Kreis J, Schuler YB, Kolsch H, Kaiser T. Reporting bias in medical research—a narrative review. Trials. 2010;11:37.
62. Smith R. Medical journals are an extension of the marketing arm of pharmaceutical companies. PLoS Med. 2005;2(5):e138.

63. Horwitz AV. How an age of anxiety became an age of depression. Milbank Q. 2010;88(1):112–38.
64. Hyman SE. The diagnosis of mental disorders: the problem of reification. Annu Rev Clin Psychol. 2010;6:155–79.
65. Wakefield JC. The concept of mental disorder: diagnostic implications of the harmful dysfunction analysis. World Psychiatry. 2007;6(3):149–56.
66. Ebeling M. 'Get with the program!': pharmaceutical marketing, symptom checklists and self-diagnosis. Soc Sci Med. 2011;73(6):825–32.
67. Healy D. The latest mania: selling bipolar disorder. PLoS Med. 2006;3(4):e185.
68. Angst J, Hengartner MP, Ajdacic-Gross V, Roessler W. [Is two weeks the optimum duration criterion for major depression?]. Actas espanolas de psiquiatria. 2014;42(1):18–27.
69. Angst J, Hengartner MP, Gamma A, von Zerssen D, Angst F. Mortality of 403 patients with mood disorders 48 to 52 years after their psychiatric hospitalisation. Eur Arch Psychiatry Clin Neurosci. 2013;263(5):425–34.
70. Hengartner MP, Angst F, Ajdacic-Gross V, Rossler W, Angst J. Treated versus non-treated subjects with depression from a 30-year cohort study: prevalence and clinical covariates. Eur Arch Psychiatry Clin Neurosci. 2016;266(2):173–80.
71. Hengartner MP, Ajdacic-Gross V, Wyss C, Angst J, Rossler W. Relationship between personality and psychopathology in a longitudinal community study: a test of the predisposition model. Psychol Med. 2016;46(8):1693–705.
72. Hengartner MP, Kruger THC, Geraedts K, Tronci E, Mancini T, Ille F, et al. Negative affect is unrelated to fluctuations in hormone levels across the menstrual cycle: evidence from a multisite observational study across two successive cycles. J Psychosom Res. 2017;99:21–7.
73. Rodgers S, Ajdacic-Gross V, Muller M, Hengartner MP, Grosse Holtforth M, Angst J, et al. The role of sex on stability and change of depression symptom subtypes over 20 years: a latent transition analysis. Eur Arch Psychiatry Clin Neurosci. 2014;264(7):577–88.
74. Rodgers S, Grosse Holtforth M, Muller M, Hengartner MP, Rossler W, Ajdacic-Gross V. Symptom-based subtypes of depression and their psychosocial correlates: a person-centered approach focusing on the influence of sex. J Affect Disord. 2014;156:92–103.

75. Rossler W, Hengartner MP, Ajdacic-Gross V, Angst J. Predictors of burnout: results from a prospective community study. Eur Arch Psychiatry Clin Neurosci. 2015;265(1):19–25.
76. Rossler W, Ajdacic-Gross V, Riecher-Rossler A, Angst J, Hengartner MP. Does menopausal transition really influence mental health? Findings from the prospective long-term Zurich study. World Psychiatry. 2016;15(2):146–54.
77. Rottenberg J, Devendorf AR, Kashdan TB, Disabato DJ. The curious neglect of high functioning after psychopathology: the case of depression. Perspect Psychol Sci. 2018;13(5):549–66.
78. Healy D, Cattell D. Interface between authorship, industry and science in the domain of therapeutics. Br J Psychiatry. 2003;183:22–7.
79. Perlis RH, Perlis CS, Wu Y, Hwang C, Joseph M, Nierenberg AA. Industry sponsorship and financial conflict of interest in the reporting of clinical trials in psychiatry. Am J Psychiatry. 2005;162(10):1957–60.
80. Moncrieff J. The myth of the chemical cure. London: Palgrave Macmillan; 2008.
81. de Vries YA, Roest AM, Beijers L, Turner EH, de Jonge P. Bias in the reporting of harms in clinical trials of second-generation antidepressants for depression and anxiety: a meta-analysis. Eur Neuropsychopharmacol. 2016;26(11):1752–9.
82. Eyding D, Lelgemann M, Grouven U, Harter M, Kromp M, Kaiser T, et al. Reboxetine for acute treatment of major depression: systematic review and meta-analysis of published and unpublished placebo and selective serotonin reuptake inhibitor controlled trials. BMJ. 2010;341:c4737.
83. Maund E, Tendal B, Hrobjartsson A, Jorgensen KJ, Lundh A, Schroll J, et al. Benefits and harms in clinical trials of duloxetine for treatment of major depressive disorder: comparison of clinical study reports, trial registries, and publications. BMJ. 2014;348:g3510.
84. Bero LA, Rennie D. Influences on the quality of published drug studies. Int J Technol Assess Health Care. 1996;12(2):209–37.
85. Chan AW, Hrobjartsson A, Haahr MT, Gotzsche PC, Altman DG. Empirical evidence for selective reporting of outcomes in randomized trials: comparison of protocols to published articles. JAMA. 2004;291(20):2457–65.
86. Dwan K, Gamble C, Williamson PR, Kirkham JJ, Reporting Bias G. Systematic review of the empirical evidence of study publication bias

and outcome reporting bias—an updated review. PLoS One. 2013;8(7):e66844.

87. Golder S, Loke YK, Wright K, Norman G. Reporting of adverse events in published and unpublished studies of health care interventions: a systematic review. PLoS Med. 2016;13(9):e1002127.
88. Hemminki E. Study of information submitted by drug companies to licensing authorities. Br Med J. 1980;280(6217):833–6.
89. Rising K, Bacchetti P, Bero L. Reporting bias in drug trials submitted to the Food and Drug Administration: review of publication and presentation. PLoS Med. 2008;5(11):e217.
90. Riveros C, Dechartres A, Perrodeau E, Haneef R, Boutron I, Ravaud P. Timing and completeness of trial results posted at ClinicalTrials.gov and published in journals. PLoS Med. 2013;10(12):e1001566.
91. Feighner JP. Mechanism of action of antidepressant medications. J Clin Psychiatry. 1999;60 (Suppl 4):4–11.
92. Harmer CJ, Duman RS, Cowen PJ. How do antidepressants work? New perspectives for refining future treatment approaches. Lancet Psychiatry. 2017;4(5):409–18.
93. Healy D. The antidepressant era. Cambridge, MA: Harvard University Press; 1997.
94. Zanos P, Gould TD. Mechanisms of ketamine action as an antidepressant. Mol Psychiatry. 2018;23(4):801–11.
95. Lieberman JA. History of the use of antidepressants in primary care. Primary Care Companion J Clin Psychiatry. 2003;5(suppl 7):6–10.
96. Aarts N, Noordam R, Hofman A, Tiemeier H, Stricker BH, Visser LE. Self-reported indications for antidepressant use in a population-based cohort of middle-aged and elderly. Int J Clin Pharm. 2016;38(5):1311–7.
97. Maust DT, Blow FC, Wiechers IR, Kales HC, Marcus SC. National trends in antidepressant, benzodiazepine, and other sedative-hypnotic treatment of older adults in psychiatric and primary care. J Clin Psychiatry. 2017;78(4):e363–71.
98. Noordam R, Aarts N, Verhamme KM, Sturkenboom MC, Stricker BH, Visser LE. Prescription and indication trends of antidepressant drugs in the Netherlands between 1996 and 2012: a dynamic population-based study. Eur J Clin Pharmacol. 2015;71(3):369–75.

99. Wong J, Motulsky A, Eguale T, Buckeridge DL, Abrahamowicz M, Tamblyn R. Treatment indications for antidepressants prescribed in primary care in Quebec, Canada, 2006–2015. JAMA. 2016;315(20):2230–2.
100. Gardarsdottir H, Heerdink ER, van Dijk L, Egberts AC. Indications for antidepressant drug prescribing in general practice in the Netherlands. J Affect Disord. 2007;98(1–2):109–15.
101. Palmer J. After the boom, no reason to smile. The Wall Street Journal. May 20, 2002.
102. Ioannidis JP. Effectiveness of antidepressants: an evidence myth constructed from a thousand randomized trials? Philos Ethics Humanit Med. 2008;3:14.
103. Olfson M, Marcus SC, Druss B, Elinson L, Tanielian T, Pincus HA. National trends in the outpatient treatment of depression. JAMA. 2002;287(2):203–9.
104. Marcus SC, Olfson M. National trends in the treatment for depression from 1998 to 2007. Arch Gen Psychiatry. 2010;67(12):1265–73.
105. Olfson M, Blanco C, Marcus SC. Treatment of adult depression in the United States. JAMA Intern Med. 2016;176(10):1482–91.
106. Mojtabai R. Increase in antidepressant medication in the US adult population between 1990 and 2003. Psychother Psychosom. 2008;77(2):83–92.
107. Pratt LA, Brody DJ, Gu Q. Antidepressant use in persons aged 12 and over: United States, 2011–2014. Hyattsville, MD: National Center for Health Statistics; 2017.
108. Gusmao R, Quintao S, McDaid D, Arensman E, Van Audenhove C, Coffey C, et al. Antidepressant utilization and suicide in Europe: an ecological multi-national study. PLoS One. 2013;8(6):e66455.
109. OECD. Health at a glance 2017: OECD indicators. Paris: OECD Publishing; 2017.
110. Vilhelmsson A. Depression and antidepressants: a nordic perspective. Front Public Health. 2013;1:30.
111. Middleton N, Gunnell D, Whitley E, Dorling D, Frankel S. Secular trends in antidepressant prescribing in the UK, 1975–1998. J Public Health Med. 2001;23(4):262–7.
112. Mars B, Heron J, Kessler D, Davies NM, Martin RM, Thomas KH, et al. Influences on antidepressant prescribing trends in the UK: 1995–2011. Soc Psychiatry Psychiatr Epidemiol. 2017;52(2):193–200.
113. Marsden J, White M, Annand F, Burkinshaw P, Carville S, Eastwood B, et al. Medicines associated with dependence or withdrawal: a mixed-

methods public health review and national database study in England. Lancet Psychiatry. 2019;6(11):935–50.

114. Martinez C, Rietbrock S, Wise L, Ashby D, Chick J, Moseley J, et al. Antidepressant treatment and the risk of fatal and non-fatal self harm in first episode depression: nested case-control study. BMJ. 2005;330(7488):389.
115. Coupland C, Hill T, Morriss R, Arthur A, Moore M, Hippisley-Cox J. Antidepressant use and risk of suicide and attempted suicide or self harm in people aged 20 to 64: cohort study using a primary care database. BMJ. 2015;350:h517.
116. Ferrari AJ, Charlson FJ, Norman RE, Patten SB, Freedman G, Murray CJ, et al. Burden of depressive disorders by country, sex, age, and year: findings from the global burden of disease study 2010. PLoS Med. 2013;10(11):e1001547.
117. Mojtabai R. Clinician-identified depression in community settings: concordance with structured-interview diagnoses. Psychother Psychosom. 2013;82(3):161–9.
118. Bachmann CJ, Aagaard L, Burcu M, Glaeske G, Kalverdijk LJ, Petersen I, et al. Trends and patterns of antidepressant use in children and adolescents from five western countries, 2005–2012. Eur Neuropsychopharmacol. 2016;26(3):411–9.
119. Wesselhoeft R, Jensen PB, Talati A, Reutfors J, Furu K, Strandberg-Larsen K, et al. Trends in antidepressant use among children and adolescents: a Scandinavian drug utilization study. Acta Psychiatr Scand. 2020;141(1):34–42.
120. Whitely M, Raven M, Jureidini J. Antidepressant prescribing and suicide/self-harm by young Australians: regulatory warnings, contradictory advice, and long-term trends. Front Psychiatry. 2020;11:478.
121. Zito JM, Pennap D, Safer DJ. Antidepressant use in medicaid-insured youth: trends, covariates, and future research needs. Front Psychiatry. 2020;11:113.
122. Lagerberg T, Molero Y, D'Onofrio BM, Fernandez de la Cruz L, Lichtenstein P, Mataix-Cols D, et al. Antidepressant prescription patterns and CNS polypharmacy with antidepressants among children, adolescents, and young adults: a population-based study in Sweden. Eur Child Adolesc Psychiatry. 2019;28(8):1137–45.
123. Aarts N, Noordam R, Hofman A, Tiemeier H, Stricker BH, Visser LE. Utilization patterns of antidepressants between 1991 and 2011 in a

population-based cohort of middle-aged and elderly. Eur Psychiatry. 2014;29(6):365–70.

124. Mojtabai R, Olfson M. National trends in long-term use of antidepressant medications: results from the U.S. National Health and Nutrition Examination Survey. J Clin Psychiatry. 2014;75(2):169–77.
125. Moore M, Yuen HM, Dunn N, Mullee MA, Maskell J, Kendrick T. Explaining the rise in antidepressant prescribing: a descriptive study using the general practice research database. BMJ. 2009;339:b3999.
126. Huijbregts KM, Hoogendoorn A, Slottje P, van Balkom A, Batelaan NM. Long-term and short-term antidepressant use in general practice: data from a large cohort in the Netherlands. Psychother Psychosom. 2017;86(6):362–9.
127. Johnson CF, Macdonald HJ, Atkinson P, Buchanan AI, Downes N, Dougall N. Reviewing long-term antidepressants can reduce drug burden: a prospective observational cohort study. Br J Gen Pract. 2012;62(604):e773–9.
128. Mojtabai R, Olfson M. National trends in psychotropic medication polypharmacy in office-based psychiatry. Arch Gen Psychiatry. 2010;67(1):26–36.
129. John A, Marchant AL, Fone DL, McGregor JI, Dennis MS, Tan JO, et al. Recent trends in primary-care antidepressant prescribing to children and young people: an e-cohort study. Psychol Med. 2016;46(16):3315–27.
130. Verhaak PFM, de Beurs D, Spreeuwenberg P. What proportion of initially prescribed antidepressants is still being prescribed chronically after 5 years in general practice? A longitudinal cohort analysis. BMJ Open. 2019;9(2):e024051.
131. Schroder C, Dorks M, Kollhorst B, Blenk T, Dittmann RW, Garbe E, et al. Outpatient antidepressant drug use in children and adolescents in Germany between 2004 and 2011. Pharmacoepidemiol Drug Saf. 2017;26(2):170–9.
132. Medawar C. The antidepressant web: marketing depression and making medicines work. Int J Risk Saf Med. 1997;10(2):75–126.
133. Jakobsen JC, Gluud C, Kirsch I. Should antidepressants be used for major depressive disorder? BMJ Evid Based Med. 2020;25(4):130–6.
134. Moncrieff J. What does the latest meta-analysis really tell us about antidepressants? Epidemiol Psychiatr Sci. 2018;27(5):430–2.

135. Warren JB. The trouble with antidepressants: why the evidence overplays benefits and underplays risks. BMJ. 2020;370:m3200.
136. Cole JO. Therapeutic efficacy of antidepressant drugs. A review. JAMA. 1964;190:448–55.
137. Cipriani A, Salanti G, Furukawa TA, Egger M, Leucht S, Ruhe HG, et al. Antidepressants might work for people with major depression: where do we go from here? Lancet Psychiatry. 2018;5(6):461–3.
138. Goodwin GM, Nutt D. Antidepressants; what's the beef? Acta Neuropsychiatr. 2019;31(1):59–60.
139. Hieronymus F, Jauhar S, Ostergaard SD, Young AH. One (effect) size does not fit at all: interpreting clinical significance and effect sizes in depression treatment trials. J Psychopharmacol. 2020;34(10):1074–8.
140. McCormack J, Korownyk C. Effectiveness of antidepressants. BMJ. 2018;360:k1073.
141. Cipriani A, Furukawa TA, Salanti G, Chaimani A, Atkinson LZ, Ogawa Y, et al. Comparative efficacy and acceptability of 21 antidepressant drugs for the acute treatment of adults with major depressive disorder: a systematic review and network meta-analysis. Lancet. 2018;391(10128):1357–66.
142. Cosgrove L, Erlich D, Shaughnessy AF. No magic pill: a prescription for enhanced shared decision-making for depression treatment. J Am Board Fam Med. 2019;32(1):6–9.
143. Ghaemi SN. Antidepressants work for major depression! Not so fast. Medscape. June 13, 2018.
144. Naudet F, Millet B, Reymann JM, Falissard B. Improving study design for antidepressant effectiveness assessment. Int J Methods Psychiatr Res. 2013;22(3):217–31.
145. Montgomery SA, Moller HJ. Is the significant superiority of escitalopram compared with other antidepressants clinically relevant? Int Clin Psychopharmacol. 2009;24(3):111–8.
146. Harris G. Debate resumes on the safety of depression's wonder drugs. The New York Times. August 7, 2003.
147. Gotzsche PC. Deadly psychiatry and organised denial. Copenhagen: People's Press; 2015.
148. Abraham J, Davis C. A comparative analysis of drug safety withdrawals in the UK and the US (1971–1992): implications for current regulatory thinking and policy. Soc Sci Med. 2005;61(5):881–92.

149. Abraham J, Davis C. Drug evaluation and the permissive principle: continuities and contradictions between standards and practices in antidepressant regulation. Soc Stud Sci. 2009;39(4):569–98.
150. Spielmans GI, Kirsch I. Drug approval and drug effectiveness. Annu Rev Clin Psychol. 2014;10:741–66.
151. Hypericum Depression Trial Study Group. Effect of Hypericum perforatum (St John's wort) in major depressive disorder: a randomized controlled trial. JAMA. 2002;287(14):1807–14.
152. Lewis G, Duffy L, Ades A, Amos R, Araya R, Brabyn S, et al. The clinical effectiveness of sertraline in primary care and the role of depression severity and duration (PANDA): a pragmatic, double-blind, placebo-controlled randomised trial. Lancet Psychiatry. 2019;6(11):903–14.
153. Webb CA, Trivedi MH, Cohen ZD, Dillon DG, Fournier JC, Goer F, et al. Personalized prediction of antidepressant v. placebo response: evidence from the EMBARC study. Psychol Med. 2019;49(7):1118–27.
154. Cosgrove L, Vannoy S, Mintzes B, Shaughnessy AF. Under the influence: the interplay among industry, publishing, and drug regulation. Account Res. 2016;23(5):257–79.
155. Gastaldon C, Papola D, Ostuzzi G, Barbui C. Esketamine for treatment resistant depression: a trick of smoke and mirrors? Epidemiol Psychiatr Sci. 2019;29:e79.
156. Turner EH. Esketamine for treatment-resistant depression: seven concerns about efficacy and FDA approval. Lancet Psychiatry. 2019;6(12):977–9.
157. Man-Son-Hing M, Laupacis A, O'Rourke K, Molnar FJ, Mahon J, Chan KB, et al. Determination of the clinical importance of study results. J Gen Intern Med. 2002;17(6):469–76.
158. Wasserstein RL, Lazar NA. The ASA's statement on p-values: context, process, and purpose. Am Stat. 2016;70(2):129–33.
159. Cumming G. Replication and p intervals: p values predict the future only vaguely, but confidence intervals do much better. Perspect Psychol Sci. 2008;3(4):286–300.
160. Greenland S, Senn SJ, Rothman KJ, Carlin JB, Poole C, Goodman SN, et al. Statistical tests, P values, confidence intervals, and power: a guide to misinterpretations. Eur J Epidemiol. 2016;31(4):337–50.
161. Siddiqui O, Hung HM, O'Neill R. MMRM vs. LOCF: a comprehensive comparison based on simulation study and 25 NDA datasets. J Biopharm Stat. 2009;19(2):227–46.

162. Streiner DL. Missing data and the trouble with LOCF. Evid Based Ment Health. 2008;11(1):3–5.
163. Woolley SB, Cardoni AA, Goethe JW. Last-observation-carried-forward imputation method in clinical efficacy trials: review of 352 antidepressant studies. Pharmacotherapy. 2009;29(12):1408–16.
164. van Ravenzwaaij D, Ioannidis JP. A simulation study of the strength of evidence in the recommendation of medications based on two trials with statistically significant results. PLoS One. 2017;12(3):e0173184.
165. Downing NS, Aminawung JA, Shah ND, Krumholz HM, Ross JS. Clinical trial evidence supporting FDA approval of novel therapeutic agents, 2005–2012. JAMA. 2014;311(4):368–77.
166. Walsh BT, Seidman SN, Sysko R, Gould M. Placebo response in studies of major depression: variable, substantial, and growing. JAMA. 2002;287(14):1840–7.
167. Boesen K, Gotzsche PC, Ioannidis JPA. EMA and FDA psychiatric drug trial guidelines: assessment of guideline development and trial design recommendations. Epidemiol Psychiatr Sci. 2021;30:e35.
168. Barbui C, Bighelli I. A new approach to psychiatric drug approval in Europe. PLoS Med. 2013;10(10):e1001530.
169. Pignatti F, Aronsson B, Gate N, Vamvakas S, Wade G, Moulon I, et al. The review of drug applications submitted to the European Medicines Evaluation Agency: frequently raised objections, and outcome. Eur J Clin Pharmacol. 2002;58(9):573–80.
170. Erhel F, Scanff A, Naudet F. The evidence base for psychotropic drugs approved by the European Medicines Agency: a meta-assessment of all European Public Assessment Reports. Epidemiol Psychiatr Sci. 2020;29:e120.
171. Light DW, Lexchin J, Darrow JJ. Institutional corruption of pharmaceuticals and the myth of safe and effective drugs. J Law Med Ethics. 2013;41(3):590–600.
172. Naci H, Ioannidis JP. How good is "evidence" from clinical studies of drug effects and why might such evidence fail in the prediction of the clinical utility of drugs? Annu Rev Pharmacol Toxicol. 2015;55:169–89.
173. Wieseler B, McGauran N, Kaiser T. New drugs: where did we go wrong and what can we do better? BMJ. 2019;366:l4340.
174. de Vries YA, Roest AM, de Jonge P, Cuijpers P, Munafo MR, Bastiaansen JA. The cumulative effect of reporting and citation biases on the apparent

efficacy of treatments: the case of depression. Psychol Med. 2018;48(15):2453–5.

175. Khin NA, Chen YF, Yang Y, Yang P, Laughren TP. Exploratory analyses of efficacy data from major depressive disorder trials submitted to the US Food and Drug Administration in support of new drug applications. J Clin Psychiatry. 2011;72(4):464–72.
176. Duhoux A, Fournier L, Gauvin L, Roberge P. What is the association between quality of treatment for depression and patient outcomes? A cohort study of adults consulting in primary care. J Affect Disord. 2013;151(1):265–74.
177. Hengartner MP. Is there a genuine placebo effect in acute depression treatments? A reassessment of regression to the mean and spontaneous remission. BMJ Evid Based Med. 2020;25(2):46–8.
178. Posternak MA, Solomon DA, Leon AC, Mueller TI, Shea MT, Endicott J, et al. The naturalistic course of unipolar major depression in the absence of somatic therapy. J Nerv Ment Dis. 2006;194(5):324–9.
179. Ten Have M, Penninx B, Tuithof M, van Dorsselaer S, Kleinjan M, Spijker J, et al. Duration of major and minor depressive episodes and associated risk indicators in a psychiatric epidemiological cohort study of the general population. Acta Psychiatr Scand. 2017;136(3):300–12.
180. Whiteford HA, Harris MG, McKeon G, Baxter A, Pennell C, Barendregt JJ, et al. Estimating remission from untreated major depression: a systematic review and meta-analysis. Psychol Med. 2013;43(8):1569–85.
181. Baumeister H. Inappropriate prescriptions of antidepressant drugs in patients with subthreshold to mild depression: time for the evidence to become practice. J Affect Disord. 2012;139(3):240–3.
182. Cuijpers P, Cristea IA. What if a placebo effect explained all the activity of depression treatments? World Psychiatry. 2015;14(3):310–1.
183. Hollon SD. Is cognitive therapy enduring or antidepressant medications iatrogenic? Depression as an evolved adaptation. Am Psychol. 2020;75(9):1207–18.
184. Posternak MA, Zimmerman M. Therapeutic effect of follow-up assessments on antidepressant and placebo response rates in antidepressant efficacy trials: meta-analysis. Br J Psychiatry. 2007;190:287–92.
185. McKay KM, Imel ZE, Wampold BE. Psychiatrist effects in the psychopharmacological treatment of depression. J Affect Disord. 2006;92(2–3):287–90.

186. Zilcha-Mano S, Roose SP, Barber JP, Rutherford BR. Therapeutic alliance in antidepressant treatment: cause or effect of symptomatic levels? Psychother Psychosom. 2015;84(3):177–82.
187. Brown WA. Treatment response in melancholia. Acta Psychiatr Scand Suppl. 2007(433):125–9.
188. Zimmerman M, Clark HL, Multach MD, Walsh E, Rosenstein LK, Gazarian D. Have treatment studies of depression become even less generalizable? A review of the inclusion and exclusion criteria used in placebo-controlled antidepressant efficacy trials published during the past 20 years. Mayo Clin Proc. 2015;90(9):1180–6.
189. Zimmerman M, Balling C, Chelminski I, Dalrymple K. Understanding the severity of depression: which symptoms of depression are the best indicators of depression severity? Compr Psychiatry. 2018;87:84–8.
190. Ten Have M, de Graaf R, van Dorsselaer S, Tuithof M, Kleinjan M, Penninx B. Recurrence and chronicity of major depressive disorder and their risk indicators in a population cohort. Acta Psychiatr Scand. 2018;137(6):503–15.
191. Salanti G, Chaimani A, Furukawa TA, Higgins JPT, Ogawa Y, Cipriani A, et al. Impact of placebo arms on outcomes in antidepressant trials: systematic review and meta-regression analysis. Int J Epidemiol. 2018;47(5):1454–64.
192. Furukawa TA, Cipriani A, Atkinson LZ, Leucht S, Ogawa Y, Takeshima N, et al. Placebo response rates in antidepressant trials: a systematic review of published and unpublished double-blind randomised controlled studies. Lancet Psychiatry. 2016;3(11):1059–66.
193. Arroll B, Elley CR, Fishman T, Goodyear-Smith FA, Kenealy T, Blashki G, et al. Antidepressants versus placebo for depression in primary care. Cochrane Database Syst Rev. 2009(3):CD007954.
194. Undurraga J, Baldessarini RJ. Randomized, placebo-controlled trials of antidepressants for acute major depression: thirty-year meta-analytic review. Neuropsychopharmacol. 2012;37(4):851–64.
195. Kirsch I, Moncrieff J. Clinical trials and the response rate illusion. Contemp Clin Trials. 2007;28(4):348–51.
196. Rabinowitz J, Werbeloff N, Mandel FS, Menard F, Marangell L, Kapur S. Initial depression severity and response to antidepressants v. placebo: patient-level data analysis from 34 randomised controlled trials. Br J Psychiatry. 2016;209(5):427–8.

197. Kraemer HC, Kupfer DJ. Size of treatment effects and their importance to clinical research and practice. Biol Psychiatry. 2006;59(11):990–6.
198. Kirsch I, Deacon BJ, Huedo-Medina TB, Scoboria A, Moore TJ, Johnson BT. Initial severity and antidepressant benefits: a meta-analysis of data submitted to the Food and Drug Administration. PLoS Med. 2008;5(2):e45.
199. Norman GR, Sloan JA, Wyrwich KW. Interpretation of changes in health-related quality of life: the remarkable universality of half a standard deviation. Med Care. 2003;41(5):582–92.
200. Turner D, Schunemann HJ, Griffith LE, Beaton DE, Griffiths AM, Critch JN, et al. The minimal detectable change cannot reliably replace the minimal important difference. J Clin Epidemiol. 2010;63(1):28–36.
201. Appleton KM, Sallis HM, Perry R, Ness AR, Churchill R. Omega-3 fatty acids for depression in adults. Cochrane Database Syst Rev. 2015(11):CD004692.
202. Gartlehner G, Gaynes BN, Amick HR, Asher GN, Morgan LC, Coker-Schwimmer E, et al. Comparative benefits and harms of antidepressant, psychological, complementary, and exercise treatments for major depression: an evidence report for a clinical practice guideline from the American College of Physicians. Ann Intern Med. 2016;164(5):331–41.
203. Linde K, Berner MM, Kriston L. St John's wort for major depression. Cochrane Database Syst Rev. 2008(4):CD000448.
204. Cuijpers P, Noma H, Karyotaki E, Vinkers CH, Cipriani A, Furukawa TA. A network meta-analysis of the effects of psychotherapies, pharmacotherapies and their combination in the treatment of adult depression. World Psychiatry. 2020;19(1):92–107.
205. De Maat S, Dekker J, Schoevers R, De Jonghe F. Relative efficacy of psychotherapy and pharmacotherapy in the treatment of depression: a meta-analysis. Psychother Res. 2006;16(5):566–78.
206. Spielmans GI, Berman MI, Usitalo AN. Psychotherapy versus second-generation antidepressants in the treatment of depression: a meta-analysis. J Nerv Ment Dis. 2011;199(3):142–9.
207. Cuijpers P, Weitz E, Lamers F, Penninx BW, Twisk J, DeRubeis RJ, et al. Melancholic and atypical depression as predictor and moderator of outcome in cognitive behavior therapy and pharmacotherapy for adult depression. Depress Anxiety. 2017;34(3):246–56.
208. Weitz ES, Hollon SD, Twisk J, van Straten A, Huibers MJ, David D, et al. Baseline depression severity as moderator of depression outcomes

between cognitive behavioral therapy vs pharmacotherapy: an individual patient data meta-analysis. JAMA Psychiatry. 2015;72(11):1102–9.

209. Biesheuvel-Leliefeld KE, Kok GD, Bockting CL, Cuijpers P, Hollon SD, van Marwijk HW, et al. Effectiveness of psychological interventions in preventing recurrence of depressive disorder: meta-analysis and meta-regression. J Affect Disord. 2015;174:400–10.
210. Cuijpers P, Hollon SD, van Straten A, Bockting C, Berking M, Andersson G. Does cognitive behaviour therapy have an enduring effect that is superior to keeping patients on continuation pharmacotherapy? A meta-analysis. BMJ Open. 2013;3(4):e002542.
211. Kuyken W, Warren FC, Taylor RS, Whalley B, Crane C, Bondolfi G, et al. Efficacy of mindfulness-based cognitive therapy in prevention of depressive relapse: an individual patient data meta-analysis from randomized trials. JAMA Psychiatry. 2016;73(6):565–74.
212. Furukawa TA, Shinohara K, Sahker E, Karyotaki E, Miguel C, Ciharova M, et al. Initial treatment choices to achieve sustained response in major depression: a systematic review and network meta-analysis. World Psychiatry. 2021;20:387–96.
213. Karyotaki E, Smit Y, Holdt Henningsen K, Huibers MJ, Robays J, de Beurs D, et al. Combining pharmacotherapy and psychotherapy or monotherapy for major depression? A meta-analysis on the long-term effects. J Affect Disord. 2016;194:144–52.
214. Hengartner MP. How effective are antidepressants for depression over the long term? A critical review of relapse prevention trials and the issue of withdrawal confounding. Ther Adv Psychopharmacol. 2020;10:2045125320921694.
215. Deshauer D, Moher D, Fergusson D, Moher E, Sampson M, Grimshaw J. Selective serotonin reuptake inhibitors for unipolar depression: a systematic review of classic long-term randomized controlled trials. CMAJ. 2008;178(10):1293–301.
216. Henssler J, Kurschus M, Franklin J, Bschor T, Baethge C. Long-term acute-phase treatment with antidepressants, 8 weeks and beyond: a systematic review and meta-analysis of randomized, placebo-controlled trials. J Clin Psychiatry. 2018;79(1):60–8.
217. Andrews PW, Kornstein SG, Halberstadt LJ, Gardner CO, Neale MC. Blue again: perturbational effects of antidepressants suggest monoaminergic homeostasis in major depression. Front Psychol. 2011;2:159.

218. Fava GA. May antidepressant drugs worsen the conditions they are supposed to treat? The clinical foundations of the oppositional model of tolerance. Ther Adv Psychopharmacol. 2020;10:2045125320970325.
219. Pigott HE, Leventhal AM, Alter GS, Boren JJ. Efficacy and effectiveness of antidepressants: current status of research. Psychother Psychosom. 2010;79(5):267–79.
220. Hengartner MP, Angst J, Rossler W. Antidepressant use prospectively relates to a poorer long-term outcome of depression: results from a prospective community cohort study over 30 years. Psychother Psychosom. 2018;87(3):181–3.
221. Vittengl JR. Poorer long-term outcomes among persons with major depressive disorder treated with medication. Psychother Psychosom. 2017;86(5):302–4.
222. Rush AJ, Trivedi M, Carmody TJ, Biggs MM, Shores-Wilson K, Ibrahim H, et al. One-year clinical outcomes of depressed public sector outpatients: a benchmark for subsequent studies. Biol Psychiatry. 2004;56(1):46–53.
223. Fava GA, Offidani E. The mechanisms of tolerance in antidepressant action. Prog Neuropsychopharmacol Biol Psychiatry. 2011;35(7):1593–602.
224. Fornaro M, Anastasia A, Novello S, Fusco A, Pariano R, De Berardis D, et al. The emergence of loss of efficacy during antidepressant drug treatment for major depressive disorder: an integrative review of evidence, mechanisms, and clinical implications. Pharmacol Res. 2019;139:494–502.
225. Kinrys G, Gold AK, Pisano VD, Freeman MP, Papakostas GI, Mischoulon D, et al. Tachyphylaxis in major depressive disorder: a review of the current state of research. J Affect Disord. 2019;245:488–97.
226. Leykin Y, Amsterdam JD, DeRubeis RJ, Gallop R, Shelton RC, Hollon SD. Progressive resistance to a selective serotonin reuptake inhibitor but not to cognitive therapy in the treatment of major depression. J Consult Clin Psychol. 2007;75(2):267–76.
227. Fava GA, Cosci F, Guidi J, Rafanelli C. The deceptive manifestations of treatment resistance in depression: a new look at the problem. Psychother Psychosom. 2020;89(5):265–73.
228. El-Mallakh RS, Briscoe B. Studies of long-term use of antidepressants: how should the data from them be interpreted? CNS Drugs. 2012;26(2):97–109.

229. Kendrick T. Long-term antidepressant treatment: time for a review? Prescriber. 2015;26(19):7–10.
230. Ghaemi SN. Why antidepressants are not antidepressants: STEP-BD, STAR*D, and the return of neurotic depression. Bipolar Disord. 2008;10(8):957–68.
231. American Psychiatric Association. Practice guideline for the treatment of patients with major depressive disorder. Washington, DC: American Psychiatric Association; 2010.
232. DGPPN. S3-leitlinie/Nationale Versorgungsleitlinie unipolare Depression. Berlin: DGPPN; 2015.
233. National Institute for Health and Care Excellence. Depression in adults: recognition and management. London: NICE; 2009.
234. Ghaemi SN, Selker HP. Maintenance efficacy designs in psychiatry: randomized discontinuation trials—enriched but not better. J Clin Transl Sci. 2017;1(3):198–204.
235. Greenhouse JB, Stangl D, Kupfer DJ, Prien RF. Methodologic issues in maintenance therapy clinical trials. Arch Gen Psychiatry. 1991;48(4):313–8.
236. Moncrieff J. Why is it so difficult to stop psychiatric drug treatment? It may be nothing to do with the original problem. Med Hypotheses. 2006;67(3):517–23.
237. Recalt AM, Cohen D. Withdrawal confounding in randomized controlled trials of antipsychotic, antidepressant, and stimulant drugs, 2000–2017. Psychother Psychosom. 2019;88(2):105–13.
238. Van Leeuwen E, van Driel ML, Horowitz MA, Kendrick T, Donald M, De Sutter AI, et al. Approaches for discontinuation versus continuation of long-term antidepressant use for depressive and anxiety disorders in adults. Cochrane Database Syst Rev. 2021;4:CD013495.
239. Hengartner MP, Plöderl M. Prophylactic effects or withdrawal reactions? An analysis of time-to-event data from antidepressant relapse prevention trials submitted to the FDA. Ther Adv Psychopharmacol. 2021;11:1–12.
240. Senn S. Mastering variation: variance components and personalised medicine. Stat Med. 2016;35(7):966–77.
241. Angst J. Severity of depression and benzodiazepine comedication in relationship to efficacy of antidepressants in acute trials. Hum Psychopharm Clin. 1993;8(6):401–7.
242. Senn S. Individual response to treatment: is it a valid assumption? BMJ. 2004;329(7472):966–8.

243. Maslej MM, Furukawa TA, Cipriani A, Andrews PW, Sanches M, Tomlinson A, et al. Individual differences in response to antidepressants: a meta-analysis of placebo-controlled randomized clinical trials. JAMA Psychiatry. 2021;78(5):490–7.
244. Munkholm K, Winkelbeiner S, Homan P. Individual response to antidepressants for depression in adults-a meta-analysis and simulation study. PLoS One. 2020;15(8):e0237950.
245. Plöderl M, Hengartner MP. What are the chances for personalised treatment with antidepressants? Detection of patient-by-treatment interaction with a variance ratio meta-analysis. BMJ Open. 2019;9(12):e034816.
246. Volkmann C, Volkmann A, Muller CA. On the treatment effect heterogeneity of antidepressants in major depression: a Bayesian meta-analysis and simulation study. PLoS One. 2020;15(11):e0241497.
247. Joyner MJ, Paneth N. Promises, promises, and precision medicine. J Clin Invest. 2019;129(3):946–8.
248. Prasad V, Fojo T, Brada M. Precision oncology: origins, optimism, and potential. Lancet Oncol. 2016;17(2):e81–6.
249. Ruppel J. "Now is a time for optimism": the politics of personalized medicine in mental health research. Sci Technol Hum Val. 2019;44(4):581–611.
250. Senn S. Statistical pitfalls of personalized medicine. Nature. 2018;563(7733):619–21.
251. Winkelbeiner S, Leucht S, Kane JM, Homan P. Evaluation of differences in individual treatment response in schizophrenia spectrum disorders: a meta-analysis. JAMA Psychiatry. 2019;76(10):1063–73.
252. Nierenberg AA, Ostacher MJ, Huffman JC, Ametrano RM, Fava M, Perlis RH. A brief review of antidepressant efficacy, effectiveness, indications, and usage for major depressive disorder. J Occup Environ Med. 2008;50(4):428–36.
253. Valerio MP, Szmulewicz AG, Martino DJ. A quantitative review on outcome-to-antidepressants in melancholic unipolar depression. Psychiatry Res. 2018;265:100–10.
254. Imai H, Noma H, Furukawa TA. Melancholic features (DSM-IV) predict but do not moderate response to antidepressants in major depression: an individual participant data meta-analysis of 1219 patients. Eur Arch Psychiatry Clin Neurosci. 2021;271(3):521–6.

255. Parker G, Fink M, Shorter E, Taylor MA, Akiskal H, Berrios G, et al. Issues for DSM-5: whither melancholia? The case for its classification as a distinct mood disorder. Am J Psychiatry. 2010;167(7):745–7.
256. Fournier JC, DeRubeis RJ, Hollon SD, Dimidjian S, Amsterdam JD, Shelton RC, et al. Antidepressant drug effects and depression severity: a patient-level meta-analysis. JAMA. 2010;303(1):47–53.
257. Furukawa TA, Maruo K, Noma H, Tanaka S, Imai H, Shinohara K, et al. Initial severity of major depression and efficacy of new generation antidepressants: individual participant data meta-analysis. Acta Psychiatr Scand. 2018;137(6):450–8.
258. Hieronymus F, Lisinski A, Nilsson S, Eriksson E. Influence of baseline severity on the effects of SSRIs in depression: an item-based, patient-level post-hoc analysis. Lancet Psychiatry. 2019;6(9):745–52.
259. Plöderl M, Hengartner MP. Guidelines for the pharmacological acute treatment of major depression: conflicts with current evidence as demonstrated with the German S3-guidelines. BMC Psychiatry. 2019;19(1):265.
260. Fried EI, Nesse RM. Depression sum-scores don't add up: why analyzing specific depression symptoms is essential. BMC Med. 2015;13:72.
261. Barbui C, Cipriani A, Patel V, Ayuso-Mateos JL, van Ommeren M. Efficacy of antidepressants and benzodiazepines in minor depression: systematic review and meta-analysis. Br J Psychiatry. 2011;198(1):11–6.
262. Cameron IM, Reid IC, MacGillivray SA. Efficacy and tolerability of antidepressants for sub-threshold depression and for mild major depressive disorder. J Affect Disord. 2014;166:48–58.
263. Hermens ML, van Hout HP, Terluin B, Ader HJ, Penninx BW, van Marwijk HW, et al. Clinical effectiveness of usual care with or without antidepressant medication for primary care patients with minor or mild-major depression: a randomized equivalence trial. BMC Med. 2007;5:36.
264. Iglesias-Gonzalez M, Aznar-Lou I, Penarrubia-Maria MT, Gil-Girbau M, Fernandez-Vergel R, Alonso J, et al. Effectiveness of watchful waiting versus antidepressants for patients diagnosed of mild to moderate depression in primary care: a 12-month pragmatic clinical trial (INFAP study). Eur Psychiatry. 2018;53:66–73.
265. Hegerl U, Mergl R. The clinical significance of antidepressant treatment effects cannot be derived from placebo-verum response differences. J Psychopharmacol. 2010;24(4):445–8.
266. Bschor T, Kern H, Henssler J, Baethge C. Switching the antidepressant after nonresponse in adults with major depression: a systematic literature search and meta-analysis. J Clin Psychiatry. 2018;79(1):16r10749.

267. Papakostas GI, Fava M. Does the probability of receiving placebo influence clinical trial outcome? A meta-regression of double-blind, randomized clinical trials in MDD. Eur Neuropsychopharmacol. 2009;19(1):34–40.
268. Braun C, Adams A, Rink L, Bschor T, Kuhr K, Baethge C. In search of a dose-response relationship in SSRIs-a systematic review, meta-analysis, and network meta-analysis. Acta Psychiatr Scand. 2020;142(6):430–42.
269. Furukawa TA, Salanti G, Cowen PJ, Leucht S, Cipriani A. No benefit from flexible titration above minimum licensed dose in prescribing antidepressants for major depression: systematic review. Acta Psychiatr Scand. 2020;141(5):401–9.
270. Furukawa TA, Cipriani A, Cowen PJ, Leucht S, Egger M, Salanti G. Optimal dose of selective serotonin reuptake inhibitors, venlafaxine, and mirtazapine in major depression: a systematic review and dose-response meta-analysis. Lancet Psychiatry. 2019;6(7):601–9.
271. Dold M, Bartova L, Rupprecht R, Kasper S. Dose escalation of antidepressants in unipolar depression: a meta-analysis of double-blind, randomized controlled trials. Psychother Psychosom. 2017;86(5):283–91.
272. Rink L, Braun C, Bschor T, Henssler J, Franklin J, Baethge C. Dose increase versus unchanged continuation of antidepressants after initial antidepressant treatment failure in patients with major depressive disorder: a systematic review and meta-analysis of randomized, double-blind trials. J Clin Psychiatry. 2018;79(3):17r11693.
273. Bostwick JM. A generalist's guide to treating patients with depression with an emphasis on using side effects to tailor antidepressant therapy. Mayo Clin Proc. 2010;85(6):538–50.
274. Moncrieff J, Cohen D. Do antidepressants cure or create abnormal brain states? PLoS Med. 2006;3(7):e240.
275. Ferguson JM. SSRI antidepressant medications: adverse effects and tolerability. Prim Care Companion J Clin Psychiatry. 2001;3(1):22–7.
276. Goldsmith L, Moncrieff J. The psychoactive effects of antidepressants and their association with suicidality. Curr Drug Saf. 2011;6(2):115–21.
277. Goodwin GM, Price J, De Bodinat C, Laredo J. Emotional blunting with antidepressant treatments: a survey among depressed patients. J Affect Disord. 2017;221:31–5.
278. Read J, Cartwright C, Gibson K. Adverse emotional and interpersonal effects reported by 1829 New Zealanders while taking antidepressants. Psychiatry Res. 2014;216(1):67–73.

279. Read J, Williams J. Adverse effects of antidepressants reported by a large international cohort: emotional blunting, suicidality, and withdrawal effects. Curr Drug Saf. 2018;13(3):176–86.
280. Del Re AC, Spielmans GI, Fluckiger C, Wampold BE. Efficacy of new generation antidepressants: differences seem illusory. PLoS One. 2014;8(6):e63509.
281. Gartlehner G, Hansen RA, Morgan LC, Thaler K, Lux L, Van Noord M, et al. Comparative benefits and harms of second-generation antidepressants for treating major depressive disorder: an updated meta-analysis. Ann Intern Med. 2011;155(11):772–85.
282. Undurraga J, Baldessarini RJ. Direct comparison of tricyclic and serotonin-reuptake inhibitor antidepressants in randomized head-to-head trials in acute major depression: systematic review and meta-analysis. J Psychopharmacol. 2017;31(9):1184–9.
283. Perry PJ. Pharmacotherapy for major depression with melancholic features: relative efficacy of tricyclic versus selective serotonin reuptake inhibitor antidepressants. J Affect Disord. 1996;39(1):1–6.
284. Amsterdam JD. Selective serotonin reuptake inhibitor efficacy in severe and melancholic depression. J Psychopharmacol. 1998;12(3 Suppl B):S99–111.
285. Barbui C, Hotopf M, Freemantle N, Boynton J, Churchill R, Eccles MP, et al. Selective serotonin reuptake inhibitors versus tricyclic and heterocyclic antidepressants: comparison of drug adherence. Cochrane Database Syst Rev. 2000(4):CD002791.
286. Geddes JR, Freemantle N, Mason J, Eccles MP, Boynton J. SSRIs versus other antidepressants for depressive disorder. Cochrane Database Syst Rev. 2000(2):CD001851.
287. Hirschfeld RM. Efficacy of SSRIs and newer antidepressants in severe depression: comparison with TCAs. J Clin Psychiatry. 1999;60(5):326–35.
288. Joyce PR, Mulder RT, Luty SE, McKenzie JM, Rae AM. A differential response to nortriptyline and fluoxetine in melancholic depression: the importance of age and gender. Acta Psychiatr Scand. 2003;108(1):20–3.
289. Hengartner MP. Editorial: antidepressant prescriptions in children and adolescents. Front Psychiatry. 2020;11:600282.
290. Jureidini JN, Doecke CJ, Mansfield PR, Haby MM, Menkes DB, Tonkin AL. Efficacy and safety of antidepressants for children and adolescents. BMJ. 2004;328(7444):879–83.

291. Safer DJ, Zito JM. Short- and long-term antidepressant clinical trials for major depressive disorder in youth: findings and concerns. Front Psychiatry. 2019;10:705.
292. Hetrick SE, McKenzie JE, Cox GR, Simmons MB, Merry SN. Newer generation antidepressants for depressive disorders in children and adolescents. Cochrane Database Syst Rev. 2012;11:CD004851.
293. Healy D, Le Noury J, Jureidini J. Paediatric antidepressants: benefits and risks. Int J Risk Saf Med. 2019;30(1):1–7.
294. Cipriani A, Zhou X, Del Giovane C, Hetrick SE, Qin B, Whittington C, et al. Comparative efficacy and tolerability of antidepressants for major depressive disorder in children and adolescents: a network meta-analysis. Lancet. 2016;388(10047):881–90.
295. Hetrick SE, McKenzie JE, Bailey AP, Sharma V, Moller CI, Badcock PB, et al. New generation antidepressants for depression in children and adolescents: a network meta-analysis. Cochrane Database Syst Rev. 2021;5:CD013674.
296. Krause M, Gutsmiedl K, Bighelli I, Schneider-Thoma J, Chaimani A, Leucht S. Efficacy and tolerability of pharmacological and non-pharmacological interventions in older patients with major depressive disorder: a systematic review, pairwise and network meta-analysis. Eur Neuropsychopharmacol. 2019;29(9):1003–22.
297. Tham A, Jonsson U, Andersson G, Soderlund A, Allard P, Bertilsson G. Efficacy and tolerability of antidepressants in people aged 65 years or older with major depressive disorder—a systematic review and a meta-analysis. J Affect Disord. 2016;205:1–12.
298. Banerjee S, Hellier J, Dewey M, Romeo R, Ballard C, Baldwin R, et al. Sertraline or mirtazapine for depression in dementia (HTA-SADD): a randomised, multicentre, double-blind, placebo-controlled trial. Lancet. 2011;378(9789):403–11.
299. Dudas R, Malouf R, McCleery J, Dening T. Antidepressants for treating depression in dementia. Cochrane Database Syst Rev. 2018;8:CD003944.
300. Batelaan N, Scholten W, Rhebergen D, Van Balkom A. Why we need to evaluate long-term antidepressant use in older patients with depression. Age Ageing. 2021;50(3):690–2.
301. Rhee TG, Olfson M, Nierenberg AA, Wilkinson ST. 20-year trends in the pharmacologic treatment of bipolar disorder by psychiatrists in outpatient care settings. Am J Psychiatry. 2020;177(8):706–15.

302. McGirr A, Vohringer PA, Ghaemi SN, Lam RW, Yatham LN. Safety and efficacy of adjunctive second-generation antidepressant therapy with a mood stabiliser or an atypical antipsychotic in acute bipolar depression: a systematic review and meta-analysis of randomised placebo-controlled trials. Lancet Psychiatry. 2016;3(12):1138–46.
303. Sachs GS, Nierenberg AA, Calabrese JR, Marangell LB, Wisniewski SR, Gyulai L, et al. Effectiveness of adjunctive antidepressant treatment for bipolar depression. N Engl J Med. 2007;356(17):1711–22.
304. Sidor MM, Macqueen GM. Antidepressants for the acute treatment of bipolar depression: a systematic review and meta-analysis. J Clin Psychiatry. 2011;72(2):156–67.
305. Ghaemi SN, Whitham EA, Vohringer PA, Barroilhet SA, Amerio A, Sverdlov O, et al. Citalopram for acute and preventive efficacy in bipolar depression (CAPE-BD): a randomized, double-blind, placebo-controlled trial. J Clin Psychiatry. 2021;82(1):19m13136.
306. Goldberg JF, Perlis RH, Ghaemi SN, Calabrese JR, Bowden CL, Wisniewski S, et al. Adjunctive antidepressant use and symptomatic recovery among bipolar depressed patients with concomitant manic symptoms: findings from the STEP-BD. Am J Psychiatry. 2007;164(9):1348–55.
307. Carvalho AF, Sharma MS, Brunoni AR, Vieta E, Fava GA. The safety, tolerability and risks associated with the use of newer generation antidepressant drugs: a critical review of the literature. Psychother Psychosom. 2016;85(5):270–88.
308. Hu XH, Bull SA, Hunkeler EM, Ming E, Lee JY, Fireman B, et al. Incidence and duration of side effects and those rated as bothersome with selective serotonin reuptake inhibitor treatment for depression: patient report versus physician estimate. J Clin Psychiatry. 2004;65(7):959–65.
309. Brambilla P, Cipriani A, Hotopf M, Barbui C. Side-effect profile of fluoxetine in comparison with other SSRIs, tricyclic and newer antidepressants: a meta-analysis of clinical trial data. Pharmacopsychiatry. 2005;38(2):69–77.
310. Trindade E, Menon D, Topfer LA, Coloma C. Adverse effects associated with selective serotonin reuptake inhibitors and tricyclic antidepressants: a meta-analysis. CMAJ. 1998;159(10):1245–52.
311. Coupland C, Hill T, Morriss R, Moore M, Arthur A, Hippisley-Cox J. Antidepressant use and risk of adverse outcomes in people aged 20–64

years: cohort study using a primary care database. BMC Med. 2018;16(1):36.

312. Joo JH, Lenze EJ, Mulsant BH, Begley AE, Weber EM, Stack JA, et al. Risk factors for falls during treatment of late-life depression. J Clin Psychiatry. 2002;63(10):936–41.
313. Beach SR, Kostis WJ, Celano CM, Januzzi JL, Ruskin JN, Noseworthy PA, et al. Meta-analysis of selective serotonin reuptake inhibitor-associated QTc prolongation. J Clin Psychiatry. 2014;75(5):e441–9.
314. Castro VM, Clements CC, Murphy SN, Gainer VS, Fava M, Weilburg JB, et al. QT interval and antidepressant use: a cross sectional study of electronic health records. BMJ. 2013;346:f288.
315. Weeke P, Jensen A, Folke F, Gislason GH, Olesen JB, Andersson C, et al. Antidepressant use and risk of out-of-hospital cardiac arrest: a nationwide case-time-control study. Clin Pharmacol Ther. 2012;92(1):72–9.
316. Hackam DG, Mrkobrada M. Selective serotonin reuptake inhibitors and brain hemorrhage: a meta-analysis. Neurology. 2012;79(18):1862–5.
317. Voican CS, Corruble E, Naveau S, Perlemuter G. Antidepressant-induced liver injury: a review for clinicians. Am J Psychiatry. 2014;171(4):404–15.
318. Anderson KN, Lind JN, Simeone RM, Bobo WV, Mitchell AA, Riehle-Colarusso T, et al. Maternal use of specific antidepressant medications during early pregnancy and the risk of selected birth defects. JAMA Psychiatry. 2020;77(12):1246–55.
319. De Vries C, Gadzhanova S, Sykes MJ, Ward M, Roughead E. A systematic review and meta-analysis considering the risk for congenital heart defects of antidepressant classes and individual antidepressants. Drug Saf. 2021;44(3):291–312.
320. Reefhuis J, Devine O, Friedman JM, Louik C, Honein MA. National birth defects prevention S. specific SSRIs and birth defects: Bayesian analysis to interpret new data in the context of previous reports. BMJ. 2015;351:h3190.
321. Hammad TA, Laughren T, Racoosin J. Suicidality in pediatric patients treated with antidepressant drugs. Arch Gen Psychiatry. 2006; 63(3):332–9.
322. Le Noury J, Nardo JM, Healy D, Jureidini J, Raven M, Tufanaru C, et al. Restoring Study 329: efficacy and harms of paroxetine and imipramine in treatment of major depression in adolescence. BMJ. 2015;351:h4320.

323. Sharma T, Guski LS, Freund N, Gotzsche PC. Suicidality and aggression during antidepressant treatment: systematic review and meta-analyses based on clinical study reports. BMJ. 2016;352:i65.
324. Stone M, Laughren T, Jones ML, Levenson M, Holland PC, Hughes A, et al. Risk of suicidality in clinical trials of antidepressants in adults: analysis of proprietary data submitted to US Food and Drug Administration. BMJ. 2009;339:b2880.
325. Healy D. Emergence of antidepressant induced suicidality. Primary Care Psychiatry. 2000;6(1):23–8.
326. Rothschild AJ, Locke CA. Reexposure to fluoxetine after serious suicide attempts by three patients: the role of akathisia. J Clin Psychiatry. 1991;52(12):491–3.
327. Gunnell D, Saperia J, Ashby D. Selective serotonin reuptake inhibitors (SSRIs) and suicide in adults: meta-analysis of drug company data from placebo controlled, randomised controlled trials submitted to the MHRA's safety review. BMJ. 2005;330(7488):385.
328. Aursnes I, Tvete IF, Gaasemyr J, Natvig B. Even more suicide attempts in clinical trials with paroxetine randomised against placebo. BMC Psychiatry. 2006;6:55.
329. Baldessarini RJ, Lau WK, Sim J, Sum MY, Sim K. Suicidal risks in reports of long-term controlled trials of antidepressants for major depressive disorder II. Int J Neuropsychopharmacol. 2017;20(3):281–4.
330. Fergusson D, Doucette S, Glass KC, Shapiro S, Healy D, Hebert P, et al. Association between suicide attempts and selective serotonin reuptake inhibitors: systematic review of randomised controlled trials. BMJ. 2005;330(7488):396.
331. Healy D, Whitaker C. Antidepressants and suicide: risk-benefit conundrums. J Psychiatry Neurosci. 2003;28(5):331–7.
332. Hengartner MP, Ploderl M. Newer-generation antidepressants and suicide risk in randomized controlled trials: a re-analysis of the FDA database. Psychother Psychosom. 2019;88(4):247–8.
333. Ploderl M, Hengartner MP, Bschor T, Kaminski JA. Commentary to "antidepressants and suicidality: a re-analysis of the re-analysis". J Affect Disord. 2020;273:252–3.
334. Healy D. Antidepressants and sexual dysfunction: a history. J R Soc Med. 2020;113(4):133–5.

335. Zimmerman M, Galione JN, Attiullah N, Friedman M, Toba C, Boerescu DA, et al. Underrecognition of clinically significant side effects in depressed outpatients. J Clin Psychiatry. 2010;71(4):484–90.
336. Serretti A, Chiesa A. Treatment-emergent sexual dysfunction related to antidepressants: a meta-analysis. J Clin Psychopharmacol. 2009;29(3):259–66.
337. Healy D. Post-SSRI sexual dysfunction & other enduring sexual dysfunctions. Epidemiol Psychiatr Sci. 2019;29:e55.
338. Reisman Y. Post-SSRI sexual dysfunction. BMJ. 2020;368:m754.
339. Papakostas GI. Limitations of contemporary antidepressants: tolerability. J Clin Psychiatry. 2007;68 Suppl 10:11–7.
340. Serretti A, Mandelli L. Antidepressants and body weight: a comprehensive review and meta-analysis. J Clin Psychiatry. 2010;71(10):1259–72.
341. Blier P, Tremblay P. Physiologic mechanisms underlying the antidepressant discontinuation syndrome. J Clin Psychiatry. 2006;67 Suppl 4:8–13.
342. Haahr ME, Fisher PM, Jensen CG, Frokjaer VG, Mahon BM, Madsen K, et al. Central 5-HT4 receptor binding as biomarker of serotonergic tonus in humans: a [11C]SB207145 PET study. Mol Psychiatry. 2014;19(4):427–32.
343. Hyman SE, Nestler EJ. Initiation and adaptation: a paradigm for understanding psychotropic drug action. Am J Psychiatry. 1996;153(2):151–62.
344. Lerner A, Klein M. Dependence, withdrawal and rebound of CNS drugs: an update and regulatory considerations for new drugs development. Brain Communications. 2019;1(1):fcz025.
345. Davies J, Read J. A systematic review into the incidence, severity and duration of antidepressant withdrawal effects: are guidelines evidence-based? Addict Behav. 2019;97:111–21.
346. Dilsaver SC, Greden JF, Snider RM. Antidepressant withdrawal syndromes: phenomenology and pathophysiology. Int Clin Psychopharmacol. 1987;2(1):1–19.
347. Fava GA, Gatti A, Belaise C, Guidi J, Offidani E. Withdrawal symptoms after selective serotonin reuptake inhibitor discontinuation: a systematic review. Psychother Psychosom. 2015;84(2):72–81.
348. Fava GA, Benasi G, Lucente M, Offidani E, Cosci F, Guidi J. Withdrawal symptoms after serotonin-noradrenaline reuptake inhibitor discontinuation: systematic review. Psychother Psychosom. 2018;87(4):195–203.
349. Haddad PM. Antidepressant discontinuation syndromes. Drug Saf. 2001;24(3):183–97.

350. Davies J, Read J, Hengartner MP, Cosci F, Fava G, Chouinard G, et al. Clinical guidelines on antidepressant withdrawal urgently need updating. BMJ. 2019;365:l2238.
351. Fava GA, Cosci F. Understanding and managing withdrawal syndromes after discontinuation of antidepressant drugs. J Clin Psychiatry. 2019;80(6):19com12794.
352. Haddad PM, Anderson IM. Recognising and managing antidepressant discontinuation symptoms. Adv Psychiatr Treat. 2007;13(6):447–57.
353. Bloch M, Stager SV, Braun AR, Rubinow DR. Severe psychiatric symptoms associated with paroxetine withdrawal. Lancet. 1995;346(8966):57.
354. Hengartner MP, Schulthess L, Sorensen A, Framer A. Protracted withdrawal syndrome after stopping antidepressants: a descriptive quantitative analysis of consumer narratives from a large internet forum. Ther Adv Psychopharmacol. 2020;10:2045125320980573.
355. Stone TE, Swanson C, Feldman MD. Venlafaxine discontinuation syndrome and suicidal ideation: a case series. J Clin Psychopharmacol. 2007;27(1):94–5.
356. Tint A, Haddad PM, Anderson IM. The effect of rate of antidepressant tapering on the incidence of discontinuation symptoms: a randomised study. J Psychopharmacol. 2008;22(3):330–2.
357. Hengartner MP, Davies J, Read J. Antidepressant withdrawal—the tide is finally turning. Epidemiol Psychiatr Sci. 2019;29:e52.
358. Massabki I, Abi-Jaoude E. Selective serotonin reuptake inhibitor 'discontinuation syndrome' or withdrawal. Br J Psychiatry. 2021;218(3):168–71.
359. Iacobucci G. NICE updates antidepressant guidelines to reflect severity and length of withdrawal symptoms. BMJ. 2019;367:l6103.
360. Hawkes N. Royal College of Psychiatrists adds voice to concerns over NICE guidance on depression. BMJ. 2019;365:l2399.
361. Linde K, Kriston L, Rucker G, Jamil S, Schumann I, Meissner K, et al. Efficacy and acceptability of pharmacological treatments for depressive disorders in primary care: systematic review and network meta-analysis. Ann Fam Med. 2015;13(1):69–79.
362. Bola J, Kao D, Soydan H. Antipsychotic medication for early episode schizophrenia. Cochrane Database Syst Rev. 2011(6):CD006374.
363. Kahn RS, Fleischhacker WW, Boter H, Davidson M, Vergouwe Y, Keet IP, et al. Effectiveness of antipsychotic drugs in first-episode schizophrenia and schizophreniform disorder: an open randomised clinical trial. Lancet. 2008;371(9618):1085–97.

364. Lieberman JA, Stroup TS, McEvoy JP, Swartz MS, Rosenheck RA, Perkins DO, et al. Effectiveness of antipsychotic drugs in patients with chronic schizophrenia. N Engl J Med. 2005;353(12):1209–23.
365. Harris MG, Kazdin AE, Chiu WT, Sampson NA, Aguilar-Gaxiola S, Al-Hamzawi A, et al. Findings from world mental health surveys of the perceived helpfulness of treatment for patients with major depressive disorder. JAMA Psychiatry. 2020;77(8):830–41.
366. Hughes S, Lacasse J, Fuller RR, Spaulding-Givens J. Adverse effects and treatment satisfaction among online users of four antidepressants. Psychiatry Res. 2017;255:78–86.
367. Schalkwijk S, Undurraga J, Tondo L, Baldessarini RJ. Declining efficacy in controlled trials of antidepressants: effects of placebo dropout. Int J Neuropsychopharmacol. 2014;17(8):1343–52.
368. Kampermann L, Nestoriuc Y, Shedden-Mora MC. Physicians' beliefs about placebo and nocebo effects in antidepressants—an online survey among German practitioners. PLoS One. 2017;12(5):e0178719.
369. Read J, Renton J, Harrop C, Geekie J, Dowrick C. A survey of UK general practitioners about depression, antidepressants and withdrawal: implementing the 2019 Public Health England report. Ther Adv Psychopharmacol. 2020;10:1–14.
370. Vijapura S, Laferton JA, Mintz D, Kaptchuk TJ, Wolfe D. Psychiatrists' attitudes toward non-pharmacologic factors within the context of antidepressant pharmacotherapy. Acad Psychiatry. 2016;40(5):783–9.
371. Parker G. The benefits of antidepressants: news or fake news? Br J Psychiatry. 2018;213(2):454–5.
372. Mendel R, Hamann J, Traut-Mattausch E, Buhner M, Kissling W, Frey D. 'What would you do if you were me, doctor?': randomised trial of psychiatrists' personal v. professional perspectives on treatment recommendations. Br J Psychiatry. 2010;197(6):441–7.
373. Alberts B, Kirschner MW, Tilghman S, Varmus H. Rescuing US biomedical research from its systemic flaws. Proc Natl Acad Sci U S A. 2014;111(16):5773–7.
374. Brownlee S, Chalkidou K, Doust J, Elshaug AG, Glasziou P, Heath I, et al. Evidence for overuse of medical services around the world. Lancet. 2017;390(10090):156–68.
375. Conrad P. The shifting engines of medicalization. J Health Soc Behav. 2005;46(1):3–14.

376. Gøtzsche PC. Deadly medicines and organised crime: how big pharma has corrupted healthcare. London: Radcliffe Publishing; 2013.
377. Ioannidis JP. Evidence-based medicine has been hijacked: a report to David Sackett. J Clin Epidemiol. 2016;73:82–6.
378. Jefferson T. Sponsorship bias in clinical trials: growing menace or dawning realisation? J R Soc Med. 2020;113(4):148–57.
379. Kassirer JP. On the take: how medicine's complicity with big business can endanger your health. Oxford: Oxford University Press; 2005.
380. Moynihan R, Bero L, Hill S, Johansson M, Lexchin J, Macdonald H, et al. Pathways to independence: towards producing and using trustworthy evidence. BMJ. 2019;367:l6576.
381. Mulinari S. Unhealthy marketing of pharmaceutical products: an international public health concern. J Public Health Policy. 2016;37(2):149–59.
382. O'Mahony S. Can medicine be cured? The corruption of a profession. London: Head of Zeus; 2019.
383. Stegenga J. Medical nihilism. Oxford, UK: Oxford University Press; 2018.
384. Abraham J. Pharmaceuticalization of society in context: theoretical, empirical and health dimensions. Sociology. 2010;44(4):603–22.
385. Moynihan R, Heath I, Henry D. Selling sickness: the pharmaceutical industry and disease mongering. BMJ. 2002;324(7342):886–91.
386. Brodersen J, Schwartz LM, Heneghan C, O'Sullivan JW, Aronson JK, Woloshin S. Overdiagnosis: what it is and what it isn't. BMJ Evid Based Med. 2018;23(1):1–3.
387. Morgan DJ, Brownlee S, Leppin AL, Kressin N, Dhruva SS, Levin L, et al. Setting a research agenda for medical overuse. BMJ. 2015;351:h4534.
388. Ledley FD, McCoy SS, Vaughan G, Cleary EG. Profitability of large pharmaceutical companies compared with other large public companies. JAMA. 2020;323(9):834–43.
389. Berwick DM, Hackbarth AD. Eliminating waste in US health care. JAMA. 2012;307(14):1513–6.
390. Bracken P, Thomas P, Timimi S, Asen E, Behr G, Beuster C, et al. Psychiatry beyond the current paradigm. Br J Psychiatry. 2012;201(6):430–4.
391. Cohen CI. The biomedicalization of psychiatry: a critical overview. Community Ment Health J. 1993;29(6):509–21.
392. Gardner C, Kleinman A. Medicine and the mind—the consequences of psychiatry's identity crisis. N Engl J Med. 2019;381(18):1697–9.

393. Harrington A. Mind fixers: psychiatry's troubled search for the biology of mental illness. New York: W.W. Norton & Company; 2019.
394. Scull A. A psychiatric revolution. Lancet. 2010;375(9722):1246–7.
395. Borsboom D, Cramer A, Kalis A. Brain disorders? Not really… Why network structures block reductionism in psychopathology research. Behav Brain Sci. 2018;42:1–54.
396. Miller GA. Mistreating psychology in the decades of the brain. Perspect Psychol Sci. 2010;5(6):716–43.
397. World Federation for Mental Health. Depression: a global crisis. Geneva: World Health Organization; 2012.
398. Parker G. Classifying depression: should paradigms lost be regained? Am J Psychiatry. 2000;157(8):1195–203.
399. Whitaker R. Anatomy of an epidemic. New York, NY: Crown Publishers; 2010.
400. Leyburn P. A critical look at antidepressant drug trials. Lancet. 1967;2(7526):1135–8.
401. Kline NS. The practical management of depression. JAMA. 1964;190:732–40.
402. Ayd FJ. Amitriptyline (Elavil) therapy for depressive reactions. Psychosomatics. 1960;1(6):320–5.
403. Stehr N. Biotechnology: between commerce and civil society. New Brunswick, NJ: Transaction Publishers; 2004.
404. Gerber L, Gaudilliere JP. Marketing masked depression: physicians, pharmaceutical firms, and the redefinition of mood disorders in the 1960s and 1970s. B Hist Med. 2016;90(3):455–90.
405. Moynihan R. Key opinion leaders: independent experts or drug representatives in disguise? BMJ. 2008;336(7658):1402–3.
406. Sismondo S. How to make opinion leaders and influence people. CMAJ. 2015. 187(10):759–60.
407. Sartorius N. Description and classification of depressive disorders. Contributions for the definition of the therapy-resistance and of therapy resistant depressions. Pharmakopsychiatr Neuropsychopharmakol. 1974;7(2):76–9.
408. American Psychiatric Association. Diagnostic and statistical manual of mental disorders DSM-III. 3rd ed. Washington, DC: American Psychiatric Association; 1980.

409. Davies J. How voting and consensus created the diagnostic and statistical manual of mental disorders (DSM-III). Anthropol Med. 2017;24(1):32–46.
410. Mulder RT. An epidemic of depression or the medicalization of distress? Perspect Biol Med. 2008;51(2):238–50.
411. Nesse RM, Stein DJ. Towards a genuinely medical model for psychiatric nosology. BMC Med. 2012;10:5.
412. Wakefield JC. Disorder as harmful dysfunction: a conceptual critique of DSM-III-R's definition of mental disorder. Psychol Rev. 1992;99(2):232–47.
413. Watson D, Clark LA. Clinical diagnosis at the crossroads. Clin Psychol-Sci Pr. 2006;13(3):210–5.
414. Frances A. Saving normal. New York, NY: Harper Collins; 2013.
415. Lane C. Shyness: how normal behavior became a sickness. New Haven: Yale University Press; 2007.
416. Wakefield JC, Horwitz AV, Schmitz MF. Are we overpathologizing the socially anxious? Social phobia from a harmful dysfunction perspective. Can J Psychiatry. 2005;50(6):317–9.
417. Scott S. The medicalisation of shyness: from social misfits to social fitness. Sociol Health Illn. 2006;28(2):133–53.
418. Gornall J. DSM-5: a fatal diagnosis? BMJ. 2013;346:f3256.
419. Insel T. National Institute of Mental Health. 2013. Available from: https://www.nimh.nih.gov/about/directors/thomas-insel/blog/2013/transforming-diagnosis.shtml.
420. Chmielewski M, Clark LA, Bagby RM, Watson D. Method matters: understanding diagnostic reliability in DSM-IV and DSM-5. J Abnorm Psychol. 2015;124(3):764–9.
421. Regier DA, Narrow WE, Clarke DE, Kraemer HC, Kuramoto SJ, Kuhl EA, et al. DSM-5 field trials in the United States and Canada, Part II: test-retest reliability of selected categorical diagnoses. Am J Psychiatry. 2013;170(1):59–70.
422. Lieblich SM, Castle DJ, Pantelis C, Hopwood M, Hunter Young A, Everall IP. High heterogeneity and low reliability in the diagnosis of major depression will impair the development of new drugs. BJPsych Open. 2015;1(2):e5–7.
423. Lader M. History of benzodiazepine dependence. J Subst Abuse Treat. 1991;8(1–2):53–9.

424. Regier DA, Hirschfeld RM, Goodwin FK, Burke JD, Jr., Lazar JB, Judd LL. The NIMH depression awareness, recognition, and treatment program: structure, aims, and scientific basis. Am J Psychiatry. 1988;145(11):1351–7.
425. Paykel ES, Tylee A, Wright A, Priest RG, Rix S, Hart D. The defeat depression campaign: psychiatry in the public arena. Am J Psychiatry. 1997;154(6 Suppl):59–65.
426. Moncrieff J, Hopker S, Thomas P. Psychiatry and the pharmaceutical industry: who pays the piper? Psychiatric Bulletin. 2005;29(3):84–5.
427. Conrad P, Leiter V. Medicalization, markets and consumers. J Health Soc Behav. 2004;45 Suppl:158–76.
428. Goldacre B. Bad pharma: how drug companies mislead doctors and harm patients. New York: Faber and Faber, Inc; 2013.
429. Koerner BI. Disorders, made to order. Mother Jones. 2002;27:58–63.
430. Moynihan R, Henry D. The fight against disease mongering: generating knowledge for action. PLoS Med. 2006;3(4):e191.
431. Parry V. The art of branding a condition. Medical Marketing and Media. 2003;38(5):43–9.
432. Wolinsky H. Disease mongering and drug marketing. Does the pharmaceutical industry manufacture diseases as well as drugs? EMBO Rep. 2005;6(7):612–4.
433. Schwartz LM, Woloshin S. Medical marketing in the United States, 1997–2016. JAMA. 2019;321(1):80–96.
434. Parker G. Is depression overdiagnosed? Yes. BMJ. 2007;335(7615):328.
435. Kroenke K, Spitzer RL, Williams JB. The PHQ-9: validity of a brief depression severity measure. J Gen Intern Med. 2001;16(9):606–13.
436. Thombs BD, Kwakkenbos L, Levis AW, Benedetti A. Addressing overestimation of the prevalence of depression based on self-report screening questionnaires. CMAJ. 2018;190(2):E44–9.
437. Levis B, Benedetti A, Ioannidis JPA, Sun Y, Negeri Z, He C, et al. Patient Health Questionnaire-9 scores do not accurately estimate depression prevalence: individual participant data meta-analysis. J Clin Epidemiol. 2020;122:115–28 e1.
438. Zimmerman M. Symptom severity and guideline-based treatment recommendations for depressed patients: implications of DSM-5's potential recommendation of the PHQ-9 as the measure of choice for depression severity. Psychother Psychosom. 2012;81(6):329–32.

439. Trautmann S, Beesdo-Baum K, Knappe S, Einsle F, Knothe L, Wieder G, et al. The treatment of depression in primary care: a cross-sectional epidemiological study. Dtsch Arztebl Int. 2017;114(43):721–8.
440. Mitchell AJ, Yadegarfar M, Gill J, Stubbs B. Case finding and screening clinical utility of the Patient Health Questionnaire (PHQ-9 and PHQ-2) for depression in primary care: a diagnostic meta-analysis of 40 studies. BJPsych Open. 2016;2(2):127–38.
441. Gilbody S, Sheldon T, House A. Screening and case-finding instruments for depression: a meta-analysis. CMAJ. 2008;178(8):997–1003.
442. Thombs BD, Ziegelstein RC. Does depression screening improve depression outcomes in primary care? BMJ. 2014;348:g1253.
443. Cosgrove L, Karter JM, Vaswani A, Thombs BD. Unexamined assumptions and unintended consequences of routine screening for depression. J Psychosom Res. 2018;109:9–11.
444. Thombs BD, Ziegelstein RC. Primary care doctors should not screen their patients for depression. Expert Rev Neurother. 2017;17(7):645–7.
445. Ferenchick EK, Ramanuj P, Pincus HA. Depression in primary care: part 1-screening and diagnosis. BMJ. 2019;365:l794.
446. Reynolds CFR, Patel V. Screening for depression: the global mental health context. World Psychiatry. 2017;16(3):316–7.
447. Bell G. The worried well: the depression epidemic and the medicalisation of our sorrows. Quartely Essay. 2005;18:1–74.
448. Raven M. Depression and antidepressants in Australia and beyond: a critical public health analysis. Wollongong: University of Wollongong; 2012.
449. Summerfield D. Depression: epidemic or pseudo-epidemic? J R Soc Med. 2006;99(3):161–2.
450. Mitchell AJ, Vaze A, Rao S. Clinical diagnosis of depression in primary care: a meta-analysis. Lancet. 2009;374(9690):609–19.
451. Tyrer P. Are general practitioners really unable to diagnose depression? Lancet. 2009;374(9690):589–90.
452. Macdonald S, Morrison J, Maxwell M, Munoz-Arroyo R, Power A, Smith M, et al. 'A coal face option': GPs' perspectives on the rise in antidepressant prescribing. Brit J Gen Pract. 2009;59(566):658–9.
453. Summerfield D. NHS antidepressant prescribing: what do we get for pound266m a year? BMJ. 2018;360:k1019.
454. Davies J. Sedated: how modern capitalism created our mental health crisis. London, UK: Atlantic Books; 2021.

455. Jureidini J, Tonkin A. Overuse of antidepressant drugs for the treatment of depression. CNS Drugs. 2006;20(8):623–32.
456. Davies J. Cracked: why psychiatry is doing more harm than good. London: Icon Books; 2013.
457. Rosenthal MB, Berndt ER, Donohue JM, Frank RG, Epstein AM. Promotion of prescription drugs to consumers. New Engl J Med. 2002;346(7):498–505.
458. Angell M. The truth about the drug companies: how they deceive us and what to do about it. New York: Random House; 2004.
459. Healy D. Pharmageddon. Berkeley, CA: University of California Press; 2012.
460. Fauber J, Fiore K, Wynn M. For one condition, the drugs came before the disorder. Milwaukee Journal Sentinel. 2017.
461. Monroe SM, Harkness KL. Recurrence in major depression: a conceptual analysis. Psychol Rev. 2011;118(4):655–74.
462. Hollon SD, Thase ME, Markowitz JC. Treatment and prevention of depression. Psychol Sci. 2002:39–77.
463. Steffen A, Holstiege J, Akmatov MK, Bätzing J. Zeitliche trends in der Diagnoseprävalenz depressiver Störungen: Eine analyse auf basis bundesweiter vertragsärztlicher Abrechnungsdaten der Jahre 2009 bis 2017. Berlin: Zentralinstitut für die kassenärztliche Versorgung in Deutschland; 2019.
464. Berardi D, Leggieri G, Ceroni GB, Rucci P, Pezzoli A, Paltrinieri E, et al. Depression in primary care. A nationwide epidemiological survey. Fam Pract. 2002;19(4):397–400.
465. Coupland C, Dhiman P, Morriss R, Arthur A, Barton G, Hippisley-Cox J. Antidepressant use and risk of adverse outcomes in older people: population based cohort study. BMJ. 2011;343:d4551.
466. Baer N, Schuler D, Füglister-Dousse S, Moreau-Gruet F. Depressionen in der Schweiz. Daten zur Epidemiologie, Behandlung und sozialberuflichen Integration (Obsan Bericht 56). Neuchatel: Schweizerisches Gesundheitsobservatorium; 2013.
467. Kessler RC, Birnbaum HG, Shahly V, Bromet E, Hwang I, McLaughlin KA, et al. Age differences in the prevalence and co-morbidity of DSM-IV major depressive episodes: results from the WHO World Mental Health Survey Initiative. Depress Anxiety. 2010;27(4):351–64.
468. Kessler RC, Chiu WT, Demler O, Merikangas KR, Walters EE. Prevalence, severity, and comorbidity of 12-month DSM-IV disorders in the

National Comorbidity Survey Replication. Arch Gen Psychiatry. 2005;62(6):617–27.
469. Eaton WW, Shao H, Nestadt G, Lee HB, Bienvenu OJ, Zandi P. Population-based study of first onset and chronicity in major depressive disorder. Arch Gen Psychiatry. 2008;65(5):513–20.
470. Mattisson C, Bogren M, Horstmann V, Munk-Jorgensen P, Nettelbladt P. The long-term course of depressive disorders in the Lundby Study. Psychol Med. 2007;37(6):883–91.
471. Steinert C, Hofmann M, Kruse J, Leichsenring F. The prospective long-term course of adult depression in general practice and the community. A systematic literature review. J Affect Disord. 2014:65–75.
472. Gunn J, Elliott P, Densley K, Middleton A, Ambresin G, Dowrick C, et al. A trajectory-based approach to understand the factors associated with persistent depressive symptoms in primary care. J Affect Disord. 2013;148(2–3):338–46.
473. Jackson JL, Passamonti M, Kroenke K. Outcome and impact of mental disorders in primary care at 5 years. Psychosom Med. 2007;69(3):270–6.
474. Walters K, Buszewicz M, Weich S, King M. Mixed anxiety and depressive disorder outcomes: prospective cohort study in primary care. Br J Psychiatry. 2011;198(6):472–8.
475. Bijl RV, de Graaf R, Hiripi E, Kessler RC, Kohn R, Offord DR, et al. The prevalence of treated and untreated mental disorders in five countries. Health Aff (Millwood). 2003;22(3):122–33.
476. Kessler RC, Berglund P, Demler O, Jin R, Koretz D, Merikangas KR, et al. The epidemiology of major depressive disorder: results from the National Comorbidity Survey Replication (NCS-R). JAMA. 2003;289(23):3095–105.
477. Olfson M, Wang S, Wall M, Marcus SC, Blanco C. Trends in serious psychological distress and outpatient mental health care of US adults. JAMA Psychiatry. 2019;76(2):152–61.
478. Forsell Y. A three-year follow-up of major depression, dysthymia, minor depression and subsyndromal depression: results from a population-based study. Depress Anxiety. 2007;24(1):62–5.
479. Hermens ML, van Hout HP, Terluin B, van der Windt DA, Beekman AT, van Dyck R, et al. The prognosis of minor depression in the general population: a systematic review. Gen Hosp Psychiatry. 2004;26(6):453–62.

480. Mojtabai R. Bereavement-related depressive episodes: characteristics, 3-year course, and implications for the DSM-5. Arch Gen Psychiatry. 2011;68(9):920–8.
481. Wakefield JC, Schmitz MF. When does depression become a disorder? Using recurrence rates to evaluate the validity of proposed changes in major depression diagnostic thresholds. World Psychiatry. 2013;12(1):44–52.
482. Wakefield JC, Schmitz MF. Predictive validation of single-episode uncomplicated depression as a benign subtype of unipolar major depression. Acta Psychiatr Scand. 2014;129(6):445–57.
483. Hughes S, Cohen D. A systematic review of long-term studies of drug treated and non-drug treated depression. J Affect Disord. 2009;118(1–3):9–18.
484. Goldberg D, Privett M, Ustun B, Simon G, Linden M. The effects of detection and treatment on the outcome of major depression in primary care: a naturalistic study in 15 cities. Br J Gen Pract. 1998;48(437):1840–4.
485. World Health Organization. Depression and other common mental disorders: global health estimates. Geneva: World Health Organisation; 2017.
486. GBD 2017 Disease and Injury Incidence and Prevalence Collaborators. Global, regional, and national incidence, prevalence, and years lived with disability for 354 diseases and injuries for 195 countries and territories, 1990–2017: a systematic analysis for the Global Burden of Disease Study 2017. Lancet. 2018;392(10159):1789–858.
487. Brhlikova P, Pollock AM, Manners R. Global Burden of Disease estimates of depression—how reliable is the epidemiological evidence? J R Soc Med. 2011;104(1):25–34.
488. Nordgaard J, Sass LA, Parnas J. The psychiatric interview: validity, structure, and subjectivity. Eur Arch Psychiatry Clin Neurosci. 2013;263(4):353–64.
489. Regier DA, Kaelber CT, Rae DS, Farmer ME, Knauper B, Kessler RC, et al. Limitations of diagnostic criteria and assessment instruments for mental disorders. Implications for research and policy. Arch Gen Psychiatry. 1998;55(2):109–15.
490. Salomon JA, Haagsma JA, Davis A, de Noordhout CM, Polinder S, Havelaar AH, et al. Disability weights for the Global Burden of Disease 2013 study. Lancet Glob Health. 2015;3(11):e712–23.
491. Vilhelmsson A. The devil in the details: public health and depression. Front Public Health. 2014;2:192.

492. Guze SB, Robins E. Suicide and primary affective disorders. Br J Psychiatry. 1970;117(539):437–8.
493. Border R, Johnson EC, Evans LM, Smolen A, Berley N, Sullivan PF, et al. No support for historical candidate gene or candidate gene-by-interaction hypotheses for major depression across multiple large samples. Am J Psychiatry. 2019;176(5):376–87.
494. Klein RA, Vianello M, Hasselman F, Adams BG, Adams RB, Jr., Alper S, et al. Many labs 2: investigating variation in replicability across samples and settings. Adv Meth Pract Psychol Sci. 2018;1(4):443–90.
495. Pereira TV, Horwitz RI, Ioannidis JP. Empirical evaluation of very large treatment effects of medical interventions. JAMA. 2012;308(16):1676–84.
496. Tajika A, Ogawa Y, Takeshima N, Hayasaka Y, Furukawa TA. Replication and contradiction of highly cited research papers in psychiatry: 10-year follow-up. Br J Psychiatry. 2015;207(4):357–62.
497. Blair-West GW, Mellsop GW, Eyeson-Annan ML. Down-rating lifetime suicide risk in major depression. Acta Psychiatr Scand. 1997;95(3):259–63.
498. Blair-West GW, Mellsop GW. Major depression: does a gender-based down-rating of suicide risk challenge its diagnostic validity? Aust N Z J Psychiatry. 2001;35(3):322–8.
499. Bostwick JM, Pankratz VS. Affective disorders and suicide risk: a reexamination. Am J Psychiatry. 2000;157(12):1925–32.
500. Inskip HM, Harris EC, Barraclough B. Lifetime risk of suicide for affective disorder, alcoholism and schizophrenia. Br J Psychiatry. 1998;172:35–7.
501. Chesney E, Goodwin GM, Fazel S. Risks of all-cause and suicide mortality in mental disorders: a meta-review. World Psychiatry. 2014;13(2):153–60.
502. Andreasen NC. The broken brain: the biological revolution in psychiatry. New York: Harper & Row; 1984.
503. Friedman RA. Psychiatry's identity crisis. The New York Times. July 17, 2015.
504. Harland R, Antonova E, Owen GS, Broome M, Landau S, Deeley Q, et al. A study of psychiatrists' concepts of mental illness. Psychol Med. 2009;39(6):967–76.
505. Sedler MJ. Medicalization in psychiatry: the medical model, descriptive diagnosis, and lost knowledge. Med Health Care Phil. 2016;19(2):247–52.

506. Dumas-Mallet E, Gonon F. Messaging in biological psychiatry: misrepresentations, their causes, and potential consequences. Harv Rev Psychiatry. 2020;28(6):395–403.
507. Leucht S, Leucht C, Huhn M, Chaimani A, Mavridis D, Helfer B, et al. Sixty years of placebo-controlled antipsychotic drug trials in acute schizophrenia: systematic review, Bayesian meta-analysis, and meta-regression of efficacy predictors. Am J Psychiatry. 2017;174(10):927–42.
508. Samara MT, Nikolakopoulou A, Salanti G, Leucht S. How many patients with schizophrenia do not respond to antipsychotic drugs in the short term? An analysis based on individual patient data from randomized controlled trials. Schizophrenia Bull. 2019;45(3):639–46.
509. van Os J, Kohne ACJ. It is not enough to sing its praises: the very foundations of precision psychiatry may be scientifically unsound and require examination. Psychol Med. 2021;51(9):1415–7.
510. Bastiaansen JA, Servaas MN, Marsman JB, Ormel J, Nolte IM, Riese H, et al. Filling the gap: relationship between the serotonin-transporter-linked polymorphic region and amygdala activation. Psychol Sci. 2014;25(11):2058–66.
511. Botvinik-Nezer R, Holzmeister F, Camerer CF, Dreber A, Huber J, Johannesson M, et al. Variability in the analysis of a single neuroimaging dataset by many teams. Nature. 2020;582(7810):84–8.
512. Culverhouse RC, Saccone NL, Horton AC, Ma Y, Anstey KJ, Banaschewski T, et al. Collaborative meta-analysis finds no evidence of a strong interaction between stress and 5-HTTLPR genotype contributing to the development of depression. Mol Psychiatry. 2018;23(1):133–42.
513. Dumas-Mallet E, Button K, Boraud T, Munafo M, Gonon F. Replication validity of initial association studies: a comparison between psychiatry, neurology and four somatic diseases. PLoS One. 2016;11(6):e0158064.
514. Eklund A, Nichols TE, Knutsson H. Cluster failure: why fMRI inferences for spatial extent have inflated false-positive rates. Proc Natl Acad Sci U S A. 2016;113(28):7900–5.
515. Ioannidis JP. Excess significance bias in the literature on brain volume abnormalities. Arch Gen Psychiatry. 2011;68(8):773–80.
516. Muller VI, Cieslik EC, Serbanescu I, Laird AR, Fox PT, Eickhoff SB. Altered brain activity in unipolar depression revisited: meta-analyses of neuroimaging studies. JAMA Psychiatry. 2017;74(1):47–55.
517. Samea F, Soluki S, Nejati V, Zarei M, Cortese S, Eickhoff SB, et al. Brain alterations in children/adolescents with ADHD revisited: a neuroimag-

ing meta-analysis of 96 structural and functional studies. Neurosci Biobehav Rev. 2019;100:1–8.
518. Vieira S, Gong QY, Pinaya WHL, Scarpazza C, Tognin S, Crespo-Facorro B, et al. Using machine learning and structural neuroimaging to detect first episode psychosis: reconsidering the evidence. Schizophr Bull. 2020;46(1):17–26.
519. Vul E, Harris C, Winkielman P, Pashler H. Puzzlingly high correlations in fMRI studies of emotion, personality, and social cognition. Perspect Psychol Sci. 2009;4(3):274–90.
520. Weinberger DR, Radulescu E. Finding the elusive psychiatric "Lesion" with 21st-century neuroanatomy: a note of caution. Am J Psychiat. 2016;173(1):27–33.
521. Kohne ACJ, van Os J. Precision psychiatry: promise for the future or rehash of a fossilised foundation? Psychol Med. 2021;51(9):1409–11.
522. Kendler KS. From many to one to many-the search for causes of psychiatric illness. JAMA Psychiatry. 2019;76(10):1085–91.
523. Insel TR, Quirion R. Psychiatry as a clinical neuroscience discipline. JAMA. 2005;294(17):2221–4.
524. Reynolds CF, 3rd, Lewis DA, Detre T, Schatzberg AF, Kupfer DJ. The future of psychiatry as clinical neuroscience. Acad Med. 2009;84(4):446–50.
525. Sharfstein SS. Big pharma and American psychiatry: the good, the bad, and the ugly. Psychiatric News. August 19, 2005.
526. World Health Organization. Guidance on community mental health services: promoting person-centred and rights-based approaches. Geneva: World Health Organization; June 10, 2021.
527. Langer E. Lewis Judd, psychiatrist who probed the science of the brain, dies at 88. The Washington Post. January 12, 2019.
528. Hyman SE. NIMH during the tenure of Director Steven E. Hyman, M.D. (1996–present): the now and future of NIMH. Am J Psychiatry. 1998;155(9 Suppl):36–40.
529. Engel GL. The need for a new medical model: a challenge for biomedicine. Science. 1977;196(4286):129–36.
530. Insel TR, Cuthbert BN. Brain disorders? Precisely. Science. 2015;348(6234):499–500.
531. Insel T, Cuthbert B, Garvey M, Heinssen R, Pine DS, Quinn K, et al. Research domain criteria (RDoC): toward a new classification frame-

work for research on mental disorders. Am J Psychiatry. 2010;167(7):748–51.
532. Frances A. RDoC is necessary, but very oversold. World Psychiatry. 2014;13(1):47–9.
533. Reardon S. NIH rethinks psychiatry trials. Nature. 2014;507(7492):288.
534. Markowitz JC, Friedman RA. NIMH's straight and neural path: the road to killing clinical psychiatric research. Psychiatr Serv. 2020;71(11):1096–97.
535. Craddock N, Antebi D, Attenburrow MJ, Bailey A, Carson A, Cowen P, et al. Wake-up call for British psychiatry. Br J Psychiatry. 2008;193(1):6–9.
536. Bullmore E, Fletcher P, Jones PB. Why psychiatry can't afford to be neurophobic. Br J Psychiatry. 2009;194(4):293–5.
537. Ross DA, Travis MJ, Arbuckle MR. The future of psychiatry as clinical neuroscience: why not now? JAMA Psychiatry. 2015;72(5):413–4.
538. Clarke J, Gawley A. The triumph of pharmaceuticals: the portrayal of depression from 1980 to 2005. Adm Policy Ment Health. 2009;36(2):91–101.
539. Deacon BJ. The biomedical model of mental disorder: a critical analysis of its validity, utility, and effects on psychotherapy research. Clin Psychol Rev. 2013;33(7):846–61.
540. Kleinman A. Rebalancing academic psychiatry: why it needs to happen—and soon. Br J Psychiatry. 2012;201(6):421–2.
541. Pescosolido BA, Martin JK, Long JS, Medina TR, Phelan JC, Link BG. "A disease like any other"? A decade of change in public reactions to schizophrenia, depression, and alcohol dependence. Am J Psychiatry. 2010;167(11):1321–30.
542. Schomerus G, Schwahn C, Holzinger A, Corrigan PW, Grabe HJ, Carta MG, et al. Evolution of public attitudes about mental illness: a systematic review and meta-analysis. Acta Psychiatr Scand. 2012;125(6):440–52.
543. Celano CM, Freudenreich O, Fernandez-Robles C, Stern TA, Caro MA, Huffman JC. Depressogenic effects of medications: a review. Dialogues Clin Neurosci. 2011;13(1):109–25.
544. Qato DM, Ozenberger K, Olfson M. Prevalence of prescription medications with depression as a potential adverse effect among adults in the United States. JAMA. 2018;319(22):2289–98.
545. Maund E, Guski LS, Gotzsche PC. Considering benefits and harms of duloxetine for treatment of stress urinary incontinence: a meta-analysis of clinical study reports. CMAJ. 2017;189(5):E194–203.

546. Fuchs E, Flugge G. Adult neuroplasticity: more than 40 years of research. Neural Plast. 2014;2014:541870.
547. Nava E, Roder B. Adaptation and maladaptation insights from brain plasticity. Prog Brain Res. 2011;191:177–94.
548. Fisher HE. Lust, attraction, and attachment in mammalian reproduction. Hum Nat. 1998;9(1):23–52.
549. Neumann ID. Oxytocin: the neuropeptide of love reveals some of its secrets. Cell Metab. 2007;5(4):231–3.
550. Schmaal L, Hibar DP, Samann PG, Hall GB, Baune BT, Jahanshad N, et al. Cortical abnormalities in adults and adolescents with major depression based on brain scans from 20 cohorts worldwide in the ENIGMA Major Depressive Disorder Working Group. Mol Psychiatry. 2017;22(6):900–9.
551. Moncrieff J. Rebuttal: depression is not a brain disease. Can J Psychiatry. 2007;52(2):100–1.
552. Hoogman M, Bralten J, Hibar DP, Mennes M, Zwiers MP, Schweren LSJ, et al. Subcortical brain volume differences in participants with attention deficit hyperactivity disorder in children and adults: a cross-sectional mega-analysis. Lancet Psychiatry 2017;4(4):310–9.
553. Whitely M, Raven M, Timimi S, Jureidini J, Phillimore J, Leo J, et al. Attention deficit hyperactivity disorder late birthdate effect common in both high and low prescribing international jurisdictions: a systematic review. J Child Psychol Psychiatry. 2019;60(4):380–91.
554. Judge TA, Cable DM. The effect of physical height on workplace success and income: preliminary test of a theoretical model. J Appl Psychol. 2004;89(3):428–41.
555. Dehue T, Bijl D, de Winter M, Scheepers F, Vanheule S, van Os J, et al. Subcortical brain volume differences in participants with attention deficit hyperactivity disorder in children and adults. Lancet Psychiatry. 2017;4(6):438–9.
556. Batstra L, Te Meerman S, Conners K, Frances A. Subcortical brain volume differences in participants with attention deficit hyperactivity disorder in children and adults. Lancet Psychiatry. 2017;4(6):439.
557. Dumas-Mallet E, Smith A, Boraud T, Gonon F. Poor replication validity of biomedical association studies reported by newspapers. PLoS One. 2017;12(2):e0172650.
558. Leo J, Lacasse JR. The media and the chemical imbalance theory of depression. Society. 2008;45(1):35–45.

559. Baldessarini RJ. The impact of psychopharmacology on contemporary psychiatry. Can J Psychiatry. 2014;59(8):401–5.
560. The Lancet Psychiatry Editors. A good enough measure. Lancet Psychiatry. 2020;7(10):825.
561. Kingdon D. Why hasn't neuroscience delivered for psychiatry? Bjpsych Bull. 2020;44(3):107–9.
562. Greden JF, Parikh SV, Rothschild AJ, Thase ME, Dunlop BW, DeBattista C, et al. Impact of pharmacogenomics on clinical outcomes in major depressive disorder in the GUIDED trial: a large, patient- and rater-blinded, randomized, controlled study. J Psychiatr Res. 2019;111:59–67.
563. Zeier Z, Carpenter LL, Kalin NH, Rodriguez CI, McDonald WM, Widge AS, et al. Clinical implementation of pharmacogenetic decision support tools for antidepressant drug prescribing. Am J Psychiatry. 2018;175(9):873–86.
564. Zubenko GS, Sommer BR, Cohen BM. On the marketing and use of pharmacogenetic tests for psychiatric treatment. JAMA Psychiatry. 2018;75(8):769–70.
565. Rogers A. Star neuroscientist Tom Insel leaves the Google-spawned verily for … A startup? Wired. November 2017.
566. Baxter AJ, Scott KM, Ferrari AJ, Norman RE, Vos T, Whiteford HA. Challenging the myth of an "epidemic" of common mental disorders: trends in the global prevalence of anxiety and depression between 1990 and 2010. Depress Anxiety. 2014;31(6):506–16.
567. Healy D, Savage M, Michael P, Harris M, Hirst D, Carter M, et al. Psychiatric bed utilization: 1896 and 1996 compared. Psychol Med. 2001;31(5):779–90.
568. Jorm AF, Patten SB, Brugha TS, Mojtabai R. Has increased provision of treatment reduced the prevalence of common mental disorders? Review of the evidence from four countries. World Psychiatry. 2017;16(1):90–9.
569. Mulder RT, Frampton CM. Outcome of mood disorders before psychopharmacology: a systematic review. Aust N Z J Psychiatry. 2014;48(3):224–36.
570. Richter D, Wall A, Bruen A, Whittington R. Is the global prevalence rate of adult mental illness increasing? Systematic review and meta-analysis. Acta Psychiatr Scand. 2019;140(5):393–407.
571. Global Burden of Disease Study Collaborators. Global, regional, and national incidence, prevalence, and years lived with disability for 301 acute and chronic diseases and injuries in 188 countries, 1990–2013: a

systematic analysis for the Global Burden of Disease Study 2013. Lancet. 2015;386(9995):743–800.
572. Lawrence D, Hancock KJ, Kisely S. The gap in life expectancy from preventable physical illness in psychiatric patients in Western Australia: retrospective analysis of population based registers. BMJ. 2013;346:f2539.
573. Lee EE, Liu J, Tu X, Palmer BW, Eyler LT, Jeste DV. A widening longevity gap between people with schizophrenia and general population: a literature review and call for action. Schizophr Res. 2018;196:9–13.
574. Viola S, Moncrieff J. Claims for sickness and disability benefits owing to mental disorders in the UK: trends from 1995 to 2014. BJPsych Open. 2016;2(1):18–24.
575. Wang PS, Aguilar-Gaxiola S, Alonso J, Angermeyer MC, Borges G, Bromet EJ, et al. Use of mental health services for anxiety, mood, and substance disorders in 17 countries in the WHO world mental health surveys. Lancet. 2007;370(9590):841–50.
576. Steel Z, Marnane C, Iranpour C, Chey T, Jackson JW, Patel V, et al. The global prevalence of common mental disorders: a systematic review and meta-analysis 1980–2013. Int J Epidemiol. 2014;43(2):476–93.
577. Ormel J, VonKorff M. Reducing common mental disorder prevalence in populations. JAMA Psychiatry. 2021;78(4):359–60.
578. United Nations. World needs "revolution" in mental health care—UN rights expert [press release]. New York, NY: United Nations; June 2017.
579. Fabbri A, Parker L, Colombo C, Mosconi P, Barbara G, Frattaruolo MP, et al. Industry funding of patient and health consumer organisations: systematic review with meta-analysis. BMJ. 2020;368:l6925.
580. McCoy MS, Carniol M, Chockley K, Urwin JW, Emanuel EJ, Schmidt H. Conflicts of interest for patient-advocacy organizations. N Engl J Med. 2017;376(9):880–5.
581. Ozieranski P, Rickard E, Mulinari S. Exposing drug industry funding of UK patient organisations. BMJ. 2019;365:l1806.
582. Rose SL, Highland J, Karafa MT, Joffe S. Patient advocacy organizations, industry funding, and conflicts of interest. JAMA Intern Med. 2017;177(3):344–50.
583. Ozieranski P, Csanadi M, Rickard E, Mulinari S. Under-reported relationship: a comparative study of pharmaceutical industry and patient organisation payment disclosures in the UK (2012–2016). BMJ Open. 2020;10(9):e037351.

584. Parker L, Fabbri A, Grundy Q, Mintzes B, Bero L. "Asset exchange"-interactions between patient groups and pharmaceutical industry: Australian qualitative study. BMJ. 2019;367:l6694.
585. Batt S, Butler J, Shannon O, Fugh-Berman A. Pharmaceutical ethics and grassroots activism in the United States: a social history perspective. J Bioeth Inq. 2020;17(1):49–60.
586. Rose SL. Patient advocacy organizations: institutional conflicts of interest, trust, and trustworthiness. J Law Med Ethics. 2013;41(3):680–7.
587. France CM, Lysaker PH, Robinson RP. The "chemical imbalance" explanation for depression: origins, lay endorsement, and clinical implications. Prof Psychol-Res Pr. 2007;38(4):411–20.
588. Leonardo Alves T, Lexchin J, Mintzes B. Medicines information and the regulation of the promotion of pharmaceuticals. Sci Eng Ethics. 2019;25(4):1167–92.
589. Mintzes B, Barer ML, Kravitz RL, Bassett K, Lexchin J, Kazanjian A, et al. How does direct-to-consumer advertising (DTCA) affect prescribing? A survey in primary care environments with and without legal DTCA. CMAJ. 2003;169(5):405–12.
590. Kravitz RL, Epstein RM, Feldman MD, Franz CE, Azari R, Wilkes MS, et al. Influence of patients' requests for direct-to-consumer advertised antidepressants: a randomized controlled trial. JAMA. 2005;293(16):1995–2002.
591. Caulfield T. The commercialisation of medical and scientific reporting. PLoS Med. 2004;1(3):e38.
592. Ahn R, Woodbridge A, Abraham A, Saba S, Korenstein D, Madden E, et al. Financial ties of principal investigators and randomized controlled trial outcomes: cross sectional study. BMJ. 2017;356:i6770.
593. Hansen C, Lundh A, Rasmussen K, Hrobjartsson A. Financial conflicts of interest in systematic reviews: associations with results, conclusions, and methodological quality. Cochrane Database Syst Rev. 2019;8:MR000047.
594. Kramer PD. Listening to Prozac. New York, NY: Penguin Books; 1993.
595. Healy D. Serotonin and depression. BMJ. 2015;350:h1771.
596. Mulinari S. Monoamine theories of depression: historical impact on biomedical research. J Hist Neurosci. 2012;21(4):366–92.
597. Nemeroff CB. The state of our understanding of the pathophysiology and optimal treatment of depression: glass half full or half empty? Am J Psychiatry. 2020;177(8):671–85.

598. Thomas-MacLean R, Stoppard JM. Physicians' constructions of depression: inside/outside the boundaries of medicalization. Health (London). 2004;8(3):275–93.
599. Baumeister AA, Hawkins MF, Uzelac SM. The myth of reserpine-induced depression: role in the historical development of the monoamine hypothesis. J Hist Neurosci. 2003;12(2):207–20.
600. Schildkraut JJ. The catecholamine hypothesis of affective disorders: a review of supporting evidence. Am J Psychiatry. 1965;122(5):509–22.
601. Coppen A. The biochemistry of affective disorders. Br J Psychiatry. 1967;113(504):1237–64.
602. Katz MM, Secunda SK, Hirschfeld RM, Koslow SH. NIMH clinical research branch collaborative program on the psychobiology of depression. Arch Gen Psychiatry. 1979;36(7):765–71.
603. Maas JW, Koslow SH, Davis JM, Katz MM, Mendels J, Robins E, et al. Biological component of the NIMH clinical research branch collaborative program on the psychobiology of depression: I. Background and theoretical considerations. Psychol Med. 1980;10(4):759–76.
604. Freemantle N, Anderson IM, Young P. Predictive value of pharmacological activity for the relative efficacy of antidepressant drugs. Meta-regression analysis. Br J Psychiatry. 2000;177:292–302.
605. Kirsch I. Antidepressants and the placebo effect. Z Psychol. 2014;222(3):128–34.
606. Ruhe HG, Mason NS, Schene AH. Mood is indirectly related to serotonin, norepinephrine and dopamine levels in humans: a meta-analysis of monoamine depletion studies. Mol Psychiatr. 2007;12(4):331–59.
607. Zetterqvist AV, Mulinari S. Misleading advertising for antidepressants in Sweden: a failure of pharmaceutical industry self-regulation. PLoS One. 2013;8(5):e62609.
608. Mulinari S. Regulating drug information in Europe: a pyrrhic victory for pharmaceutical industry critics? Sociol Health Illn. 2013;35(5):761–77.
609. Read J, Cartwright C, Gibson K, Shiels C, Magliano L. Beliefs of people taking antidepressants about the causes of their own depression. J Affect Disord. 2015;174:150–6.
610. Aikens JE, Nease DE, Jr., Klinkman MS. Explaining patients' beliefs about the necessity and harmfulness of antidepressants. Ann Fam Med. 2008;6(1):23–9.
611. Scholten W, Batelaan N, Van Balkom A. Barriers to discontinuing antidepressants in patients with depressive and anxiety disorders: a review of

the literature and clinical recommendations. Ther Adv Psychopharmacol. 2020;10:2045125320933404.

612. Eveleigh R, Speckens A, van Weel C, Oude Voshaar R, Lucassen P. Patients' attitudes to discontinuing not-indicated long-term antidepressant use: barriers and facilitators. Ther Adv Psychopharmacol. 2019;9:2045125319872344.
613. Maund E, Dewar-Haggart R, Williams S, Bowers H, Geraghty AWA, Leydon G, et al. Barriers and facilitators to discontinuing antidepressant use: a systematic review and thematic synthesis. J Affect Disord. 2019;245:38–62.
614. Andrews PW, Thomson JA, Jr., Amstadter A, Neale MC. Primum non nocere: an evolutionary analysis of whether antidepressants do more harm than good. Front Psychol. 2012;3:117.
615. Moret C, Isaac M, Briley M. Problems associated with long-term treatment with selective serotonin reuptake inhibitors. J Psychopharmacol. 2009;23(8):967–74.
616. Bann CM, Parker CB, Bradwejn J, Davidson JR, Vitiello B, Gadde KM. Assessing patient beliefs in a clinical trial of Hypericum perforatum in major depression. Depress Anxiety. 2004;20(3):114–22.
617. Schroder HS, Duda JM, Christensen K, Beard C, Bjorgvinsson T. Stressors and chemical imbalances: beliefs about the causes of depression in an acute psychiatric treatment sample. J Affect Disord. 2020;276:537–45.
618. Watson LM, Beshai S. Causal explanations of depression on perceptions of and likelihood to choose cognitive behavioural therapy and antidepressant medications as depression treatments. Psychol Psychother. 2021;94(2):201–16.
619. Angermeyer MC, Holzinger A, Carta MG, Schomerus G. Biogenetic explanations and public acceptance of mental illness: systematic review of population studies. Br J Psychiatry. 2011;199(5):367–72.
620. Larkings JS, Brown PM. Do biogenetic causal beliefs reduce mental illness stigma in people with mental illness and in mental health professionals? A systematic review. Int J Ment Health Nurs. 2018;27(3):928–41.
621. Kvaale EP, Gottdiener WH, Haslam N. Biogenetic explanations and stigma: a meta-analytic review of associations among laypeople. Soc Sci Med. 2013;96:95–103.

622. Lebowitz MS, Appelbaum PS. Biomedical explanations of psychopathology and their implications for attitudes and beliefs about mental disorders. Annu Rev Clin Psychol. 2019;15:555–77.
623. McHenry L. Ethical issues in psychopharmacology. J Med Ethics. 2006;32(7):405–10.
624. Pies R. Psychiatry's new brain-mind and the legend of the "chemical imbalance". Psychiatric Times. July 11, 2011.
625. Pilkington PD, Reavley NJ, Jorm AF. The Australian public's beliefs about the causes of depression: associated factors and changes over 16 years. J Affect Disord. 2013;150(2):356–62.
626. Pies R. Proposed model for self-injurious behavior. Am J Psychiatry. 1992;149(3):420.
627. Lacasse JR, Leo J. Antidepressants and the chemical imbalance theory of depression: a reflection and update on the discourse. Behavior Therapist. 2015;38(7):206–13.
628. Cole S, Raju M, Barrett J, Gerrity M, Dietrich A. The MacArthur foundation depression education program for primary care physicians: background and rationale. Gen Hosp Psychiatry. 2000;22(5):299–358.
629. Friedrichs J, Padberg T. Depressionen. Aus dem Schatten ans Licht. Zeit Magazin. June 9, 2016.
630. Hegerl U. Prevention of suicidal behavior. Dialogues Clin Neurosci. 2016;18(2):183–90.
631. Nowotny M, Kern D, Breyer E, Bengough T, Griebler R. Depressionsbericht Österreich. Eine interdisziplinäre und multiperspektivische Bestandsaufnahme. Wien: Bundesministerium für Arbeit, Soziales, Gesundheit und Konsumentenschutz; 2019.
632. Sprooten E, Rasgon A, Goodman M, Carlin A, Leibu E, Lee WH, et al. Addressing reverse inference in psychiatric neuroimaging: meta-analyses of task-related brain activation in common mental disorders. Hum Brain Mapp. 2017;38(4):1846–64.
633. Fried EI, Kievit RA. The volumes of subcortical regions in depressed and healthy individuals are strikingly similar: a reinterpretation of the results by Schmaal et al. Mol Psychiatry. 2016;21(6):724–5.
634. Helm K, Viol K, Weiger TM, Tass PA, Grefkes C, Del Monte D, et al. Neuronal connectivity in major depressive disorder: a systematic review. Neuropsychiatr Dis Treat. 2018;14:2715–37.
635. Hill AB. The environment and disease: association or causation? Proc R Soc Med. 1965;58:295–300.

636. Rothman KJ, Greenland S. Causation and causal inference in epidemiology. Am J Public Health. 2005;95 Suppl 1:S144–50.
637. Moncrieff J, Cooper R, Stockmann T, Amendola S, Hengartner MP, Horowitz HA. The serotonin theory of depression: a systematic umbrella review of the evidence. Mol Psychiatry. 2021;in press.
638. Kessler RC, Demler O, Frank RG, Olfson M, Pincus HA, Walters EE, et al. Prevalence and treatment of mental disorders, 1990 to 2003. N Engl J Med. 2005;352(24):2515–23.
639. Sundquist J, Ohlsson H, Sundquist K, Kendler KS. Common adult psychiatric disorders in Swedish primary care where most mental health patients are treated. BMC Psychiatry. 2017;17(1):235.
640. Demyttenaere K, Bruffaerts R, Posada-Villa J, Gasquet I, Kovess V, Lepine JP, et al. Prevalence, severity, and unmet need for treatment of mental disorders in the World Health Organization World Mental Health Surveys. JAMA. 2004;291(21):2581–90.
641. Djulbegovic B, Guyatt GH. Progress in evidence-based medicine: a quarter century on. Lancet. 2017;390(10092):415–23.
642. Sackett DL, Rosenberg WM, Gray JA, Haynes RB, Richardson WS. Evidence based medicine: what it is and what it isn't. BMJ. 1996;312(7023):71–2.
643. Atkins D, Best D, Briss PA, Eccles M, Falck-Ytter Y, Flottorp S, et al. Grading quality of evidence and strength of recommendations. BMJ. 2004;328(7454):1490.
644. Cochrane. About us: Cochrane; 2021. Available from: https://www.cochrane.org/about-us.
645. Prasad VK, Cifu AS. Ending medical reversal: improving outcomes, saving lives. Baltimore: Johns Hopkins University Press; 2015.
646. Haslam A, Livingston C, Prasad V. Medical reversals in family practice: a review. Curr Ther Res Clin Exp. 2020;92:100579.
647. Prasad V, Vandross A, Toomey C, Cheung M, Rho J, Quinn S, et al. A decade of reversal: an analysis of 146 contradicted medical practices. Mayo Clin Proc. 2013;88(8):790–8.
648. Cardiac Arrhythmia Suppression Trial Investigators. Preliminary report: effect of encainide and flecainide on mortality in a randomized trial of arrhythmia suppression after myocardial infarction. N Engl J Med. 1989;321(6):406–12.
649. Howick J. Exploring the asymmetrical relationship between the power of finance bias and evidence. Perspect Biol Med. 2019;62(1):159–87.

650. Greenhalgh T, Howick J, Maskrey N. Evidence based medicine renaissance G. Evidence based medicine: a movement in crisis? BMJ. 2014;348:g3725.
651. Fabbri A, Lai A, Grundy Q, Bero LA. The influence of industry sponsorship on the research agenda: a scoping review. Am J Public Health. 2018;108(11):e9–16.
652. Lexchin J. Sponsorship bias in clinical research. Int J Risk Saf Med. 2012;24(4):233–42.
653. Jefferson T, Jorgensen L. Redefining the 'E' in EBM. BMJ Evid Based Med. 2018;23(2):46–7.
654. Anderson ML, Chiswell K, Peterson ED, Tasneem A, Topping J, Califf RM. Compliance with results reporting at ClinicalTrials.gov. N Engl J Med. 2015;372(11):1031–9.
655. Goldacre B, DeVito NJ, Heneghan C, Irving F, Bacon S, Fleminger J, et al. Compliance with requirement to report results on the EU Clinical Trials Register: cohort study and web resource. BMJ. 2018;362:k3218.
656. Moses H, 3rd, Matheson DH, Cairns-Smith S, George BP, Palisch C, Dorsey ER. The anatomy of medical research: US and international comparisons. JAMA. 2015;313(2):174–89.
657. Sismondo S. Ghost management: how much of the medical literature is shaped behind the scenes by the pharmaceutical industry? PLoS Med. 2007;4(9):e286.
658. Sismondo S, Doucet M. Publication ethics and the ghost management of medical publication. Bioethics. 2010;24(6):273–83.
659. Matheson A. The disposable author: how pharmaceutical marketing is embraced within medicine's scholarly literature. Hastings Cent Rep. 2016;46(4):31–7.
660. Ioannidis JPA, Stuart ME, Brownlee S, Strite SA. How to survive the medical misinformation mess. Eur J Clin Invest. 2017;47(11):795–802.
661. Prasad V, Berger VW. Hard-wired bias: how even double-blind, randomized controlled trials can be skewed from the start. Mayo Clin Proc. 2015;90(9):1171–5.
662. Dwan K, Altman DG, Clarke M, Gamble C, Higgins JP, Sterne JA, et al. Evidence for the selective reporting of analyses and discrepancies in clinical trials: a systematic review of cohort studies of clinical trials. PLoS Med. 2014;11(6):e1001666.

663. Hopewell S, Loudon K, Clarke MJ, Oxman AD, Dickersin K. Publication bias in clinical trials due to statistical significance or direction of trial results. Cochrane Database Syst Rev. 2009(1):MR000006.
664. Mathieu S, Boutron I, Moher D, Altman DG, Ravaud P. Comparison of registered and published primary outcomes in randomized controlled trials. JAMA. 2009;302(9):977–84.
665. Wieseler B, Wolfram N, McGauran N, Kerekes MF, Vervolgyi V, Kohlepp P, et al. Completeness of reporting of patient-relevant clinical trial outcomes: comparison of unpublished clinical study reports with publicly available data. PLoS Med. 2013;10(10):e1001526.
666. Cro S, Forbes G, Johnson NA, Kahan BC. Evidence of unexplained discrepancies between planned and conducted statistical analyses: a review of randomised trials. BMC Med. 2020;18(1):137.
667. Boutron I, Ravaud P. Misrepresentation and distortion of research in biomedical literature. Proc Natl Acad Sci U S A. 2018;115(11):2613–9.
668. Boutron I, Dutton S, Ravaud P, Altman DG. Reporting and interpretation of randomized controlled trials with statistically nonsignificant results for primary outcomes. JAMA. 2010;303(20):2058–64.
669. Jellison S, Roberts W, Bowers A, Combs T, Beaman J, Wayant C, et al. Evaluation of spin in abstracts of papers in psychiatry and psychology journals. BMJ Evid Based Med. 2019:178–81.
670. Stoll M, Mancini A, Hubenschmid L, Dreimuller N, Konig J, Cuijpers P, et al. Discrepancies from registered protocols and spin occurred frequently in randomized psychotherapy trials-A meta-epidemiologic study. J Clin Epidemiol. 2020;128:49–56.
671. Kane RL, Butler M, Ng W. Examining the quality of evidence to support the effectiveness of interventions: an analysis of systematic reviews. BMJ Open. 2016;6(5):e011051.
672. Howick J, Koletsi D, Pandis N, Fleming PS, Loef M, Walach H, et al. The quality of evidence for medical interventions does not improve or worsen: a metaepidemiological study of Cochrane reviews. J Clin Epidemiol. 2020;126:154–9.
673. Heres S, Davis J, Maino K, Jetzinger E, Kissling W, Leucht S. Why olanzapine beats risperidone, risperidone beats quetiapine, and quetiapine beats olanzapine: an exploratory analysis of head-to-head comparison studies of second-generation antipsychotics. Am J Psychiatry. 2006;163(2):185–94.

674. Flacco ME, Manzoli L, Boccia S, Capasso L, Aleksovska K, Rosso A, et al. Head-to-head randomized trials are mostly industry sponsored and almost always favor the industry sponsor. J Clin Epidemiol. 2015;68(7):811–20.
675. Zhang AD, Puthumana J, Downing NS, Shah ND, Krumholz HM, Ross JS. Assessment of clinical trials supporting US Food and Drug Administration approval of novel therapeutic agents, 1995–2017. JAMA Netw Open. 2020;3(4):e203284.
676. Kesselheim AS, Avorn J. The F.D.A. has reached a new low. The New York Times. June 15, 2021.
677. Loke YK, Derry S. Reporting of adverse drug reactions in randomised controlled trials—a systematic survey. BMC Clin Pharmacol. 2001;1:3.
678. Light DW, Lexchin JR. Pharmaceuticals as a market for "lemons": theory and practice. Soc Sci Med. 2021;268:113368.
679. Frieden TR. Evidence for health decision making—beyond randomized, controlled trials. N Engl J Med. 2017;377(5):465–75.
680. Button KS, Ioannidis JP, Mokrysz C, Nosek BA, Flint J, Robinson ES, et al. Power failure: why small sample size undermines the reliability of neuroscience. Nat Rev Neurosci. 2013;14(5):365–76.
681. Yarkoni T. Big correlations in little studies: inflated fMRI correlations reflect low statistical power-commentary on Vul et al. (2009). Perspect Psychol Sci. 2009;4(3):294–8.
682. Van Spall HG, Toren A, Kiss A, Fowler RA. Eligibility criteria of randomized controlled trials published in high-impact general medical journals: a systematic sampling review. JAMA. 2007;297(11):1233–40.
683. Fergusson D, Glass KC, Waring D, Shapiro S. Turning a blind eye: the success of blinding reported in a random sample of randomised, placebo controlled trials. BMJ. 2004;328(7437):432.
684. Baethge C, Assall OP, Baldessarini RJ. Systematic review of blinding assessment in randomized controlled trials in schizophrenia and affective disorders 2000–2010. Psychother Psychosom. 2013;82(3):152–60.
685. Savovic J, Turner RM, Mawdsley D, Jones HE, Beynon R, Higgins JPT, et al. Association between risk-of-bias assessments and results of randomized trials in Cochrane reviews: the ROBES meta-epidemiologic study. Am J Epidemiol. 2018;187(5):1113–22.
686. Phillips R, Hazell L, Sauzet O, Cornelius V. Analysis and reporting of adverse events in randomised controlled trials: a review. BMJ Open. 2019;9(2):e024537.

687. Pitrou I, Boutron I, Ahmad N, Ravaud P. Reporting of safety results in published reports of randomized controlled trials. Arch Intern Med. 2009;169(19):1756–61.
688. Schroll JB, Maund E, Gotzsche PC. Challenges in coding adverse events in clinical trials: a systematic review. PLoS One. 2012;7(7):e41174.
689. Mayo-Wilson E, Fusco N, Li T, Hong H, Canner JK, Dickersin K, et al. Harms are assessed inconsistently and reported inadequately Part 2: non-systematic adverse events. J Clin Epidemiol. 2019;113:11–9.
690. Berlin JA, Glasser SC, Ellenberg SS. Adverse event detection in drug development: recommendations and obligations beyond phase 3. Am J Public Health. 2008;98(8):1366–71.
691. Healy D, Mangin D. Clinical judgments, not algorithms, are key to patient safety-an essay by David Healy and Dee Mangin. BMJ. 2019;367:l5777.
692. Silverman SL. From randomized controlled trials to observational studies. Am J Med. 2009;122(2):114–20.
693. Antonuccio DO, Danton WG, DeNelsky GY, Greenberg RP, Gordon JS. Raising questions about antidepressants. Psychother Psychosom. 1999;68(1):3–14.
694. Moncrieff J. Are antidepressants overrated? A review of methodological problems in antidepressant trials. J Nerv Ment Dis. 2001;189(5):288–95.
695. Wang SM, Han C, Lee SJ, Jun TY, Patkar AA, Masand PS, et al. Efficacy of antidepressants: bias in randomized clinical trials and related issues. Expert Rev Clin Pharmacol. 2018;11(1):15–25.
696. Wisniewski SR, Rush AJ, Nierenberg AA, Gaynes BN, Warden D, Luther JF, et al. Can phase III trial results of antidepressant medications be generalized to clinical practice? A STAR*D report. Am J Psychiatry. 2009;166(5):599–607.
697. Zimmerman M, Balling C, Chelminski I, Dalrymple K. Have treatment studies of depression become even less generalizable? Applying the inclusion and exclusion criteria in placebo-controlled antidepressant efficacy trials published over 20 years to a clinical sample. Psychother Psychosom. 2019;88(3):165–70.
698. Zimmerman M, Mattia JI, Posternak MA. Are subjects in pharmacological treatment trials of depression representative of patients in routine clinical practice? Am J Psychiatry. 2002;159(3):469–73.
699. Zimmerman M, Chelminski I, Posternak MA. Generalizability of antidepressant efficacy trials: differences between depressed psychiatric out-

patients who would or would not qualify for an efficacy trial. Am J Psychiatry. 2005;162(7):1370–2.

700. Kornstein SG, Schneider RK. Clinical features of treatment-resistant depression. J Clin Psychiatry. 2001;62 Suppl 16:18–25.
701. Lee S, Walker JR, Jakul L, Sexton K. Does elimination of placebo responders in a placebo run-in increase the treatment effect in randomized clinical trials? A meta-analytic evaluation. Depress Anxiety. 2004;19(1):10–9.
702. Benasi G, Guidi J, Offidani E, Balon R, Rickels K, Fava GA. Benzodiazepines as a monotherapy in depressive disorders: a systematic review. Psychother Psychosom. 2018;87(2):65–74.
703. Hrobjartsson A, Thomsen AS, Emanuelsson F, Tendal B, Hilden J, Boutron I, et al. Observer bias in randomised clinical trials with binary outcomes: systematic review of trials with both blinded and non-blinded outcome assessors. BMJ. 2012;344:e1119.
704. Hrobjartsson A, Thomsen AS, Emanuelsson F, Tendal B, Hilden J, Boutron I, et al. Observer bias in randomized clinical trials with measurement scale outcomes: a systematic review of trials with both blinded and nonblinded assessors. CMAJ. 2013;185(4):E201–11.
705. Page MJ, Higgins JP, Clayton G, Sterne JA, Hrobjartsson A, Savovic J. Empirical evidence of study design biases in randomized trials: systematic review of meta-epidemiological studies. PLoS One. 2016;11(7):e0159267.
706. Savovic J, Jones HE, Altman DG, Harris RJ, Juni P, Pildal J, et al. Influence of reported study design characteristics on intervention effect estimates from randomized, controlled trials. Ann Intern Med. 2012;157(6):429–38.
707. Even C, Siobud-Dorocant E, Dardennes RM. Critical approach to antidepressant trials. Blindness protection is necessary, feasible and measurable. Br J Psychiatry. 2000;177:47–51.
708. Fisher S, Greenberg RP. How sound is the double-blind design for evaluating psychotropic drugs? J Nerv Ment Dis. 1993;181(6):345–50.
709. Khan A, Faucett J, Lichtenberg P, Kirsch I, Brown WA. A systematic review of comparative efficacy of treatments and controls for depression. PLoS One. 2012;7(7):e41778.
710. Moncrieff J, Wessely S, Hardy R. Active placebos versus antidepressants for depression. Cochrane Database Syst Rev. 2004(1):CD003012.

711. Schafer JL, Graham JW. Missing data: our view of the state of the art. Psychol Methods. 2002;7(2):147–77.
712. Vannoy S, Brodt M, Cosgrove L, Shaughnessy AF. Variation in analytic transparency in recent efficacy studies of antidepressant medication. BMJ Evid Based Med. 2018;23(5):177–82.
713. Johnson VE. Revised standards for statistical evidence. Proc Natl Acad Sci U S A. 2013;110(48):19313–7.
714. Tsang R, Colley L, Lynd LD. Inadequate statistical power to detect clinically significant differences in adverse event rates in randomized controlled trials. J Clin Epidemiol. 2009;62(6):609–16.
715. Healy D. Did regulators fail over selective serotonin reuptake inhibitors? BMJ. 2006;333(7558):92–5.
716. Whitaker R. An FDA whistleblower's documents: commerce, corruption, and death. Mad in America; August 23, 2020.
717. Jonville-Bera AP, Giraudeau B, Autret-Leca E. Reporting of drug tolerance in randomized clinical trials: when data conflict with authors' conclusions. Ann Intern Med. 2006;144(4):306–7.
718. Amrhein V, Greenland S, McShane B. Scientists rise up against statistical significance. Nature. 2019;567(7748):305–7.
719. Altman DG, Bland JM. Absence of evidence is not evidence of absence. BMJ. 1995;311(7003):485.
720. Holbrook AM, Crowther R, Lotter A, Cheng C, King D. Meta-analysis of benzodiazepine use in the treatment of insomnia. CMAJ. 2000;162(2):225–33.
721. Gomez AF, Barthel AL, Hofmann SG. Comparing the efficacy of benzodiazepines and serotonergic anti-depressants for adults with generalized anxiety disorder: a meta-analytic review. Expert Opin Pharmacother. 2018;19(8):883–94.
722. Montane E, Arellano AL, Sanz Y, Roca J, Farre M. Drug-related deaths in hospital inpatients: a retrospective cohort study. Br J Clin Pharmacol. 2018;84(3):542–52.
723. Pirmohamed M, James S, Meakin S, Green C, Scott AK, Walley TJ, et al. Adverse drug reactions as cause of admission to hospital: prospective analysis of 18,820 patients. BMJ. 2004;329(7456):15–9.
724. Katon WJ. Epidemiology and treatment of depression in patients with chronic medical illness. Dialogues Clin Neurosci. 2011;13(1):7–23.
725. Haller E, Watzke B, Blozik E, Rosemann T, Reich O, Huber CA, et al. Antidepressant prescription practice and related factors in Switzerland: a

cross-sectional analysis of health claims data. BMC Psychiatry. 2019;19(1):196.

726. Geddes JR, Carney SM, Davies C, Furukawa TA, Kupfer DJ, Frank E, et al. Relapse prevention with antidepressant drug treatment in depressive disorders: a systematic review. Lancet. 2003;361(9358):653–61.

727. Borges S, Chen YF, Laughren TP, Temple R, Patel HD, David PA, et al. Review of maintenance trials for major depressive disorder: a 25-year perspective from the US Food and Drug Administration. J Clin Psychiatry. 2014;75(3):205–14.

728. Hansen R, Gaynes B, Thieda P, Gartlehner G, Deveaugh-Geiss A, Krebs E, et al. Meta-analysis of major depressive disorder relapse and recurrence with second-generation antidepressants. Psychiat Serv. 2008;59(10):1121–30.

729. Baldessarini RJ. Risks in discontinuation trials with antidepressants. J Clin Psychiatry. 2014;75(12):e1443.

730. Tondo L, Baldessarini RJ. Discontinuing psychotropic drug treatment. BJPsych Open. 2020;6(2):e24.

731. Baldessarini RJ, Tondo L, Ghiani C, Lepri B. Illness risk following rapid versus gradual discontinuation of antidepressants. Am J Psychiatry. 2010;167(8):934–41.

732. Chouinard G, Chouinard VA. New classification of selective serotonin reuptake inhibitor withdrawal. Psychother Psychosom. 2015;84(2):63–71.

733. Fava GA, Bernardi M, Tomba E, Rafanelli C. Effects of gradual discontinuation of selective serotonin reuptake inhibitors in panic disorder with agoraphobia. Int J Neuropsychopharmacol. 2007;10(6):835–8.

734. Michelson D, Fava M, Amsterdam J, Apter J, Londborg P, Tamura R, et al. Interruption of selective serotonin reuptake inhibitor treatment. Double-blind, placebo-controlled trial. Br J Psychiatry. 2000;176:363–8.

735. Rosenbaum JF, Fava M, Hoog SL, Ascroft RC, Krebs WB. Selective serotonin reuptake inhibitor discontinuation syndrome: a randomized clinical trial. Biol Psychiatry. 1998;44(2):77–87.

736. Khan A, Brown WA. Antidepressants versus placebo in major depression: an overview. World Psychiatry. 2015;14(3):294–300.

737. Nelson JC, Thase ME, Khan A, Nelson JC. Are antidepressants effective? What's a clinician to think? J Clin Psychiatry. 2008;69(6):1014–5.

738. Pies R. Are antidepressants effective in the acute and long-term treatment of depression? Sic et Non. Innov Clin Neurosci. 2012;9(5–6):31–40.

739. Khan A, Fahl Mar K, Faucett J, Khan Schilling S, Brown WA. Has the rising placebo response impacted antidepressant clinical trial outcome? Data from the US Food and Drug Administration 1987–2013. World Psychiatry. 2017;16(2):181–92.
740. Furukawa TA, Cipriani A, Leucht S, Atkinson LZ, Ogawa Y, Takeshima N, et al. Is placebo response in antidepressant trials rising or not? A reanalysis of datasets to conclude this long-lasting controversy. Evid Based Ment Health. 2018;21(1):1–3.
741. Parker G, Ricciardi T, Hadzi-Pavlovic D. Placebo response rates in trials of antidepressant drugs in adults with clinical depression: increasing, decreasing, constant or all of the above? J Affect Disord. 2020;271:139–44.
742. Kirsch I, Sapirstein G. Listening to Prozac but hearing placebo: a meta-analysis of antidepressant medication. Prev Treat. 1998;1(2):0002a.
743. Hrobjartsson A, Gotzsche PC. Placebo interventions for all clinical conditions. Cochrane Database Syst Rev. 2010(1):CD003974.
744. Kienle GS, Kiene H. The powerful placebo effect: fact or fiction? J Clin Epidemiol. 1997;50(12):1311–8.
745. McDonald CJ, Mazzuca SA, McCabe GP, Jr. How much of the placebo 'effect' is really statistical regression? Stat Med. 1983;2(4):417–27.
746. Bagby RM, Ryder AG, Schuller DR, Marshall MB. The Hamilton Depression rating scale: has the gold standard become a lead weight? Am J Psychiatry. 2004;161(12):2163–77.
747. Carrozzino D, Patierno C, Fava GA, Guidi J. The Hamilton rating scales for depression: a critical review of clinimetric properties of different versions. Psychother Psychosom. 2020;89(3):133–50.
748. Bech P. Rating scales in depression: limitations and pitfalls. Dialogues Clin Neurosci. 2006;8(2):207–15.
749. Ostergaard SD. Do not blame the SSRIs: blame the Hamilton Depression rating scale. Acta Neuropsychiatr. 2018;30(5):241–3.
750. Hofmann SG, Curtiss J, Carpenter JK, Kind S. Effect of treatments for depression on quality of life: a meta-analysis. Cogn Behav Ther. 2017;46(4):265–86.
751. Kamenov K, Twomey C, Cabello M, Prina AM, Ayuso-Mateos JL. The efficacy of psychotherapy, pharmacotherapy and their combination on functioning and quality of life in depression: a meta-analysis. Psychol Med. 2017;47(3):414–25.
752. Fried EI. Are more responsive depression scales really superior depression scales? J Clin Epidemiol. 2016;77:4–6.

753. Antonuccio D, Healy D. Relabeling the medications we call antidepressants. Scientifica (Cairo). 2012;2012:965908.
754. Engelhardt N, Feiger AD, Cogger KO, Sikich D, DeBrota DJ, Lipsitz JD, et al. Rating the raters: assessing the quality of Hamilton rating scale for depression clinical interviews in two industry-sponsored clinical drug trials. J Clin Psychopharmacol. 2006;26(1):71–4.
755. Kobak KA, Feiger AD, Lipsitz JD. Interview quality and signal detection in clinical trials. Am J Psychiatry. 2005;162(3):628.
756. Khan A, Faucett J, Brown WA. Magnitude of change with antidepressants and placebo in antidepressant clinical trials using structured, taped and appraised rater interviews (SIGMA-RAPS) compared to trials using traditional semi-structured interviews. Psychopharmacology (Berl). 2014;231(22):4301–7.
757. Greenberg RP, Bornstein RF, Greenberg MD, Fisher S. A meta-analysis of antidepressant outcome under "blinder" conditions. J Consult Clin Psychol. 1992;60(5):664–9; discussion 70–7.
758. Spielmans GI, Gerwig K. The efficacy of antidepressants on overall well-being and self-reported depression symptom severity in youth: a meta-analysis. Psychother Psychosom. 2014;83(3):158–64.
759. Jones CW, Keil LG, Holland WC, Caughey MC, Platts-Mills TF. Comparison of registered and published outcomes in randomized controlled trials: a systematic review. BMC Med. 2015;13:282.
760. Vedula SS, Bero L, Scherer RW, Dickersin K. Outcome reporting in industry-sponsored trials of gabapentin for off-label use. N Engl J Med. 2009;361(20):1963–71.
761. Hartung DM, Zarin DA, Guise JM, McDonagh M, Paynter R, Helfand M. Reporting discrepancies between the ClinicalTrials.gov results database and peer-reviewed publications. Ann Intern Med. 2014;160(7):477–83.
762. Papanikolaou PN, Churchill R, Wahlbeck K, Ioannidis JP. Safety reporting in randomized trials of mental health interventions. Am J Psychiatry. 2004;161(9):1692–7.
763. Hughes S, Cohen D, Jaggi R. Differences in reporting serious adverse events in industry sponsored clinical trial registries and journal articles on antidepressant and antipsychotic drugs: a cross-sectional study. BMJ Open. 2014;4(7):e005535.

764. DeVito NJ, Bacon S, Goldacre B. Compliance with legal requirement to report clinical trial results on ClinicalTrials.gov: a cohort study. Lancet. 2020;395(10221):361–9.
765. Gotzsche PC, Hrobjartsson A, Johansen HK, Haahr MT, Altman DG, Chan AW. Ghost authorship in industry-initiated randomised trials. PLoS Med. 2007;4(1):e19.
766. Ross JS, Hill KP, Egilman DS, Krumholz HM. Guest authorship and ghostwriting in publications related to rofecoxib: a case study of industry documents from rofecoxib litigation. JAMA. 2008;299(15):1800–12.
767. Spielmans GI, Parry PI. From evidence-based medicine to marketing-based medicine: evidence from internal industry documents. J Bioethic Inq. 2010;7(1):13–29.
768. Every-Palmer S, Howick J. How evidence-based medicine is failing due to biased trials and selective publication. J Eval Clin Pract. 2014;20(6):908–14.
769. Spielmans GI, Biehn TL, Sawrey DL. A case study of salami slicing: pooled analyses of duloxetine for depression. Psychother Psychosom. 2010;79(2):97–106.
770. Healy D, Le Noury J, Wood J. Children of the cure: missing data, lost lives and antidepressants: Samizdat Health; 2020.
771. Lancet Editors. Depressing research. Lancet. 2004;363(9418):1335.
772. Ebrahim S, Bance S, Athale A, Malachowski C, Ioannidis JP. Meta-analyses with industry involvement are massively published and report no caveats for antidepressants. J Clin Epidemiol. 2016;70:155–63.
773. Pompili M, Serafini G, Innamorati M, Ambrosi E, Giordano G, Girardi P, et al. Antidepressants and suicide risk: a comprehensive overview. Pharmaceuticals (Basel). 2010;3(9):2861–83.
774. Kramer JC, Klein DF, Fink M. Withdrawal symptoms following dicontinuation of imipramine therapy. Am J Psychiatry. 1961;118:549–50.
775. Shatan C. Withdrawal symptoms after abrupt termination of imipramine. Can Psychiatr Assoc J. 1966;11:Suppl:150–8.
776. Teicher MH, Glod C, Cole JO. Emergence of intense suicidal preoccupation during fluoxetine treatment. Am J Psychiatry. 1990;147(2):207–10.
777. Beasley CM, Jr., Dornseif BE, Bosomworth JC, Sayler ME, Rampey AH, Jr., Heiligenstein JH, et al. Fluoxetine and suicide: a meta-analysis of controlled trials of treatment for depression. BMJ. 1991;303(6804):685–92.

778. Khan A, Khan S, Kolts R, Brown WA. Suicide rates in clinical trials of SSRIs, other antidepressants, and placebo: analysis of FDA reports. Am J Psychiatry. 2003;160(4):790–2.
779. Storosum JG, van Zwieten BJ, van den Brink W, Gersons BP, Broekmans AW. Suicide risk in placebo-controlled studies of major depression. Am J Psychiatry. 2001;158(8):1271–5.
780. Mosholder AD, Willy M. Suicidal adverse events in pediatric randomized, controlled clinical trials of antidepressant drugs are associated with active drug treatment: a meta-analysis. J Child Adolesc Psychopharmacol. 2006;16(1–2):25–32.
781. Reichenpfader U, Gartlehner G, Morgan LC, Greenblatt A, Nussbaumer B, Hansen RA, et al. Sexual dysfunction associated with second-generation antidepressants in patients with major depressive disorder: results from a systematic review with network meta-analysis. Drug Saf. 2014;37(1):19–31.
782. March J, Silva S, Petrycki S, Curry J, Wells K, Fairbank J, et al. Fluoxetine, cognitive-behavioral therapy, and their combination for adolescents with depression: Treatment for Adolescents with Depression Study (TADS) randomized controlled trial. JAMA. 2004;292(7):807–20.
783. March JS, Silva S, Petrycki S, Curry J, Wells K, Fairbank J, et al. The Treatment for Adolescents with Depression Study (TADS): long-term effectiveness and safety outcomes. Arch Gen Psychiatry. 2007;64(10):1132–43.
784. Jureidini JN, McHenry LB. Key opinion leaders and paediatric antidepressant overprescribing. Psychother Psychosom. 2009;78(4):197–201.
785. Jureidini JN, McHenry LB, Mansfield PR. Clinical trials and drug promotion: selective reporting of study 329. Int J Risk Saf Med. 2008;20:73–81.
786. McGoey L, Jackson E. Seroxat and the suppression of clinical trial data: regulatory failure and the uses of legal ambiguity. J Med Ethics. 2009;35(2):107–12.
787. Keller MB, Ryan ND, Strober M, Klein RG, Kutcher SP, Birmaher B, et al. Efficacy of paroxetine in the treatment of adolescent major depression: a randomized, controlled trial. J Am Acad Child Adolesc Psychiatry. 2001;40(7):762–72.
788. Kondro W, Sibbald B. Drug company experts advised staff to withhold data about SSRI use in children. CMAJ. 2004;170(5):783.

789. Rosack J. FDA warns of suicide risk with paroxetine. Psychiatric News. July 18, 2003.
790. Roehr B. GlaxoSmithKline is fined record $3bn in US. BMJ. 2012;345:e4568.
791. Doshi P. No correction, no retraction, no apology, no comment: paroxetine trial reanalysis raises questions about institutional responsibility. BMJ. 2015;351:h4629.
792. Johnson CF, Williams B, MacGillivray SA, Dougall NJ, Maxwell M. 'Doing the right thing': factors influencing GP prescribing of antidepressants and prescribed doses. BMC Fam Pract. 2017;18(1):72.
793. Mercier A, Auger-Aubin I, Lebeau JP, Van Royen P, Peremans L. Understanding the prescription of antidepressants: a qualitative study among French GPs. BMC Fam Pract. 2011;12:99.
794. Bekelman JE, Li Y, Gross CP. Scope and impact of financial conflicts of interest in biomedical research: a systematic review. JAMA. 2003;289(4):454–65.
795. Lundh A, Lexchin J, Mintzes B, Schroll JB, Bero L. Industry sponsorship and research outcome. Cochrane Database Syst Rev. 2017;2:MR000033.
796. Mitchell AP, Trivedi NU, Gennarelli RL, Chimonas S, Tabatabai SM, Goldberg J, et al. Are financial payments from the pharmaceutical industry associated with physician prescribing? A systematic review. Ann Intern Med. 2021;174(3):353–61.
797. Psaty BM, Kronmal RA. Reporting mortality findings in trials of rofecoxib for Alzheimer disease or cognitive impairment: a case study based on documents from rofecoxib litigation. JAMA. 2008;299(15):1813–7.
798. Spurling GK, Mansfield PR, Montgomery BD, Lexchin J, Doust J, Othman N, et al. Information from pharmaceutical companies and the quality, quantity, and cost of physicians' prescribing: a systematic review. PLoS Med. 2010;7(10):e1000352.
799. Wang AT, McCoy CP, Murad MH, Montori VM. Association between industry affiliation and position on cardiovascular risk with rosiglitazone: cross sectional systematic review. BMJ. 2010;340:c1344.
800. Macdonald H, McCartney M, Heneghan C, Godlee F. Doctors' conflicts of interest. BMJ. 2020;370:m3247.
801. Camilleri M, Cortese DA. Managing conflict of interest in clinical practice. Mayo Clin Proc. 2007;82(5):607–14.
802. Brody H. Clarifying conflict of interest. Am J Bioeth. 2011;11(1):23–8.

803. Wiersma M, Kerridge I, Lipworth W. Dangers of neglecting non-financial conflicts of interest in health and medicine. J Med Ethics. 2018;44(5):319–22.
804. Rice DB, Raffoul H, Ioannidis JPA, Moher D. Academic criteria for promotion and tenure in biomedical sciences faculties: cross sectional analysis of international sample of universities. BMJ. 2020;369:m2081.
805. Aarts AA, Anderson JE, Anderson CJ, Attridge PR, Attwood A, Axt J, et al. Estimating the reproducibility of psychological science. Science. 2015;349(6251):aac4716.
806. Luborsky L, Diguer L, Seligman DA, Rosenthal R, Krause ED, Johnson S, et al. The researcher's own therapy allegiances: a "wild card" in comparisons of treatment efficacy. Clin Psychol-Sci Pr. 1999;6(1):95–106.
807. Munder T, Brutsch O, Leonhart R, Gerger H, Barth J. Researcher allegiance in psychotherapy outcome research: an overview of reviews. Clin Psychol Rev. 2013;33(4):501–11.
808. Chervenak FA, McCullough LB, Hale RW. Guild interests: an insidious threat to professionalism in obstetrics and gynecology. Am J Obstet Gynecol. 2018;219(6):581–4.
809. Minkoff H, Ecker J. When guild interests and professional obligations collide. Obstet Gynecol. 2017;130(2):454–7.
810. Krumholz HM. A note to my younger colleagues…be brave. Circ Cardiovasc Qual Outcomes. 2012;5(3):245–6.
811. Bennett CL, Hoque S, Olivieri N, Taylor MA, Aboulafia D, Lubaczewski C, et al. Consequences to patients, clinicians, and manufacturers when very serious adverse drug reactions are identified (1997–2019): a qualitative analysis from the Southern Network on Adverse Reactions (SONAR). EClinicalMedicine. 2021;31:100693.
812. Schafer A. Biomedical conflicts of interest: a defence of the sequestration thesis-learning from the cases of Nancy Olivieri and David Healy. J Med Ethics. 2004;30(1):8–24.
813. Cumberlege J. First do no harm: the report of the Independent Medicines and Medical Devices Safety Review. July 8, 2020.
814. Haskell H. Cumberlege review exposes stubborn and dangerous flaws in healthcare. BMJ. 2020;370:m3099.
815. Allen M, Pierce O, Zamora A. The voices of patient harm. ProPublica; July 19, 2013.

816. Golomb BA, McGraw JJ, Evans MA, Dimsdale JE. Physician response to patient reports of adverse drug effects: implications for patient-targeted adverse effect surveillance. Drug Saf. 2007;30(8):669–75.
817. Hohl CM, Small SS, Peddie D, Badke K, Bailey C, Balka E. Why clinicians don't report adverse drug events: qualitative study. JMIR Public Health Surveill. 2018;4(1):e21.
818. Hazell L, Shakir SA. Under-reporting of adverse drug reactions: a systematic review. Drug Saf. 2006;29(5):385–96.
819. Zed PJ, Abu-Laban RB, Balen RM, Loewen PS, Hohl CM, Brubacher JR, et al. Incidence, severity and preventability of medication-related visits to the emergency department: a prospective study. CMAJ. 2008;178(12):1563–9.
820. Lazarou J, Pomeranz BH, Corey PN. Incidence of adverse drug reactions in hospitalized patients—a meta-analysis of prospective studies. JAMA. 1998;279(15):1200–5.
821. Furberg CD, Levin AA, Gross PA, Shapiro RS, Strom BL. The FDA and drug safety: a proposal for sweeping changes. Arch Intern Med. 2006;166(18):1938–42.
822. Kesselheim AS, Avorn J. The role of litigation in defining drug risks. JAMA. 2007;297(3):308–11.
823. Abraham J. Transnational industrial power, the medical profession and the regulatory state: adverse drug reactions and the crisis over the safety of Halcion in the Netherlands and the UK. Soc Sci Med. 2002;55(9):1671–90.
824. Krumholz HM, Ross JS, Presler AH, Egilman DS. What have we learnt from Vioxx? BMJ. 2007;334(7585):120–3.
825. Abraham J, Davis C. International and temporal comparative analysis of UK and US drug safety regulation in changing political contexts. Soc Sci Med. 2020;255:113005.
826. Lasser KE, Allen PD, Woolhandler SJ, Himmelstein DU, Wolfe SM, Bor DH. Timing of new black box warnings and withdrawals for prescription medications. JAMA. 2002;287(17):2215–20.
827. Lexchin J. New drugs and safety: what happened to new active substances approved in Canada between 1995 and 2010? Arch Intern Med. 2012;172(21):1680–1.
828. Braslow JT, Marder SR. History of psychopharmacology. Annu Rev Clin Psychol. 2019;15:25–50.

829. Cristea IA, Naudet F. Defending psychiatry or defending the trivial effects of therapeutic interventions? A citation content analysis of an influential paper. Epidemiol Psychiatr Sci. 2018;27(3):230–9.
830. Lowry F. APA blasts 60 minutes program on antidepressants. Medscape. March 20, 2012.
831. Whitaker R. Psychiatry defends its antipsychotics: a case study of institutional corruption. Mad in America; May 21, 2017.
832. Dharmawardene V, Menkes DB. Responding to the UN Special Rapporteur's anti-psychiatry bias. Aust N Z J Psychiatry. 2019;53(4):282–3.
833. Hengartner MP. Targeting the replication crisis and improving the credibility of research findings in clinical psychology. A commentary on Pittelkow et al. Clin Psychol Sci Prac. 2021;28(2):226–8.
834. Davies J. Calling someone 'anti-psychiatry' is not an argument—and for many it feels abusive. Mad in the UK; February 22, 2020.
835. Mark TL, Levit KR, Buck JA. Datapoints: psychotropic drug prescriptions by medical specialty. Psychiatr Serv. 2009;60(9):1167.
836. Kirsch I, Moore TJ, Scoboria A, Nicholls SS. The emperor's new drugs: an analysis of antidepressant medication data submitted to the U.S. Food and Drug Administration. Prev Treat. 2002;5(1):23.
837. Fountoulakis KN, Moller HJ. Efficacy of antidepressants: a re-analysis and re-interpretation of the Kirsch data. Int J Neuropsychopharmacol. 2011;14(3):405–12.
838. Klein DF. Listening to meta-analysis but hearing bias. Prev Treat. 1998;1(2):6c.
839. Horder J, Matthews P, Waldmann R. Placebo, prozac and PLoS: significant lessons for psychopharmacology. J Psychopharmacol. 2011;25(10):1277–88.
840. Moncrieff J. Against the stream: antidepressants are not antidepressants—an alternative approach to drug action and implications for the use of antidepressants. Bjpsych Bull. 2018;42(1):42–4.
841. Hengartner MP, Passalacqua S, Andreae A, Heinsius T, Hepp U, Rossler W, et al. Antidepressant use during acute inpatient care is associated with an increased risk of psychiatric rehospitalisation over a 12-month follow-up after discharge. Front Psychiatry. 2019;10:79.
842. Seifritz E. Commentary: antidepressant use during acute inpatient care is associated with an increased risk of psychiatric rehospitalisation over a 12-month follow-up after discharge. Front Psychiatry. 2019;10:990.

843. Brugha TS, Bebbington PE, MacCarthy B, Sturt E, Wykes T. Antidepressants may not assist recovery in practice: a naturalistic prospective survey. Acta Psychiatr Scand. 1992;86(1):5–11.
844. Mass R, Backhaus K, Hestermann D, Balzer C, Szelies M. Inpatient treatment decreases depression but antidepressants may not contribute. A prospective quasi-experimental study. Compr Psychiatry. 2019;94:152124.
845. Hengartner MP, Davies J, Read J. How long does antidepressant withdrawal typically last? Am J Psychiatry. 2019;176(6):487.
846. Hengartner MP, Ploderl M. Starting two antidepressants to prevent suicide: a potentially dangerous recommendation? Aust N Z J Psychiatry. 2018:4867418816811.
847. Volkmann C, Ploderl M, Hengartner MP. Comment on Osler et al: misinterpretation of pre-post differences invalidates the authors' conclusions. Acta Psychiatr Scand. 2019;140(6):589–90.
848. Ongur D, Bauchner H. Notice of retraction: Maslej et al. individual differences in response to antidepressants: a meta-analysis of placebo-controlled randomized clinical trials. JAMA Psychiatry. 2020;77(6):607–617. JAMA Psychiatry. 2020;77(8):786.
849. Volkmann C, Volkmann A, Hengartner MP, Plöderl M. Commentary on Maslej et al: no evidence of individual differences in response to antidepressants. Researchgate.net;2020.
850. Gossweiler A. Kreuzzug für umstrittene Psychopillen. Gesundheitstipp. February, 2020:22–3.
851. Anderegg S, Huwiler S. Diese Ärzte kassieren am meisten. Tagesanzeiger. August 28, 2020.
852. International Committee of Medical Journal Editors. Recommendations for the conduct, reporting, editing, and publication of scholarly work in medical journals. International Committee of Medical Journal Editors. December 2019.
853. Reichmuth A. Selbst Alltagsstress gilt als unerkannte depression. Tagesanzeiger. November 28, 2019.
854. Alberti S, Chiesa A, Andrisano C, Serretti A. Insomnia and somnolence associated with second-generation antidepressants during the treatment of major depression: a meta-analysis. J Clin Psychopharmacol. 2015;35(3):296–303.
855. Hengartner MP, Plöderl M. Reply to the letter to the editor: "newer-generation antidepressants and suicide risk: thoughts on Hengartner and Ploderl's re-analysis". Psychother Psychosom. 2019;88(6):373–4.

856. Tungaraza T, Poole R. Influence of drug company authorship and sponsorship on drug trial outcomes. Br J Psychiatry. 2007;191:82–3.
857. Meschenmoser M. Pharma: 300‘000 Franken in Professoren-Pensionskasse. Schweizer Radio und Fernsehen (SRF); April 20, 2016.
858. O’Brien C. Addiction and dependence in DSM-V. Addiction. 2011;106(5):866–7.
859. Straumann F. Antidepressiva wirken. Tagesanzeiger. January 31, 2020.
860. Holsboer-Trachsler E, Hättenschwiler J, Beck J, Brand S, Hemmeter UM, Ekkehard Keck M, et al. Die Akutbehandlung depressiver Episoden. Swiss Medical Forum. 2016;16(35):716–24.
861. Bschor T. [Antidepressants do not prevent suicide attempts or suicides]. Nervenarzt. 2015;86(9):1168–9.
862. Hengartner MP, Amendola S, Kaminski JA, Kindler S, Bschor T, Plöderl M. Suicide risk with selective serotonin reuptake inhibitors and other new-generation antidepressants in adults: a systematic review and meta-analysis of observational studies. J Epidemiol Community Health. 2021; https://doi.org/10.1136/jech-2020-214611.
863. Safer DJ, Zito JM. Do antidepressants reduce suicide rates? Public Health. 2007;121(4):274–7.
864. Spielmans GI, Spence-Sing T, Parry P. Duty to warn: antidepressant black box suicidality warning is empirically justified. Front Psychiatry. 2020;11:18.
865. Horowitz MA, Taylor D. Tapering of SSRI treatment to mitigate withdrawal symptoms. Lancet Psychiatry. 2019;6(6):538–46.
866. American Academy of Pain Medicine, American Pain Society, American Society of Addiction Medicine. Definitions related to the use of opioids for the treatment of pain. American Academy of Pain Medicine, American Pain Society, American Society of Addiction Medicine; 2001.
867. National Institute on Drug Abuse. Tolerance, dependence, addiction: what’s the difference? National Institute on Drug Abuse; January 12, 2017.
868. Nielsen M, Hansen EH, Gotzsche PC. What is the difference between dependence and withdrawal reactions? A comparison of benzodiazepines and selective serotonin re-uptake inhibitors. Addiction. 2012;107(5):900–8.
869. Balon R, Silberman EK, Starcevic V, Cosci F, Freire RC, Nardi AE, et al. Benzodiazepines, antidepressants and addiction: a plea for conceptual rigor and consistency. J Psychopharmacol. 2019;33(11):1467–70.

870. Meyer JH, Kapur S, Eisfeld B, Brown GM, Houle S, DaSilva J, et al. The effect of paroxetine on 5-HT(2A) receptors in depression: an [(18) F]setoperone PET imaging study. Am J Psychiatry. 2001;158(1):78–85.
871. Glenmullen J. The antidepressant solution. New York, NY: Simon & Schuster; 2006.
872. Royal College of Psychiatrists. Position statement on antidepressants and depression. November 25, 2019. Available from: https://www.rcpsych.ac.uk/docs/default-source/improving-care/better-mh-policy/position-statements/ps04_19%2D%2D-antidepressants-and-depression.pdf?sfvrsn=ddea9473_5.
873. Hengartner MP, Plöderl M. False beliefs in academic psychiatry: the case of antidepressant drugs. Ethical Hum Psychol Psychiatry. 2018;20(1):6–16.
874. Nielsen M, Hansen EH, Gotzsche PC. Dependence and withdrawal reactions to benzodiazepines and selective serotonin reuptake inhibitors. How did the health authorities react? Int J Risk Saf Med. 2013;25(3):155–68.
875. Medawar C. Through the doors of deception? Nature. 1994;368:369–70.
876. Freeman H. Listening to Prozac. Nature. 1994;369:178.
877. Schatzberg AF, Haddad P, Kaplan EM, Lejoyeux M, Rosenbaum JF, Young AH, et al. Serotonin reuptake inhibitor discontinuation syndrome: a hypothetical definition. Discontinuation Consensus panel. J Clin Psychiatry. 1997;58(Suppl 7):5–10.
878. Fava GA, Belaise C. Discontinuing antidepressant drugs: lesson from a failed trial and extensive clinical experience. Psychother Psychosom. 2018;87(5):257–67.
879. Lane C. Antidepressant withdrawal and scientific consensus. Psychology Today. August 26, 2019.
880. Guy A, Brown M, Lewis S, Horowitz M. The 'patient voice': patients who experience antidepressant withdrawal symptoms are often dismissed, or misdiagnosed with relapse, or a new medical condition. Ther Adv Psychopharmacol. 2020;10:2045125320967183.
881. Framer A. What I have learnt from helping thousands of people taper off antidepressants and other psychotropic medications. Ther Adv Psychopharmacol. 2021;11:2045125321991274.
882. Kessing LV, Hansen HV, Demyttenaere K, Bech P. Depressive and bipolar disorders: patients' attitudes and beliefs towards depression and antidepressants. Psychol Med. 2005;35(8):1205–13.

883. Carey B, Gebeloff B. Many people taking antidepressants discover they cannot quit. New York Times. April 7, 2018.
884. Baldwin DS, Montgomery SA, Nil R, Lader M. Discontinuation symptoms in depression and anxiety disorders. Int J Neuropsychopharmacol. 2007;10(1):73–84.
885. Stockmann T, Odegbaro D, Timimi S, Moncrieff J. SSRI and SNRI withdrawal symptoms reported on an internet forum. Int J Risk Saf Med. 2018;29(3–4):175–80.
886. Perlis RH. Anxiety about antidepressants. Am J Psychiatry. 2018;175(6):500–1.
887. Calling S, Midlov P, Johansson SE, Sundquist K, Sundquist J. Longitudinal trends in self-reported anxiety. Effects of age and birth cohort during 25 years. BMC Psychiatry. 2017;17(1):119.
888. Hedegaard H, Curtin SC, Warner M. Suicide mortality in the United States, 1999–2017. Hyattsville, MD: National Center for Health Statistics; 2018.
889. Mojtabai R, Jorm AF. Trends in psychological distress, depressive episodes and mental health treatment-seeking in the United States: 2001–2012. J Affect Disord. 2015;174:556–61.
890. Weinberger AH, Gbedemah M, Martinez AM, Nash D, Galea S, Goodwin RD. Trends in depression prevalence in the USA from 2005 to 2015: widening disparities in vulnerable groups. Psychol Med. 2017:1–10.
891. Ormel J, Kessler RC, Schoevers R. Depression: more treatment but no drop in prevalence: how effective is treatment? And can we do better? Curr Opin Psychiatry. 2019;32(4):348–54.
892. Judge R, Parry MG, Quail D, Jacobson JG. Discontinuation symptoms: comparison of brief interruption in fluoxetine and paroxetine treatment. Int Clin Psychopharmacol. 2002;17(5):217–25.
893. Sir A, D'Souza RF, Uguz S, George T, Vahip S, Hopwood M, et al. Randomized trial of sertraline versus venlafaxine XR in major depression: efficacy and discontinuation symptoms. J Clin Psychiatry. 2005;66(10):1312–20.
894. Groot PC, van Os J. How user knowledge of psychotropic drug withdrawal resulted in the development of person-specific tapering medication. Ther Adv Psychopharmacol. 2020;10:2045125320932452.

895. Horowitz MA. Peer-support groups were right, guidelines were wrong: Dr. Mark Horowitz on tapering off antidepressants. Mad in America; 2019.
896. Stockmann T. What it was like to stop an antidepressant. Ther Adv Psychopharmacol. 2019;9:2045125319884834.
897. White E, Read J, Julo S. The role of Facebook groups in the management and raising of awareness of antidepressant withdrawal: is social media filling the void left by health services? Ther Adv Psychopharmacol. 2021;11:2045125320981174.
898. Hogberg G, Antonuccio DO, Healy D. Suicidal risk from TADS study was higher than it first appeared. Int J Risk Saf Med. 2015;27(2):85–91.
899. Isacsson G, Rich CL, Jureidini J, Raven M. The increased use of antidepressants has contributed to the worldwide reduction in suicide rates. Br J Psychiatry. 2010;196(6):429–33.
900. Sparks JA, Duncan BL. Outside the black box: re-assessing pediatric antidepressant prescription. J Can Acad Child Adolesc Psychiatry. 2013;22(3):240–6.
901. Stone MB. The FDA warning on antidepressants and suicidality—why the controversy? N Engl J Med. 2014;371(18):1668–71.
902. Khan A, Warner HA, Brown WA. Symptom reduction and suicide risk in patients treated with placebo in antidepressant clinical trials—an analysis of the food and drug administration database. Arch Gen Psychiat. 2000;57(4):311–7.
903. Pharmacovigilance Working Party. Antidepressants and suicidal thoughts and behaviour. MHRA; January 2008.
904. Zalsman G, Hawton K, Wasserman D, van Heeringen K, Arensman E, Sarchiapone M, et al. Suicide prevention strategies revisited: 10-year systematic review. Lancet Psychiatry. 2016;3(7):646–59.
905. Amendola S, Plöderl M, Hengartner MP. Did the introduction and increased prescribing of antidepressants lead to changes in long-term trends of suicide rates? Eur J Public Health. 2021;31(2):291–7.
906. Hengartner MP, Amendola S, Kaminski JA, Kindler S, Bschor T, Plöderl M. Suicide risk with selective serotonin reuptake inhibitors and other new-generation antidepressants in adults: a systematic review and meta-analysis of observational studies. J Epidemiol Community Health. 2021;in press.
907. Teicher MH, Glod CA, Cole JO. Antidepressant drugs and the emergence of suicidal tendencies. Drug Saf. 1993;8(3):186–212.

908. Mathews AW. In debate over antidepressants, FDA weighed risk of false alarm. Doubting data on suicide and kids, officials stopped presentation by staffer. The Wall Street Journal. May 25, 2004.
909. Alliance for Human Research Protection. Letter of complaint to FDA Commissioner, 2007. Alliance for Human Research Protection. November 30, 2007.
910. Medawar C, Herxheimer A, Bell A, Jofre S. Paroxetine, Panorama and user reporting of ADRs: consumer intelligence matters in clinical practice and post-marketing drug surveillance. Int J Risk Saf Med. 2002;15(3–4):161–9.
911. Bruder C, Bulliard JL, Germann S, Konzelmann I, Bochud M, Leyvraz M, et al. Estimating lifetime and 10-year risk of lung cancer. Prev Med Rep. 2018;11:125–30.
912. Olfson M, Shaffer D. SSRI prescriptions and the rate of suicide. Am J Psychiatry. 2007;164(12):1907–8.
913. Stone MB. In search of a Pony: sources, methods, outcomes, and motivated reasoning. Med Care. 2018;56(5):375–81.
914. Wheeler BW, Gunnell D, Metcalfe C, Stephens P, Martin RM. The population impact on incidence of suicide and non-fatal self harm of regulatory action against the use of selective serotonin reuptake inhibitors in under 18s in the United Kingdom: ecological study. BMJ. 2008;336(7643):542–5.
915. Wheeler BW, Metcalfe C, Martin RM, Gunnell D. International impacts of regulatory action to limit antidepressant prescribing on rates of suicide in young people. Pharmacoepidemiol Drug Saf. 2009;18(7):579–88.
916. Greenland S, Morgenstern H. Ecological bias, confounding, and effect modification. Int J Epidemiol. 1989;18(1):269–74.
917. Dahlberg M, Lundin D. Antidepressants and the suicide rate: is there really a connection? Adv Health Econ Health Serv Res. 2005;16:121–41.
918. Zahl PH, De Leo D, Ekeberg O, Hjelmeland H, Dieserud G. The relationship between sales of SSRI, TCA and suicide rates in the Nordic countries. BMC Psychiatry. 2010;10:62.
919. Baldessarini RJ, Tondo L, Strombom IM, Dominguez S, Fawcett J, Licinio J, et al. Ecological studies of antidepressant treatment and suicidal risks. Harv Rev Psychiatry. 2007;15(4):133–45.
920. Kamat MA, Edgar L, Niblock P, McDowell C, Kelly CB. Association between antidepressant prescribing and suicide rates in OECD countries: an ecological study. Pharmacopsychiatry. 2014;47(1):18–21.

921. Barnhorst A. The empty promise of suicide prevention. The New York Times. April 26, 2019.
922. Whitaker R, Blumke D. Screening + drug treatment = increase in veteran suicides. Mad in America; November 10, 2019.
923. Fava GA. The cult of mediocrity. Psychother Psychosom. 2005;74(1):1–2.
924. Kuhn TS. The structure of scientific revolutions. 3rd ed. Chicago: University of Chicago Press; 1996.
925. Arnold DG, Stewart OJ, Beck T. Financial penalties imposed on large pharmaceutical firms for illegal activities. JAMA. 2020;324(19):1995–7.
926. Almashat S, Lang R, Wolfe SM, Carome M. Twenty-seven years of pharmaceutical industry criminal and civil penalties: 1991 through 2017. Public Citizen; March 14, 2018.
927. Outterson K. Punishing health care fraud—is the GSK settlement sufficient? N Engl J Med. 2012;367(12):1082–5.
928. Marks JH. Lessons from corporate influence in the opioid epidemic: toward a norm of separation. J Bioethic Inq. 2020;17(2):173–89.
929. Healton C, Pack R, Galea S. The opioid crisis, corporate responsibility, and lessons from the tobacco Master Settlement Agreement. JAMA. 2019;322(21):2071–2.
930. Kolodny A, Courtwright DT, Hwang CS, Kreiner P, Eadie JL, Clark TW, et al. The prescription opioid and heroin crisis: a public health approach to an epidemic of addiction. Annu Rev Public Health. 2015;36:559–74.
931. Van Zee A. The promotion and marketing of oxycontin: commercial triumph, public health tragedy. Am J Public Health. 2009;99(2):221–7.
932. Hoffman J, Benner K. Purdue Pharma pleads guilty to criminal charges for opioid sales. The New York Times. October 21, 2020.
933. Chimonas S, Stahl F, Rothman DJ. Exposing conflict of interest in psychiatry: does transparency matter? Int J Law Psychiatry. 2012;35(5–6):490–5.
934. Blackwell B. International Network for the History of Neuropsychopharmacology. 2017. Available from: http://inhn.org/controversies/barry-blackwell-corporate-corruption-in-the-psychopharmaceutical-industry-revised.html.
935. Amsterdam JD, McHenry LB, Jureidini JN. Industry-corrupted psychiatric trials. Psychiatr Pol. 2017;51(6):993–1008.
936. Kelly RE, Jr., Cohen LJ, Semple RJ, Bialer P, Lau A, Bodenheimer A, et al. Relationship between drug company funding and outcomes of clinical psychiatric research. Psychol Med. 2006;36(11):1647–56.

937. Raven M, Parry P. Psychotropic marketing practices and problems: implications for DSM-5. J Nerv Ment Dis. 2012;200(6):512–6.
938. Healy D, Thase ME. Is academic psychiatry for sale? Br J Psychiatry. 2003;182:388–90.
939. Brennan TA, Rothman DJ, Blank L, Blumenthal D, Chimonas SC, Cohen JJ, et al. Health industry practices that create conflicts of interest—a policy proposal for academic medical centers. JAMA. 2006;295(4):429–33.
940. DeAngelis CD, Fontanarosa PB. Impugning the integrity of medical science—the adverse effects of industry influence. JAMA. 2008;299(15):1833–5.
941. De Jesus-Morales K, Prasad V. Closed financial loops: when they happen in government, they're called corruption; in medicine, they're just a footnote. Hastings Cent Rep. 2017;47(3):9–14.
942. Steinbrook R, Kassirer JP, Angell M. Justifying conflicts of interest in medical journals: a very bad idea. BMJ. 2015;350:h2942.
943. Brax H, Fadlallah R, Al-Khaled L, Kahale LA, Nas H, El-Jardali F, et al. Association between physicians' interaction with pharmaceutical companies and their clinical practices: a systematic review and meta-analysis. Plos One. 2017;12(4):e0175493.
944. Kjaergard LL, Als-Nielsen B. Association between competing interests and authors' conclusions: epidemiological study of randomised clinical trials published in the BMJ. BMJ. 2002;325(7358):249.
945. Lin DH, Lucas E, Murimi IB, Kolodny A, Alexander GC. Financial conflicts of interest and the Centers for Disease Control and Prevention's 2016 guideline for prescribing opioids for chronic pain. JAMA Intern Med. 2017;177(3):427–8.
946. Nejstgaard CH, Bero L, Hrobjartsson A, Jorgensen AW, Jorgensen KJ, Le M, et al. Association between conflicts of interest and favourable recommendations in clinical guidelines, advisory committee reports, opinion pieces, and narrative reviews: systematic review. BMJ. 2020;371:m4234.
947. Stelfox HT, Chua G, O'Rourke K, Detsky AS. Conflict of interest in the debate over calcium-channel antagonists. N Engl J Med. 1998;338(2):101–6.
948. Yank V, Rennie D, Bero LA. Financial ties and concordance between results and conclusions in meta-analyses: retrospective cohort study. BMJ. 2007;335(7631):1202–5.

949. Abraham J. Sociology of pharmaceuticals development and regulation: a realist empirical research programme. Sociol Health Ill. 2008;30(6):869–85.
950. Piller C. FDA's own documents reveal agency's lax, slow, and secretive oversight of clinical research. Science; October 1, 2020.
951. Dal-Re R, Kesselheim AS, Bourgeois FT. Increasing access to FDA inspection reports on irregularities and misconduct in clinical trials. JAMA. 2020;323(19):1903–4.
952. Abraham J. Partial progress: governing the pharmaceutical industry and the NHS, 1948–2008. J Health Polit Policy Law. 2009;34(6):931–77.
953. Lenzer J. FDA bars own expert from evaluating risks of painkillers. BMJ. 2004;329(7476):1203.
954. Fromer MJ. Survey of FDA scientists shows they feel pressure to exclude or alter findings: fear retaliation for voicing safety concerns. Oncology Times. 2006;28(16):12–6.
955. Darrow JJ, Avorn J, Kesselheim AS. FDA approval and regulation of pharmaceuticals, 1983–2018. JAMA. 2020;323(2):164–76.
956. Davis C, Abraham J. Unhealthy pharmaceutical regulation: innovation, politics and promissory science. London: Palgrave Macmillan; 2013.
957. Carpenter D, Chattopadhyay J, Moffitt S, Nall C. The complications of controlling agency time discretion: FDA review deadlines and postmarket drug safety. Am J Pol Sci. 2012;56(1):98–114.
958. Ledford H. Physician with drug-industry ties is Trump's FDA pick. Nature. March 10, 2017.
959. LaVito A. Former FDA Commissioner Scott Gottliebt joins Pfizer's board of directors. CNBC. June 27, 2019.
960. Piller C. FDA's revolving door: companies often hire agency staffers who managed their successful drug reviews. Science. July 5, 2018.
961. Hayes MJ, Prasad V. Financial conflicts of interest at FDA Drug Advisory Committee meetings. Hastings Cent Rep. 2018;48(2):10–3.
962. Pham-Kanter G. Revisiting financial conflicts of interest in FDA advisory committees. The Milbank Quarterly. 2014;92(3):446–70.
963. Steinbrook R. Financial conflicts of interest and the Food and Drug Administration's Advisory Committees. N Engl J Med. 2005;353(2):116–8.
964. Piller C. Hidden conflicts? Science. 2018;361(6397):16–20.
965. Testoni FE, Garcia Carrillo M, Gagnon MA, Rikap C, Blaustein M. Whose shoulders is health research standing on? Determining the key

actors and contents of the prevailing biomedical research agenda. PLoS One. 2021;16(4):e0249661.

966. Lundbeckfonden. Six brain professors receive DKK 232 million. Lundbeck Foundation; December 10, 2019.
967. Anderson TS, Dave S, Good CB, Gellad WF. Academic medical center leadership on pharmaceutical company boards of directors. JAMA. 2014;311(13):1353–5.
968. Anderson TS, Good CB, Gellad WF. Prevalence and compensation of academic leaders, professors, and trustees on publicly traded US healthcare company boards of directors: cross sectional study. BMJ. 2015;351:h4826.
969. Campbell EG, Weissman JS, Ehringhaus S, Rao SR, Moy B, Feibelmann S, et al. Institutional academic industry relationships. JAMA. 2007;298(15):1779–86.
970. Dorsey ER, de Roulet J, Thompson JP, Reminick JI, Thai A, White-Stellato Z, et al. Funding of US biomedical research, 2003–2008. JAMA. 2010;303(2):137–43.
971. Rottingen JA, Regmi S, Eide M, Young AJ, Viergever RF, Ardal C, et al. Mapping of available health research and development data: what's there, what's missing, and what role is there for a global observatory? Lancet. 2013;382(9900):1286–307.
972. Rasmussen K, Schroll J, Gotzsche PC, Lundh A. Under-reporting of conflicts of interest among trialists: a cross-sectional study. J R Soc Med. 2015;108(3):101–7.
973. Tau N, Shochat T, Gafter-Gvili A, Amir E, Shepshelovich D. Undisclosed financial conflicts of interest of authors of clinical drug trials published in influential medical journals: a cohort study. Mayo Clin Proc. 2019;94(11):2272–6.
974. Rush AJ, Trivedi MH, Wisniewski SR, Nierenberg AA, Stewart JW, Warden D, et al. Acute and longer-term outcomes in depressed outpatients requiring one or several treatment steps: a STAR*D report. Am J Psychiatry. 2006;163(11):1905–17.
975. Thacker PD. A few tiny steps towards transparency: how the Sunshine Act shone light on industry's influence in medicine. BMJ. 2020;370:m3229.
976. Norris SL, Holmer HK, Ogden LA, Burda BU, Fu R. Characteristics of physicians receiving large payments from pharmaceutical companies and the accuracy of their disclosures in publications: an observational study. BMC Med Ethics. 2012;13:24.

977. Harris G. Drug maker told studies would aid it, papers say. The New York Times. March 19, 2009.
978. Harris G. Top psychiatrist didn't report drug makers' pay. The New York Times. October 3, 2008.
979. Smith R. Medical journals and pharmaceutical companies: uneasy bedfellows. BMJ. 2003;326(7400):1202–5.
980. Lexchin J, Light DW. Commercial influence and the content of medical journals. BMJ. 2006;332(7555):1444–7.
981. Glassman PA, Hunter-Hayes J, Nakamura T. Pharmaceutical advertising revenue and physician organizations: how much is too much? West J Med. 1999;171(4):234–8.
982. Smith R. Lapses at the New England Journal of Medicine. J Roy Soc Med. 2006;99(8):380–2.
983. Lundh A, Barbateskovic M, Hrobjartsson A, Gotzsche PC. Conflicts of interest at medical journals: the influence of industry-supported randomised trials on journal impact factors and revenue—cohort study. PLoS Med. 2010;7(10):e1000354.
984. Liu JJ, Bell CM, Matelski JJ, Detsky AS, Cram P. Payments by US pharmaceutical and medical device manufacturers to US medical journal editors: retrospective—observational study. BMJ. 2017;359.
985. Haque W, Minhajuddin A, Gupta A, Agrawal D. Conflicts of interest of editors of medical journals. PLoS One. 2018;13(5):e0197141.
986. Dal-Re R, Bouter LM, Moher D, Marusic A. Mandatory disclosure of financial interests of journals and editors. BMJ. 2020;370:j4619.
987. Ozieranski P, Csanadi M, Rickard E, Tchilingirian J, Mulinari S. Analysis of pharmaceutical industry payments to UK Health Care Organizations in 2015. JAMA Netw Open. 2019;2(6):e196253.
988. Moynihan R, Albarqouni L, Nangla C, Dunn AG, Lexchin J, Bero L. Financial ties between leaders of influential US professional medical associations and industry: cross sectional study. BMJ. 2020;369:m1505.
989. Lurie P, Tran T, Wolfe SM, Goodman R. Violations of exhibiting and FDA rules at an American Psychiatric Association annual meeting. J Public Health Policy. 2005;26(4):389–99.
990. Cosgrove L, Wheeler EE. Drug firms, the codification of diagnostic categories, and bias in clinical guidelines. J Law Med Ethics. 2013;41(3):644–53.

991. Cosgrove L, Krimsky S. A comparison of DSM-IV and DSM-5 panel members' financial associations with industry: a pernicious problem persists. PLoS Med. 2012;9(3):e1001190.
992. Cosgrove L, Bursztajn HJ, Krimsky S, Anaya M, Walker J. Conflicts of interest and disclosure in the American Psychiatric Association's clinical practice guidelines. Psychother Psychosom. 2009;78(4):228–32.
993. Cosgrove L, Shaughnessy AF, Peters SM, Lexchin JR, Bursztajn H, Bero L. Conflicts of interest and the presence of methodologists on guideline development panels: a cross-sectional study of clinical practice guidelines for major depressive disorder. Psychother Psychosom. 2017;86(3):168–70.
994. Norris SL, Holmer HK, Ogden LA, Burda BU. Conflict of interest in clinical practice guideline development: a systematic review. PLoS One. 2011;6(10):e25153.
995. Choudhry NK, Stelfox HT, Detsky AS. Relationships between authors of clinical practice guidelines and the pharmaceutical industry. JAMA. 2002;287(5):612–7.
996. Kung J, Miller RR, Mackowiak PA. Failure of clinical practice guidelines to meet institute of medicine standards: two more decades of little, if any, progress. Arch Intern Med. 2012;172(21):1628–33.
997. Khan R, Scaffidi MA, Rumman A, Grindal AW, Plener IS, Grover SC. Prevalence of financial conflicts of interest among authors of clinical guidelines related to high-revenue medications. JAMA Intern Med. 2018;178(12):1712–5.
998. Neuman J, Korenstein D, Ross JS, Keyhani S. Prevalence of financial conflicts of interest among panel members producing clinical practice guidelines in Canada and United States: cross sectional study. BMJ. 2011;343:d5621.
999. Campsall P, Colizza K, Straus S, Stelfox HT. Financial relationships between organizations that produce clinical practice guidelines and the biomedical industry: a cross-sectional study. PLoS Med. 2016;13(5):e1002029.
1000. Elder K, Turner KA, Cosgrove L, Lexchin J, Shnier A, Moore A, et al. Reporting of financial conflicts of interest by Canadian clinical practice guideline producers: a descriptive study. CMAJ. 2020;192(23):E617–25.
1001. Bindslev JB, Schroll J, Gotzsche PC, Lundh A. Underreporting of conflicts of interest in clinical practice guidelines: cross sectional study. BMC Med Ethics. 2013;14:19.

1002. Zafra-Tanaka JH, Goicochea-Lugo S, Villarreal-Zegarra D, Taype-Rondan A. Characteristics and quality of clinical practice guidelines for depression in adults: a scoping review. BMC Psychiatry. 2019;19(1):76.
1003. Bennett K, Courtney D, Duda S, Henderson J, Szatmari P. An appraisal of the trustworthiness of practice guidelines for depression and anxiety in children and youth. Depress Anxiety. 2018;35(6):530–40.
1004. Cosgrove L, Bursztajn HJ, Erlich DR, Wheeler EE, Shaughnessy AF. Conflicts of interest and the quality of recommendations in clinical guidelines. J Eval Clin Pract. 2013;19(4):674–81.
1005. Birmaher B, Brent D, Issues AWGoQ, Bernet W, Bukstein O, Walter H, et al. Practice parameter for the assessment and treatment of children and adolescents with depressive disorders. J Am Acad Child Adolesc Psychiatry. 2007;46(11):1503–26.
1006. Lexchin J. Clinical practice guidelines and managing financial conflicts of interest. eLS. 2020;1:263–9.
1007. Taylor R, Giles J. Cash interests taint drug advice. Nature. 2005;437(7062):1070–1.
1008. Shaneyfelt TM, Centor RM. Reassessment of clinical practice guidelines: go gently into that good night. JAMA. 2009;301(8):868–9.
1009. Ioannidis JPA. Professional societies should abstain from authorship of guidelines and disease definition statements. Circ Cardiovasc Qual Outcomes. 2018;11(10):e004889.
1010. Fickweiler F, Fickweiler W, Urbach E. Interactions between physicians and the pharmaceutical industry generally and sales representatives specifically and their association with physicians' attitudes and prescribing habits: a systematic review. BMJ Open. 2017;7(9):e016408.
1011. Wazana A. Physicians and the pharmaceutical industry: is a gift ever just a gift? JAMA. 2000;283(3):373–80.
1012. Fugh-Berman A. Industry-funded medical education is always promotion-an essay by Adriane Fugh-Berman. BMJ. 2021;373:n1273.
1013. Barnes B. Financial conflicts of interest in continuing medical education: implications and accountability. JAMA. 2017;317(17):1741–2.
1014. Golestaneh L, Cowan E. Hidden conflicts of interest in continuing medical education. Lancet. 2017;390(10108):2128–30.
1015. Schofferman J. The medical-industrial complex, professional medical associations, and continuing medical education. Pain Med. 2011;12(12):1713–9.

1016. Steinman MA, Bero LA, Chren MM, Landefeld CS. Narrative review: the promotion of gabapentin: an analysis of internal industry documents. Ann Intern Med. 2006;145(4):284–93.
1017. Tabas JA, Boscardin C, Jacobsen DM, Steinman MA, Volberding PA, Baron RB. Clinician attitudes about commercial support of continuing medical education: results of a detailed survey. Arch Intern Med. 2011;171(9):840–6.
1018. Sismondo S. Key opinion leaders and the corruption of medical knowledge: what the Sunshine Act will and won't cast light on. J Law Med Ethics. 2013;41(3):635–43.
1019. Marshall DC, Tarras ES, Rosenzweig K, Korenstein D, Chimonas S. Trends in industry payments to physicians in the United States from 2014 to 2018. JAMA. 2020;324(17):1785–8.
1020. Gagnon MA, Lexchin J. The cost of pushing pills: a new estimate of pharmaceutical promotion expenditures in the United States. PLoS Med. 2008;5(1):e1.
1021. Mintzes B, Lexchin J, Sutherland JM, Beaulieu MD, Wilkes MS, Durrieu G, et al. Pharmaceutical sales representatives and patient safety: a comparative prospective study of information quality in Canada, France and the United States. J Gen Intern Med. 2013;28(10):1368–75.
1022. Roughead EE, Gilbert AL, Harvey KJ. Self-regulatory codes of conduct: are they effective in controlling pharmaceutical representatives' presentations to general medical practitioners? Int J Health Serv. 1998;28(2):269–79.
1023. Chimonas S, Brennan TA, Rothman DJ. Physicians and drug representatives: exploring the dynamics of the relationship. J Gen Intern Med. 2007;22(2):184–90.
1024. Riese F, Guloksuz S, Roventa C, Fair JD, Haravuori H, Rolko T, et al. Pharmaceutical industry interactions of psychiatric trainees from 20 European countries. Eur Psychiatry. 2015;30(2):284–90.
1025. Avorn J, Chen M, Hartley R. Scientific versus commercial sources of influence on the prescribing behavior of physicians. Am J Med. 1982;73(1):4–8.
1026. Molloy W, Strang D, Guyatt G, Lexchin J, Bedard M, Dubois S, et al. Assessing the quality of drug detailing. J Clin Epidemiol. 2002;55(8):825–32.
1027. Sah S, Fugh-Berman A. Physicians under the influence: social psychology and industry marketing strategies. J Law Med Ethics. 2013;41(3):665–72.

1028. Gibson SA. New Jersey/Pennsylvania doctor indicted for accepting bribes and kickbacks in exchange for prescribing powerful fentanyl drug. Drug Enforcement Administration. New Jersey; 2019.
1029. Morgenson G. It was his dream job. He never thought he'd be bribing doctors and waring a wire for the feds. NBC News. July 7, 2020.
1030. Turone F. Italian doctors face criminal allegations over bribes. BMJ. 2004;328(7452):1333.
1031. Steinman MA, Shlipak MG, McPhee SJ. Of principles and pens: attitudes and practices of medicine housestaff toward pharmaceutical industry promotions. Am J Med. 2001;110(7):551–7.
1032. Dana J, Loewenstein G. A social science perspective on gifts to physicians from industry. JAMA. 2003;290(2):252–5.
1033. DeJong C, Aguilar T, Tseng CW, Lin GA, Boscardin WJ, Dudley RA. Pharmaceutical industry-sponsored meals and physician prescribing patterns for medicare beneficiaries. JAMA Intern Med. 2016;176(8):1114–22.
1034. Fleischman W, Agrawal S, King M, Venkatesh AK, Krumholz HM, McKee D, et al. Association between payments from manufacturers of pharmaceuticals to physicians and regional prescribing: cross sectional ecological study. BMJ. 2016;354:i4189.
1035. Goupil B, Balusson F, Naudet F, Esvan M, Bastian B, Chapron A, et al. Association between gifts from pharmaceutical companies to French general practitioners and their drug prescribing patterns in 2016: retrospective study using the French Transparency in Healthcare and National Health Data System databases. BMJ. 2019;367:l6015.
1036. Mehta HB, Moore TJ, Alexander GC. Association of pharmaceutical industry payments to physicians with prescription and medicare expenditures for pimavanserin. Psychiatr Serv. 2021;72(1):77–80.
1037. Nguyen TD, Bradford WD, Simon KI. Pharmaceutical payments to physicians may increase prescribing for opioids. Addiction. 2019;114(6):1051–9.
1038. Goldberg DS. The shadows of sunlight: why disclosure should not be a priority in addressing conflicts of interest. Public Health Eth-Uk. 2019;12(2):202–12.
1039. Braillon A, Lexchin J, Blumsohn A, Hengartner MP. The "pharmaceuticalisation" of life. BMJ. 2019;365:l1972.

1040. Vilhelmsson A, Svensson T, Meeuwisse A. A pill for the ill? Patients' reports of their experience of the medical encounter in the treatment of depression. PLoS One. 2013;8(6):e66338.
1041. Hengartner MP. Eine methodenkritische evaluation der bio-medizinischen Depressionsforschung: Wie zuverlässig und praxisrelevant sind vielbeachtete neurobiogenetische Befunde? Psychotherapeutenjournal. 2019;2:110–7.
1042. Kennis M, Gerritsen L, van Dalen M, Williams A, Cuijpers P, Bockting C. Prospective biomarkers of major depressive disorder: a systematic review and meta-analysis. Mol Psychiatry. 2020;25(2):321–38.
1043. Greenslit NP, Kaptchuk TJ. Antidepressants and advertising: psychopharmaceuticals in crisis. Yale J Biol Med. 2012;85(1):153–8.
1044. Melander H, Salmonson T, Abadie E, van Zwieten-Boot B. A regulatory Apologia—a review of placebo-controlled studies in regulatory submissions of new-generation antidepressants. Eur Neuropsychopharmacol. 2008;18(9):623–7.
1045. Bolling MY, Kohlenberg RJ. Reasons for quitting serotonin reuptake inhibitor therapy: paradoxical psychological side effects and patient satisfaction. Psychother Psychosom. 2004;73(6):380–5.
1046. Price J, Cole V, Goodwin GM. Emotional side-effects of selective serotonin reuptake inhibitors: qualitative study. Br J Psychiatry. 2009;195(3):211–7.
1047. Kales HC, Gitlin LN, Lyketsos CG. When less is more, but still not enough: why focusing on limiting antipsychotics in people with dementia is the wrong policy imperative. J Am Med Dir Assoc. 2019;20(9):1074–9.
1048. Maust DT, Mavandadi S, Eakin A, Streim JE, Difillipo S, Snedden T, et al. Telephone-based behavioral health assessment for older adults starting a new psychiatric medication. Am J Geriatr Psychiatry. 2011;19(10):851–8.
1049. Maust DT, Sirey JA, Kales HC. Antidepressant prescribing in primary care to older adults without major depression. Psychiatr Serv. 2017;68(5):449–55.
1050. Wong J, Motulsky A, Abrahamowicz M, Eguale T, Buckeridge DL, Tamblyn R. Off-label indications for antidepressants in primary care: descriptive study of prescriptions from an indication based electronic prescribing system. BMJ. 2017;356:j603.

1051. Doshi P, Jefferson T, Del Mar C. The imperative to share clinical study reports: recommendations from the Tamiflu experience. PLoS Med. 2012;9(4):e1001201.
1052. Vargesson N. Thalidomide-induced teratogenesis: history and mechanisms. Birth Defects Res C Embryo Today. 2015;105(2):140–56.
1053. Blume S. Anti-vaccination movements and their interpretations. Soc Sci Med. 2006;62(3):628–42.
1054. Yaqub O, Castle-Clarke S, Sevdalis N, Chataway J. Attitudes to vaccination: a critical review. Soc Sci Med. 2014;112:1–11.
1055. Goldstein J. Univ. of Cincinnati psychiatrist under more scrutiny over funding. The Wall Street Journal. April 21, 2008.
1056. Harris G, Carey B, Roberts J. Psychiatrists, children and drug industry's role. The New York Times. May 10, 2007.
1057. Naish J. Revealed: doctors pushing new drugs don't have to admit they are funded by the pill's makers … and a treatment for depression using Class B drug ketamine is just the latest example. The Daily Mail. August 26, 2019.
1058. Petersen M. Undisclosed financial ties prompt reproval of doctor. The New York Times. August 3, 2003.
1059. American Psychiatric Association. Diagnostic and statistical manual of mental disorders DSM-5. Washington, DC: American Psychiatric Association; 2013.
1060. Wichniak A, Wierzbicka A, Walecka M, Jernajczyk W. Effects of antidepressants on sleep. Curr Psychiatry Rep. 2017;19(9):63.
1061. Gafoor R, Booth HP, Gulliford MC. Antidepressant utilisation and incidence of weight gain during 10 years' follow-up: population based cohort study. BMJ. 2018;361:k1951.
1062. Wakefield JC, Schmitz MF, First MB, Horwitz AV. Extending the bereavement exclusion for major depression to other losses: evidence from the National Comorbidity Survey. Arch Gen Psychiatry. 2007;64(4):433–40.
1063. Wakefield JC, Schmitz MF. Can the DSM's major depression bereavement exclusion be validly extended to other stressors? Evidence from the NCS. Acta Psychiatr Scand. 2013;128(4):294–305.
1064. Wakefield JC. The DSM-5 debate over the bereavement exclusion: psychiatric diagnosis and the future of empirically supported treatment. Clin Psychol Rev. 2013;33(7):825–45.

1065. Morres ID, Hatzigeorgiadis A, Stathi A, Comoutos N, Arpin-Cribbie C, Krommidas C, et al. Aerobic exercise for adult patients with major depressive disorder in mental health services: a systematic review and meta-analysis. Depress Anxiety. 2019;36(1):39–53.
1066. Schuch FB, Vancampfort D, Richards J, Rosenbaum S, Ward PB, Stubbs B. Exercise as a treatment for depression: a meta-analysis adjusting for publication bias. J Psychiatr Res. 2016;77:42-–51.
1067. Jerant A, Kravitz RL, Fernandez YGE, Feldman MD, Cipri C, Nishio D, et al. Potential antidepressant overtreatment associated with office use of brief depression symptom measures. J Am Board Fam Med. 2014;27(5):611–20.
1068. Irving G, Neves AL, Dambha-Miller H, Oishi A, Tagashira H, Verho A, et al. International variations in primary care physician consultation time: a systematic review of 67 countries. BMJ Open. 2017;7(10):e017902.
1069. Loh A, Simon D, Hennig K, Hennig B, Harter M, Elwyn G. The assessment of depressive patients' involvement in decision making in audio-taped primary care consultations. Patient Educ Couns. 2006;63(3):314–8.
1070. Young HN, Bell RA, Epstein RM, Feldman MD, Kravitz RL. Physicians' shared decision-making behaviors in depression care. Arch Intern Med. 2008;168(13):1404–8.
1071. Couet N, Desroches S, Robitaille H, Vaillancourt H, Leblanc A, Turcotte S, et al. Assessments of the extent to which health-care providers involve patients in decision making: a systematic review of studies using the OPTION instrument. Health Expect. 2015;18(4):542–61.
1072. Demasi M, Gotzsche PC. Presentation of benefits and harms of antidepressants on websites: a cross-sectional study. Int J Risk Saf Med. 2020;31(2):53–65.
1073. Lebowitz MS, Ahn WK, Nolen-Hoeksema S. Fixable or fate? Perceptions of the biology of depression. J Consult Clin Psychol. 2013;81(3):518–27.
1074. Kvaale EP, Haslam N, Gottdiener WH. The 'side effects' of medicalization: a meta-analytic review of how biogenetic explanations affect stigma. Clin Psychol Rev. 2013;33(6):782–94.
1075. Lewis-Fernandez R, Rotheram-Borus MJ, Betts VT, Greenman L, Essock SM, Escobar JI, et al. Rethinking funding priorities in mental health research. Br J Psychiatry. 2016;208(6):507–9.
1076. Ortigue S, Bianchi-Demicheli F, Patel N, Frum C, Lewis JW. Neuroimaging of love: fMRI meta-analysis evidence toward new perspectives in sexual medicine. J Sex Med. 2010;7(11):3541–52.

1077. Kendler KS, Hettema JM, Butera F, Gardner CO, Prescott CA. Life event dimensions of loss, humiliation, entrapment, and danger in the prediction of onsets of major depression and generalized anxiety. Arch Gen Psychiatry. 2003;60(8):789–96.
1078. Stegenga BT, Nazareth I, Grobbee DE, Torres-Gonzalez F, Svab I, Maaroos HI, et al. Recent life events pose greatest risk for onset of major depressive disorder during mid-life. J Affect Disord. 2012;136(3):505–13.
1079. Glasziou P, Altman DG, Bossuyt P, Boutron I, Clarke M, Julious S, et al. Reducing waste from incomplete or unusable reports of biomedical research. Lancet. 2014;383(9913):267–76.
1080. Demyttenaere K, Donneau AF, Albert A, Ansseau M, Constant E, van Heeringen K. What is important in being cured from depression? Discordance between physicians and patients (1). J Affect Disord. 2015;174:390–6.
1081. Zimmermann TM, Clouth J, Elosge M, Heurich M, Schneider E, Wilhelm S, et al. Patient preferences for outcomes of depression treatment in Germany: a choice-based conjoint analysis study. J Affect Disord. 2013;148(2–3):210–9.
1082. Amick HR, Gartlehner G, Gaynes BN, Forneris C, Asher GN, Morgan LC, et al. Comparative benefits and harms of second generation antidepressants and cognitive behavioral therapies in initial treatment of major depressive disorder: systematic review and meta-analysis. BMJ. 2015;351:h6019.
1083. Cooney GM, Dwan K, Greig CA, Lawlor DA, Rimer J, Waugh FR, et al. Exercise for depression. Cochrane Database Syst Rev. 2013(9):CD004366.
1084. Cuijpers P, Sijbrandij M, Koole SL, Andersson G, Beekman AT, Reynolds CF, 3rd. The efficacy of psychotherapy and pharmacotherapy in treating depressive and anxiety disorders: a meta-analysis of direct comparisons. World Psychiatry. 2013;12(2):137–48.
1085. Loewenstein G, Sah S, Cain DM. The unintended consequences of conflict of interest disclosure. JAMA. 2012;307(7):669–70.
1086. PLoS Medicine Editors. Does conflict of interest disclosure worsen bias? PLoS Med. 2012;9(4):e1001210.
1087. Altman DG. The scandal of poor medical research. BMJ. 1994;308(6924):283–4.

Index

M. P. Hengartner, *Evidence-biased Antidepressant Prescription*,
https://doi.org/10.1007/978-3-030-82587-4

www.ingramcontent.com/pod-product-compliance
Lightning Source LLC
Chambersburg PA
CBHW021551190925
32866CB00001B/1
* 9 7 8 3 0 3 0 8 2 5 8 6 7 *